MAJOR PROBLEMS IN
CHILDHOOD CANCER

MAJOR PROBLEMS IN
CHILDHOOD CANCER

Edited by

CARL POCHEDLY, M.D.

Director, Pediatric Hematology
Nassau County Medical Center
East Meadow, Long Island, New York

and

THOMAS F. NECHELES, M.D., Ph.D.

Chief, Pediatric Hematology
New England Medical Center Hospitals
Associate Professor of Pediatrics
Tufts University School of Medicine
Boston, Massachusetts

With a Foreword by

Sydney S. Gellis, M.D.

Professor and Chairman
Department of Pediatrics
Tufts University School of Medicine
Medford, Massachusetts
Pediatrician-in-Chief
The New England Medical Center Hospitals
Boston, Massachusetts

THOMAS BOOKS · SYMBOL OF LEADERSHIP

CHARLES C THOMAS · PUBLISHER
Springfield · Illinois · U.S.A.

Published and Distributed Throughout the World by

CHARLES C THOMAS • PUBLISHER
BANNERSTONE HOUSE
301-327 East Lawrence Avenue, Springfield, Illinois, U.S.A.

ISBN 0-398-02713-7

Library of Congress Catalog Card Number: 72-88466

With THOMAS BOOKS *careful attention is given to all details of manufacturing and design. It is the Publisher's desire to present books that are satisfactory as to their physical qualities and artistic possibilities and appropriate for their particular use.* THOMAS BOOKS *will be true to those laws of quality that assure a good name and good will.*

Printed in the United States of America

N-1

CONTRIBUTORS

Janet Cuttner, M.D.

Assistant Professor of Medicine
Mt. Sinai School of Medicine
City University of New York
New York, New York

Jerry Z. Finklestein, M.D., C.M.

Chief, Division of Pediatric Hematology
Harbor General Hospital
Torrance, California
Assistant Professor of Pediatrics
School of Medicine
University of California at Los Angeles
Los Angeles, California

Gerald S. Gilchrist, M.B., C.Ch.

Mayo Clinic and Mayo Foundation
Rochester, Minnesota

Evan M. Hersh, M.D.

Associate Professor of Medicine
Chief, Section of Immunology
Department of Developmental Therapeutics
M. D. Anderson Hospital and Tumor Institute
Houston, Texas

Barbara Jones, M.D.

Professor of Pediatrics
School of Medicine
West Virginia University
Morgantown, West Virginia

Thomas F. Necheles, M.D., Ph.D.

Chief, Pediatric Hematology
New England Medical Center Hospitals
Associate Professor of Pediatrics
Tufts University School of Medicine
Boston, Massachusetts

Carl Pochedly, M.D.

Director, Pediatric Hematology
Nassau County Medical Center
East Meadow, Long Island, New York

Marilyn J. Sonley, M.D.

Chief, Department of Pediatrics
The Princess Margaret Hospital
(Ontario Cancer Institute)
Pediatrician, The Hospital for Sick Children
Toronto, Ontario, Canada

Seymour Zimbler, M.D.

New England Medical Center Hospitals
Associate Professor of Orthopedics
Tufts University School of Medicine
Boston, Massachusetts

Jordan U. Gutterman, M.D.

Assistant Professor of Medicine, Section of Immunology
Department of Developmental Therapeutics
M. D. Anderson Hospital and Tumor Institute
Houston, Texas

Giora Mavligit, M.D.

Assistant Professor of Medicine, Section of Immunology
Department of Developmental Therapeutics
M. D. Anderson Hospital and Tumor Institute
Houston, Texas

FOREWORD

ONE OUT OF EVERY SIX DEATHS in children under the age of fourteen years is due to cancer. Malignancy is *the* leading cause of death from disease in the childhood years. As the practicing pediatrician or general physician finds more and more of infectious disease states yielding to immunization procedures or antimicrobial therapy, the early diagnosis of malignancy becomes a relatively more frequent problem than it has in the past. Accordingly, he must become more sensitive to the great variety of clinical expressions of cancer in the younger individual.

Only a few short years ago, the practicing physician usually deliberately chose to avoid this area of medicine. The outlook for children with cancer was almost uniformly hopeless and the physician found that his involvement with these pathetic patients was so depressing that he was only too glad to refer their total care to the hematologist or oncologist at the nearest medical center. Care was frequently fragmented between the surgeon, radiotherapist and hematologist with no one formulating an organized plan of care or maintaining communication with the primary physician. The latter frequently lost track of the patient or when the family did turn to him for advice or counsel, he was unaware of the current status of the patient or his therapy.

New drugs, new approaches and the combination of various modalities of therapy have led to a marked improvement in the prognosis in a number of types of childhood malignancies. This improvement, in many cases, is predicated on the close cooperation between the hematologist-oncologist, the radiotherapist and the surgeon. The participation of the primary physician in this cooperative effort becomes increasingly important. Not only may he be called upon to administer various aspects of the patients' chemotherapy and to recognize possible side effects, but he must also be able to communicate with the family, discussing the child's condition, care and prognosis, as well as providing the personal support so important for any family faced with a catastrophic illness.

Close participation of the pediatrician or generalist in the care of these children necessitates a fairly comprehensive knowledge of current techniques in the diagnosis, therapy and prognosis of the various types of malignancies. Unfortunately, this information is not readily available; many of the current texts are outdated, and review articles are scattered throughout the medical literature. Drs. Pochedly and Necheles have gathered together contributions from a number of clinicians active in this field into a monograph which encompasses the more common forms of childhood cancer. Included is a review of immunotherapy which, although without immediate clinical utility, may well represent the most dramatic prospect for the eventual control of cancer.

For most affected children, cancer is still a fatal disease. However, the increasing numbers of children with acute leukemia, Hodgkin's disease, or Wilms' tumor who survive for five years or longer with no evidence of disease provide the basis for realistic hope for the eventual control of most varieties of malignant disease. Even now, the application of present knowledge in this field can improve the life of practically every patient.

SYDNEY S. GELLIS

PREFACE

Knowledge in the field of childhood cancer has grown at an ever-increasing rate in the past twenty years. The impetus has been successful therapy, with surgery, x-ray therapy and chemotherapy. Progress in many other areas of pediatrics has kept pace and has enabled the pediatrician to build a meaningful interest in the child with cancer and to participate importantly in therapy.

The material contained in the various chapters was selected on the basis of its clinical relevance and its value to the practitioner. The chapters are clinically oriented and are not intended to be comprehensive reviews of the topics discussed.

The editors are very grateful to the many contributors for their diligence in preparing the various chapters and for meeting a reasonable time schedule. The editors are also grateful to Dr. Guilio D'Angio, of Memorial Hospital for Cancer and Allied Diseases, for reviewing the chapter on Wilms' tumor, and to Dr. E. Omer Burgert, of Mayo Clinic, for reviewing the chapter on bone tumors.

Carl Pochedly
Thomas F. Necheles

CONTENTS

MAJOR PROBLEMS IN

CHILDHOOD CANCER

Chapter 1

ACUTE LEUKEMIA

JANET CUTTNER

ACUTE LEUKEMIA is the commonest of the childhood malignancies, accounting for approximately 50 percent of the deaths from childhood cancer in the United States from 1950 to 1959.[1] This is a disease of unknown etiology characterized by infiltration of primitive white cells, mainly blasts, into the marrow and peripheral blood. It generally terminates months to years after onset with the death of the child. In the past two decades important gains, attributable to intensive research in many different disciplines, have brought about an increase in the survival time of afflicted children. Considerable progress has been made in the field of chemotherapy, but the disease remains fatal in the great majority of affected children. Of prime importance in helping to extend the life span of leukemic children is the necessity of recognizing complications early so that supportive care can be given.

ETIOLOGY

The etiology of leukemia is unknown. Many investigators believe that this disease is caused by an infectious agent. There have been several reports of so-called leukemic clusters, in which an unusually high incidence of leukemia has been reported within a relatively small area.[2,3] Of those who consider an infectious etiology for leukemia, most believe the infectious agent to be a virus. There are diseases in chickens, mice and cats which resemble the human leukemias and which are definitely known to be caused by viruses.[4-6]

Note: This study was aided in part by United States Public Health Service Grants number CA 04457, CA 08866 and CA 11816 from the National Cancer Institute and from the Albert A. List, Frederick Machlin and Anna Ruth Lowenberg funds.

Electron microscopic studies on human acute leukemia patients have been reported to show virus-like particles similar to those found to induce the animal leukemias.[7] There are other factors which may point to a viral etiology: one is the presence of the Australia antigen and another is the finding of RNA-dependent DNA polymerases. The Australian antigen, which originally was found in the blood of an Australian patient with hepatitis, has also been found in many patients with acute leukemia. The Australian antigen has also been found in patients with Down's syndrome in which there is an increased incidence of both leukemia and hepatitis.[8,9] More recently Temin[10] and Baltimore[11] reported an RNA-dependent DNA polymerase in several RNA oncogenic viruses. In addition, an RNA-dependent polymerase analogous to that of RNA tumor viruses was found in the lymphoblasts of patients with acute lymphocytic leukemia.[12] RNA-dependent DNA polymerases have subsequently been found in the blood of patients with acute myelocytic leukemia.[13] It remains to be determined whether this enzyme is of viral origin.

The relationship of genetics to leukemia is uncertain. Families have been reported in which there appears to be an unusually high incidence of leukemia and lymphoma.[14-16] Chromosome abnormalities have been reported in several cases of acute leukemia.[17,18] However there is doubt as to their etiological significance. The only consistent chromosome abnormality is that of trisomy[21] found in Down's syndrome.[19,20] These children definitely have an increased incidence of acute leukemia. Bloom's syndrome, which is inherited through an autosomal recessive gene, shows an increased susceptibility to acute leukemia.[21] The apparent association of acute leukemia with a variety of chromosomal disorders suggests that genetic mechanisms may form part of the causal chain of leukemogenesis in a small proportion of cases.[22] Ionizing radiation is known to be associated with both an increased incidence of leukemia and an increase in chromosome breaks.[23,24] It may well be that in order for leukemia to be expressed several etiologic factors have to be present. Thus, certain children may have inherited, or acquired through exposure to radiation, an increased susceptibility to a leukemogenic virus. In one study the association of four factors was noted: mother's irradiation before conception, *in utero* irradiation of the child, previous history of reproductive wastage and the occurrence of viral disease in children less than four years of age. They found that any one of these factors alone was not associated with an increased incidence of leukemia but that the association of three of the four factors resulted in an increased incidence of leukemia.[25]

SYMPTOMS

The commonest symptoms observed in a leukemic child are those related to infection or bleeding. A persistent or recurrent fever with infection is often the reason the mother brings her child to the physician. The mother may observe that her child appears unusually tired. She may note that her child has developed many ecchymoses which cannot be accounted for by trauma. Joint pains resembling those seen in acute rheumatic fever can occasionally be a presenting symptom. Headache, nausea and vomiting are often present when there is involvement of the central nervous system. Proptosis can be seen as the presenting symptom in children with acute myeloblastic leukemia who initially have localized involvement, a so-called chloroma.

PHYSICAL FINDINGS

Upon examination, pallor especially of the mucous membranes is apparent. Scattered petechiae and ecchymoses are evidence of easy bruisability. Generalized lymphadenopathy varying from pea size to several centimeters in diameter frequently are found. Bone tenderness may be present. The child may develop respiratory stridor due to greatly enlarged cervical and mediastinal lymph nodes.[26] The liver and spleen are usually enlarged. Gingival hypertrophy is unusual in children but it is seen in monomyeloblastic leukemia. Cranial nerve paralysis may be seen in children with central nervous system involvement. Enlargement of the testicles may also be present.

LABORATORY FINDINGS

The diagnosis of acute leukemia usually is easily made after a complete blood count and bone marrow examination. One finds evidence of anemia in the low hemoglobin, red cell count and hematocrit. The platelet count is usually low and the white blood count may be decreased, normal or elevated. The diagnosis is made on the stained peripheral blood smear and bone marrow examination by the presence of large numbers of blasts. In children the commonest type of leukemia is acute lymphoblastic leukemia, where mainly lymphoblasts and lymphocytes are found in the marrow and the peripheral blood. The other type of leukemia which is seen, though not nearly as frequently, is acute myeloblastic leukemia. Here one sees predominantly myeloblasts and promyelocytes in the peripheral blood and bone marrow. Some of the myeloblasts contain bright red rods (Auer rods) in their cytoplasm, which are diagnostic of acute myeloblastic leukemia. Even less common are acute progranulocytic leukemia, acute monocytic leukemia and erythroleukemia.

Hyperuricemia is seen very frequently and is associated with either an elevated white blood count or hepatosplenomegaly, or both, with a concomittant increase in purine catabolism.[27] Since uric acid is the end product of nucleoprotein degradation, large quantities may be produced and may lead to uric acid nephropathy. This is especially likely to occur when the child is undergoing chemotherapy because of the great increase in cell catabolism. This danger has virtually been eliminated through the prophylactic use of allopurinol (Zyloprim®), a xanthine oxidase inhibitor which interferes with the final conversion of oxypurine by effectively blocking the conversion of hypoxanthine and xanthine to uric acid.[28]

Hypercalcemia is an uncommon complication. It is usually associated with roentgenographic evidence of bone disease.[29] Most often this complication appears coincidently with bone marrow relapse but has occasionally preceded actual bone marrow relapse by a few weeks. The hypercalcemia responds to the treatment of the leukemia; however, temporary alleviation of symptoms may also be obtained by the administration of corticosteroids or sodium sulfate.

Serum muramidase (lysozyme) is a hydrolytic enzyme commonly found in the lysosomes of granulocytes and monocytes. Its chief value lies in the differentiation of acute lymphocytic leukemia from acute myelocytic leukemia and acute monomyelocytic leukemia. There have been many papers corroborating the fact that the serum muramidase is elevated consistently in acute monocytic leukemia, acute monomyelocytic leukemia and many cases of acute myelocytic leukemia.[30,31] In acute lymphocytic leukemia the serum muramidase level has been found to be normal or low. It may prove of value in following patients with monomyelocytic leukemia as there is evidence that the serum muramidase will rise before there is evidence of peripheral blood relapse.[32]

It is well known that children with chronic myelogenous leukemia have a very elevated *fetal hemoglobin*.[33] The reason for this elevation is unknown. Perhaps this is an abortive effort to respond to the anemia or represents dyserythropoiesis secondary to the leukemic process. Elevated fetal hemoglobin levels have also been found in children with acute leukemia.[34]

Disseminated intravascular coagulation may play an important role in the bleeding diathesis which many of these patients have.[35] Coagulation studies will usually show a hypofibrinogenemia, a prolonged prothrombin time, prolonged partial thromboplastin time, and thrombocytopenia. The most definitive test is the finding of fibrin split-products in the patient's blood. Intravenous heparin administration has proved helpful for the immediate treatment of defibrination, however, one must also treat the underlying cause, namely the leukemia.

Immunoglobulin levels performed at the time of diagnosis of children with leukemia have been found to be within normal limits.[36] After the institution of chemotherapy, however, a temporary decrease in IgG levels has been noted. With each change in chemotherapy there has been a greater reduction in IgG levels with a gradual return to normal values. A significantly greater depression was found in those patients who were no longer able to respond to therapy. There have been a few case reports of children with acute leukemia who develop a monoclonal spike in the serum protein electrophoresis.[37-39] In most of these cases the abnormal immunoglobulin has been IgG. We observed a child of seven years of age with acute lymphoblastic leukemia who was found to have a monoclonal gammapathy due to IgG (Fig. 1-1). He was in remission for eighteen months when first studied because of frequent infections. When he relapsed several months later the IgG spike disappeared.

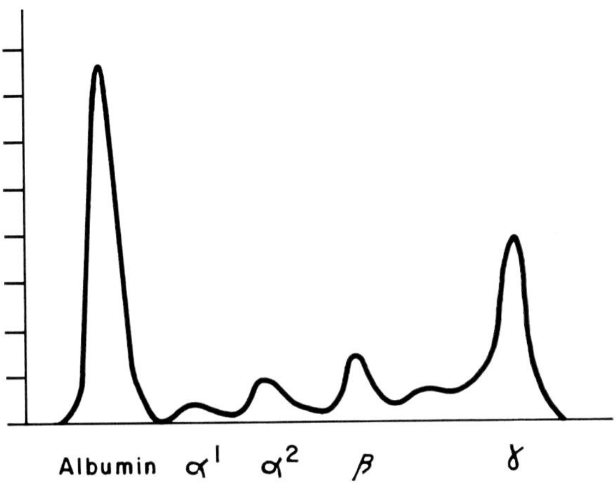

Figure 1-1. Serum protein electrophoresis showing an M spike in the region of gamma-globulin. Immunoelectrophoresis showed this to consist of IgC, type kappa.

COMPLICATIONS

Infection is the chief fatal complication in patients with acute leukemia, presumably due to the absolute granulocytopenia and lymphopenia which these patients have.[40,41] The incidence of infections can be correlated with the degree of granulocytopenia. The critical level of granulocytopenia is 1,500/mm^3. Above this level there is no further decrease in the incidence of infection.[42] At any given level of granulocyte count and lymphocyte count, the frequency of infectious episodes is greater during relapse than with the same count during remission. There is evidence that circulating granulocytes are functionally impaired, since the leukocytes of children with acute leukemia have decreased bacteriocidal activity.[43] It has also been shown that granulocytes from patients with acute leukemia are not mobilized well.[44]

The commonest type of infections are those caused by gram-negative organisms.[40,41] It is believed that the patient becomes infected with organisms that are normally present in his own gastrointestinal tract. The other bacterial infection which is commonly seen is staphylococcal. The skin is the common portal of entry for these infections. Over the last several years we have become more aware of the great danger of opportunistic infections. These are infections due to microorganisms that adapt themselves to unique circumstances offered by their environment.[45] Certainly a child with acute leukemia undergoing chemotherapy will be both immunosuppressed and granulocytopenic and therefore would be a prime candidate for such infections. The majority of these infections are caused by fungi.[45] Monilial infections may take the form of thrush which is easy to diagnose if one is alert to the frequency of this complication. More difficult to diagnose are disseminated monilial infections. Cryptococcal infections especially of the central nervous system are being seen with increasing frequency, as are aspergillus infections of the lungs.[47] *Pneumocystis carinii* infections of the lungs are seen in children both in remission as well as relapse. The possibility of such an infection should be considered in any child with shortness of breath, bilateral pulmonary infiltrates and an alveolar capillary block. Unfortunately the only reliable way of making the diagnosis is by lung biopsy. This procedure should be carried out as soon as possible so that treatment with pentamidine or stilbamidine can be instituted as soon as the diagnosis is confirmed.[48,49] Cytomegalic inclusion disease is also being seen with increasing frequency.[50,51]

Hemorrhage is a very frequent complication and, in the main, is related to thrombocytopenia. Ecchymoses especially on the extremities are the commonest manifestation of bleeding. Gingival and gastrointestinal bleeding are frequently seen. Central nervous system hemorrhage is the most serious complication and still accounts for a number of fatalities. Patients with a very high white blood count over 100,000/mm^3 have a higher incidence of central nervous system hemorrhage.[52,53]

Central nervous system involvement is usually caused by leukemic infiltration of the meninges and frequently occurs when the child is in a hematological remission. Within the last decade an increasing incidence of central nervous system leukemia has been observed.[54,55] In one study an overall incidence of 51 percent was seen.[55] This increase can best be explained by the fact that survival has been increased and there is a greater chance that this complication will develop. The child will usually complain of a headache and will have persistent nausea and vomiting, especially in the morning. These symptoms are so common that we feel that any child with acute lymphoblastic leukemia who has nausea and vomiting for more than twenty-four hours, especially if accompanied by a headache, should have a lumbar puncture to rule out central nervous system leukemia. Sometimes children will present with isolated cranial nerve involvement. Localizing neurological findings are usually sparse unless there is cranial nerve involvement. In our experience papilledema is the commonest physical finding. The diagnosis is made by lumbar puncture. The spinal fluid pressure is usually elevated. The cerebrospinal fluid protein concentration and cell count are elevated. If the CSF is centrifuged and a drop of sediment dried on a slide and stained, leukemic blasts may be identified (Fig. 1-2). The treatment is intrathecal methotrexate at a dose of 12 mg/m^2, repeated every other day until the CSF is clear. One can also give radiotherapy either to the cranium or to the entire central nervous system.[56] Promising results have recently been obtained using cranial irradiation and intrathecal methotrexate prophylactically.[57] (See section on therapy.)

A child presenting with *testicular involvement* may pose problems with differential diagnosis.[58] That this is a major problem is evident from a study in which testicular involvement was seen in 64 percent of males with acute leukemia.[59] The diagnosis is made by testicular biopsy. The treatment may be orchiectomy or local radiotherapy. What must be borne in mind is that involvement may occur when the patient is in complete hematological remission. Burchenal reported that 5 of 157 patients with acute leukemia who survived five years or longer developed local recurrences; two were due to testicular involvement.[60]

Bony involvement in acute leukemia is not uncommon.[61-64]

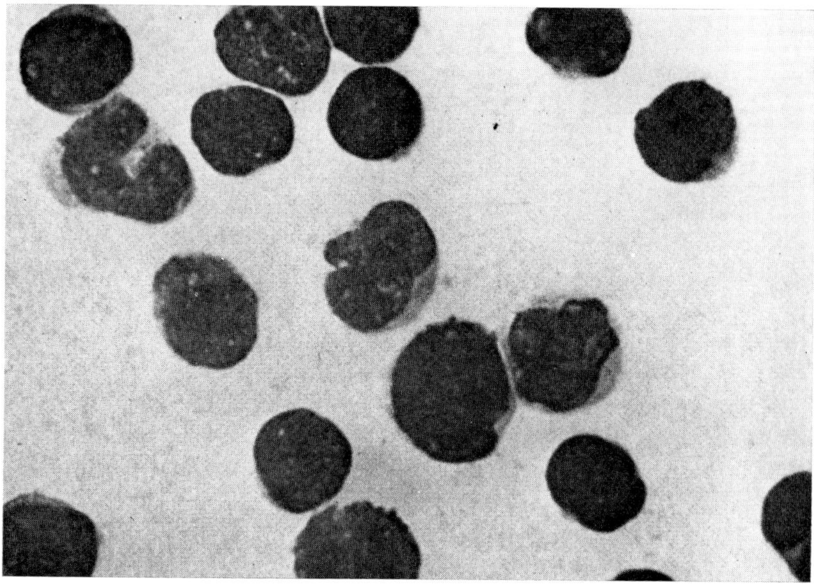

Figure 1-2. Leukemic "blasts" in the cerebrospinal fluid. (Courtesy of Dr. Rolland Skeel.)

The four commonest radiological findings of bone involvement in acute leukemia are diffuse demineralization, osteolytic lesions especially of the extremities, cortical and periosteal lesions, and metaphyseal bands (Fig. 1-3) . The osteolytic lesion starting as the punctate form is the most characteristic radiographic feature.

Occasionally the presenting sign in children with acute myeloblastic leukemia may be the so-called green tumor, or *chloroma,* which is formed from myeloid tissue. This myeloblastoma can also occur without the green pigmentation. The tumor masses are usually found in close association with bony structures, especially the skull, spine, ribs and sternum.[65]

Two types of *cutaneous lesions* may be observed. *Leukemia cutis* refers to the specific infiltrative cutaneous lesions which are nodular or papular, small in size and usually of plum color.[66] Diagnosis is made by needle aspiration or biopsy. The other common cutaneous lesion is the so-called leukemid. Clinically, this resembles nonspecific or toxic cutaneous lesions, but histologically

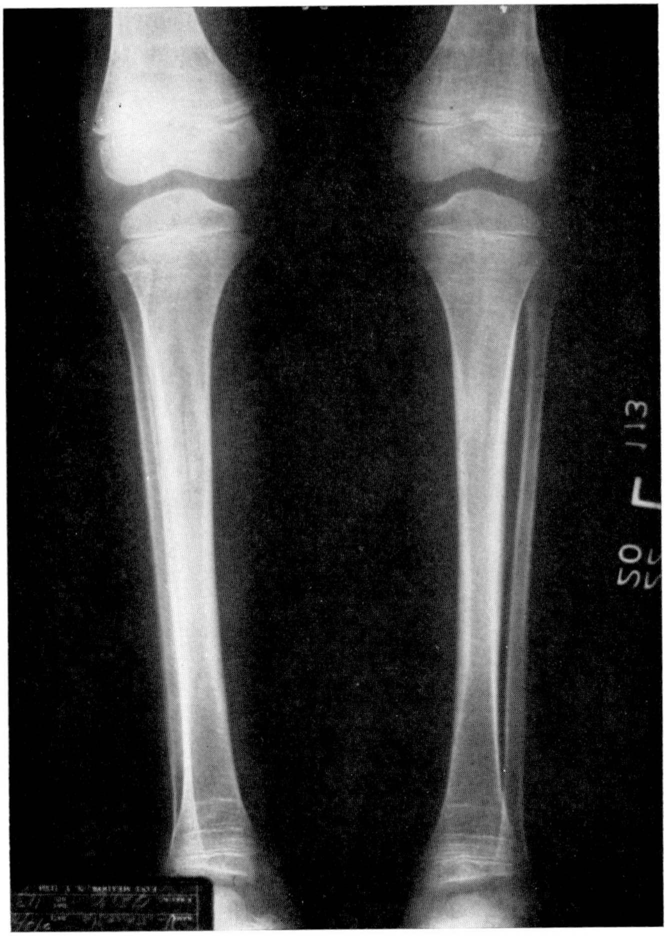

Figure 1-3. Lower legs of a child with long-standing acute leukemia showing growth-arrest lines in the metaphyses.

they appear as specific or true cutaneous infiltrates of leukemic cells.[66]

Cardiac manifestations sometimes occur. Most patients are symptomatic and EKG changes if present are nonspecific. In one study of 420 patients with acute leukemia there was a 37 percent incidence of leukemic infiltration of the heart.[67] The most frequent site of infiltration was the pericardium. The commonest cardiac lesion, however, was hemorrhage which was found in 54 percent of patients and usually was related to thrombocytopenia. In an autopsy study of children with leukemia, 44 percent were found to have at least one focus of leukemic infiltration of the heart.[68] Cardiac hypertrophy of significant degree was seen in about one-third of the children and was believed to be related to anemia.

THERAPY

Supportive Therapy

The use of packed red cells for the treatment of anemia is of great importance and should be performed to keep the child's hemoglobin above 7 gm%. Platelet transfusions when available should be given to those thrombocytopenic children who show evidence of bleeding.[69] We usually use 4 to 6 platelet units every other day. If bleeding is more severe 6 to 10 units per day may have to be administered. It is not unusual for the bleeding manifestations to stop without necessarily seeing a rise in the platelet count. We routinely start the children on allopurinol prior to the institution of chemotherapy, regardless of the serum uric acid level, to prevent hyperuricemia and urate nephropathy.

It cannot be stated too often that the leading cause of death today in acute leukemia is *infection*. This being the case we feel very strongly that all infections in children, especially when in relapse, should be treated vigorously and quickly. Children in relapse who have persistent temperatures over 101 degrees and who do not have an obvious viral exanthem should have a thorough physical examination looking for signs of infection in the throat, ears, lungs, et cetera. If an infection is found it should be treated promptly. If no infection is found then the child should have a nose, throat, urine and blood culture performed as well as a chest x-ray. He should then be started on antibiotics that are bacteriocidal for both gram-negative and staphylococcal infections. My own preference is cephalosporin (Keflin®) in combination with either gentamycin or kanomycin. One must be constantly on the lookout for opportunistic infections. Ideally it would be advantageous to use white cell transfusions, but this is not feasible as there are no adequate methods at present for harvesting the large numbers of white cells that are needed. A few studies have shown that large numbers of white blood cells from patients with chronic granulocytic leukemia may be harvested.[70] Another method which has been used is bone marrow transfusion using the marrow of closely related donors. Both of these methods can be used to temporarily increase the number of circulating granulocytes. The use of a protected environment for patients undergoing chemotherapy is currently under investigation at several hospital centers. So-called life islands and laminar air flow units are being used. In principle, air passes into these units through high efficiency filters which reduce the microbial flora. In addition most of these patients also receive oral nonabsorbable antibiotics in an effort to decrease the flora of the gastrointestinal tract.

Before going into a discussion of the specific chemotherapy of acute leukemia a brief statement on the philosophy of treatment of acute leukemia would be in order. It has been mainly through the efforts of special study groups that prolonged remissions have been obtained. Almost all the treatment regimens that are effective today have come from such protocol studies. However, this has been achieved at a certain risk which is related to the toxicity of the chemotherapeutic agents. To keep this risk at a minimum the child must be treated at a center where there are hematologists and pediatricians who are experienced in the use of these agents. The hospital must have the facilities available to give blood and platelet infusions when necessary. When the child is in remission and at home he should be cared for jointly by the pediatrician or general practitioner and the hematologist. The ultimate aim of course in such a strictly controlled protocol is to obtain more prolonged remissions, leading hopefully to a "cure."

Specific Therapy

Before discussing the use of individual agents it should be noted that all compounds, with the possible exception of corticosteroids, produce significant bone marrow depression. The dose will have to be adjusted according to the degree of bone marrow depression, particularly during the maintenance phase. Acute lymphoblastic leukemia is the commonest type of leukemia seen in children. In this disease one can usually obtain at least two or three remissions. It is known that children who obtain a complete remission have a longer survival than those who do not. It is encouraging to note that there has been an increase in survival from one to two and three years.[71-74]

In order to qualify for a complete remission status certain criteria have to be met (Table 1-1). The bone marrow must have normal granulopoiesis, erythropoiesis and megakaryocytopoiesis. In addition there should be no more than 5 percent blasts in the bone marrow. The hemoglobin should be over 10 gm% in a child under two years of age and over 11 gm% in a child over two years. The level of circulating granulocytes should be over 1000/mm^3 in children over four years. The platelet count must be over 100,000/mm^3. There should be no blasts in the peripheral blood. Physical examination should be essentially within normal limits. There should be no significant lymphadenopathy and no splenomegaly.

Chemotherapeutic Agents

Vincristine (Oncovin®) is a vinca alkaloid derived from the periwinkle plant and has been most effective in inducing remissions.[75-77] It is usually given weekly intravenously in a dose of 1.5 to 2 mg/m^2 in combination with oral prednisone (Table 1-2). Vincristine has a well-known neurotoxicity which must be kept in mind.[78] Numbness and tingling of the fingers and toes are often seen. One must check the deep tendon reflexes before each dose. Adynamic ileus which may cause constipation and obstipation is seen in children, though much less commonly than in adults. This complication can almost always be prevented by starting the patient on a laxative concomitant with the start of vincristine therapy. Cranial nerve palsies, especially involving the fifth and seventh cranial nerves, have been seen.[78] These can occasionally cause problems in differential diagnosis between vincristine toxicity and leukemic involvement of the nervous system. Alopecia to some degree is fairly common but is of a temporary nature. Bone marrow depression occurs though to a lesser extent than with many other agents.

TABLE 1-1
CRITERIA FOR EVALUATION OF RESPONSE TO THERAPY OF A CHILD WITH ACUTE LEUKEMIA

Bone Marrow (M)

M1. Blasts less than 5%
Lymphocytes less than 35%

M2. Blasts 5 to 25%
Lymphocytes 35 to 70%

M3. Blasts 25 to 50%

M4. Blasts greater than 50%

Hemogram (H)

H1. Hemoglobin greater than 10 gm
Total poly count over 1500/mm^3
Platelet count over 100,000/mm^3
No blasts.

H2. Hemoglobin 9.0–9.9 gm
Total poly count 750–1499/mm^3
Platelet count 50,000–99,000/mm^3
Blasts 0%–5%

H3. Hemoglobin 7.0–8.9 gm
Total poly count 500–750/mm^3
Platelet count 25,000–49,000/mm^3
Blasts 6%–20%

H4. Hemoglobin less than 7.0 gm
Total poly count less than 500/mm^3
Platelet count less than 25,000/mm^3
Blasts greater than 20%

Physical Findings (P)

P1. Liver spleen and lymph nodes of normal size with no evidence of leukemic infiltration

P2. Mild enlargement of liver, spleen, lymph nodes or leukemic infiltration

P3. Moderate enlargement of liver, spleen and lymph nodes or leukemic infitration

P4. Massive enlargement of liver, spleen and lymph nodes or leukemic infiltration

Clinical Symptoms (S)

S1. Asymptomatic with full normal activity

S2. Mild symptoms only, but normal activity

S3. Moderate symptoms with limited activity, but less than 50% of normal waking hours in bed

S4. Severe symptoms with more than 50% of normal waking hours in bed.

Disease Status

A. Rating of 1 in all categories (complete remission)

B. Rating of 2 in one or more categories but no rating of 3 or 4 in any catecategory (partial remission)

C. Rating of 3 in one or more categories but no rating of 4 in any category

D. Rating of 4 in one or more categories (progressive disease)

TABLE 1-2
CHEMOTHERAPEUTIC AGENTS EFFECTIVE IN TREATMENT OF ACUTE LEUKEMIA

Drug	*Usual Dose*	*Route of Administration*	*Toxic Side Effects*
Antimetabolites			
Purinethol® (6-mercaptopurine)	3 mg/kg/day	oral	At high dosage, same as methotrexate.
Methotrexate (amethopterin)	30 mg/m²/biweekly	oral, IM or IT	Oral ulcers, diarrhea, hematopoietic depression, alopecia, increased skin pigmentation. Hepatotoxicity.
Cytosar® (cytosine arabinoside, AraC)	50–100 mg/m²/day or 100 mg/m²/q12h.	IV or IM	Hematopoietic depression.
Cytotoxic agents			
Cytoxan® (cyclophosphamide)	2.5 mg/kg/day	oral	Hemorrhagic cystitis, stomatitis, diarrhea, alopecia and hematopoietic depression.
Oncovin® (vincristine)	1.5 to 2 mg/m² weekly	IV	Peripheral neuritis, cranial nerve palsy, severe constipation and alopecia.
Daunomycin (daunorubicin)	1.0 mg/kg/day for 5 days	IV	Hematopoietic depression, cardiotoxicity, alopecia.
Adriamycin	0.5 mg/kg/day for 5 days	IV	Hematopoietic depression, cardiotoxicity, alopecia.
Enzyme			
Asparaginase	1000 U/kg/day for 5 days, or 5000 U/kg/week	IV	Anaphylactic reactions, pancreatitis, hypofibrinogenemia, defibrination, hypoproteinemia, azotemia.
Adrenocorticosteroids			
Prednisone (adrenocortical hormone)	40–120 mg/m²/day	oral	Cushingoid appearance, osteoporosis, sodium and water retention, hypertension, cerebral edema and peptic ulcer.
Decadron® (dexamethasone)	6 mg/m²/day	oral	Same

Adrenocorticosteroids are almost always used in combination with another chemotherapeutic agent for remission induction. Prednisone or prednisolone can be given orally in dose of 40 mg/m^2 daily. Once the child is in remission the prednisone is tapered over a ten-day period and then stopped. The toxicity of these drugs is well known and will not be reviewed here.

The chemotherapy of acute leukemia began when Dr. Sidney Farber introduced the folate antagonists.[79] *Methotrexate* is the best known of this group. It has been used in combination with other drugs for induction of remission, but it is now mainly used in maintenance therapy. The maintenance dose is 30 mg/m^2 twice weekly either orally or intramuscularly. Biweekly methotrexate has been shown in a study of the Acute Leukemia Cooperative Group B to be definitely superior to daily oral methotrexate.[80] The use of enormous infusions of methotrexate has been advocated by Djerassi for the treatment of acute lymphoblastic leukemia both for remission induction and maintenance.[81] Although most of the treated children required intensive supportive care, especially platelet transfusions, some very prolonged remissions were obtained.[82] Intrathecal methotrexate in a dose of 12 mg/m^2 is the treatment of choice for central nervous system involvement. The lumbar puncture is repeated every two to five days depending on the child's symptoms; methotrexate is instilled until the pressure has returned to normal and there are five or less cells in the cerebrospinal fluid.

Mucosal ulcerations are a sign of methotrexate toxicity and when present call for therapy to be temporarily stopped. If ulcerations recur then the dose of methotrexate should be reduced. There have been recent reports of children in remission on methotrexate maintenance who have developed bilateral pulmonary infiltrates.[83] Some of the children have biopsy-proven infection due to *P carinii*.[84] The reason for this increased incidence of pulmonary complications is not clear. Most of the children have continued taking methotrexate without a recurrence of this complication. Alopecia is also seen. Another complication of prolonged methotrexate administration is the development of hepatic fibrosis, and treatment should be stopped if this occurs.[35] Osteoporosis can also be seen after prolonged administration of methotrexate.[86]

6-Mercaptopurine is one of the purine antagonists. When used for remission induction it is usually given in combination with prednisone. For maintenance therapy it is most frequently given alone. An oral dose of 90 mg/m^2 given daily has been shown to produce prolonged remissions.[87] The maintenance dose is the same and is given daily until relapse. If the child is receiving allopurinol concomitantly with the 6-mercaptopurine then the dose of 6-mercaptopurine must be reduced to 25 percent of the calculated dose.[88] Hepatic toxicity in the form of intrahepatic cholestasis can be seen and calls for the cessation of therapy.[89,90]

Cyclophosphamide (Cytoxan®, Endoxan®) is an alkylating agent and is useful for remission induction usually in combination with prednisone. It is also a good drug for remission maintenance.[87] The dose is 2.5 to 3 mg/kg daily by mouth both for remission induction and for maintenance. It is given continuously until relapse. A sterile chemical cystitis may be seen and usually calls for a temporary cessation of therapy. Alopecia occurs.

Daunorubicin is an antibiotic of the streptomyces family. It is believed to act by the inhibition of both DNA and RNA synthesis. It is unique in that it is effective against both acute lymphoblastic and acute myeloblastic leukemia.[91-94] It is used daily for three to five days for remission induction in acute lymphoblastic leukemia either alone or in combination with prednisone and vincristine. It is given intravenously in a dose of 30 to 60 mg/m^2. If given in combination with vincristine and prednisone then one uses a weekly schedule. A recent study in children with acute lymphoblastic leukemia resistant to conventional drugs compared daunorubicin administered intravenously for five days either alone or in combination with prednisone with a third group receiving weekly daunorubicin and vincristine plus daily prednisone. The dose of daunorubicin was 45 mg/m^2. There was no significant difference in the remission rate of any of the three schedules. An overall remission rate of 36 percent was seen.[92] In the treatment of acute myeloblastic leukemia daunorubicin can be given alone or in combination with other drugs. In one series, five complete or partial remissions occurred in a group of twelve patients with acute myeloblastic leukemia.[94]

Daunorubicin produces severe marrow depression very rapidly. It is not unusual to see a patient with a white blood count of 100,000/mm³ drop to 3,000/mm³ in forty-eight to seventy-two hours after the institution of therapy. Daunorubicin cannot be used for continuous maintenance therapy because of its cardiac toxicity.[93,95] Severe congestive heart failure resulting in death has been reported.[93] This is known to be dose related and one should not exceed a total dose of 550 mg/m².

l-Asparaginase is an experimental drug that has excited much interest among chemotherapists. It is an enzyme that catalyzes the hydrolysis of l-asparagine to aspartic acid. It is produced commercially from bacteria, especially *Escherichia coli*. This enzyme inhibits the replication of sensitive leukemic cells by catalyzing the hydrolysis of l-asparagine, which is necessary for the growth of these cells.[96,97] It is given intravenously. The most effective dose is not known, but doses varying from 50 to 5,000 international units (IU) per kilogram have been given. It can be given daily or weekly either alone or in combination with other drugs. It is effective in inducing remission in children with acute lymphoblastic leukemia.[98,99]

Since l-asparaginase is prepared from *E coli* it is very difficult to obtain in a pure form. Perhaps this may account for some of the toxicity. Allergic reactions including anaphylaxis have been seen and for this reason it is difficult to use this drug in a maintenance regimen.[99] When administering this drug we routinely have Adrenalin®, Benadryl® and hydrocortisone at the patient's bedside. Multiple coagulation defects including fibrinolysis can occur.[100] We have seen three children who had laboratory evidence of defibrination. Hypoproteinemia and hypocholesterolemia are presumably the result of decreased protein synthesis. Central nervous system depression and excitation have been reported.[101] Hyperosmolar, nonketotic acidosis occurs though infrequently. Elevations of the blood urea nitrogen can be seen.[102] We have seen one child with acute lymphoblastic leukemia of four years duration induced into remission with daily l-asparaginase who developed acute renal failure which proved fatal. Autopsy revealed bilateral renal cortical necrosis.

Cytosine arabinoside (Ara-C, Cytosar®) is the single most effective agent for the treatment of acute myeloblastic leukemia. It is a pyrimidine antemetabolite. The drug is administered intravenously in a dose of 50 to 120 mg/m^2. It may be given as a single injection, as an infusion of one hour, or longer infusions of up to twenty-four hours' duration. Our experience at Mount Sinai Hospital in several of the Acute Leukemia Group B protocols is that a dose of 50 or 100 mg/m^2 administered intravenously daily over one hour is a very effective treatment. A recent study of patients with acute myeloblastic leukemia compared treatment with cytosine arabinoside alone or combined with 6-thioguanine, 6-mercaptopurine or daunorubicin.[103] Cytosine arabinoside was given in a dose of 100 mg/m^2 in a one-hour infusion every day. The combination of cytosine arabinoside and 6-thioguanine produced the best remission rate (50 percent). Cytosine arabinoside in a daily single injection in combination with oral 6-thioguanine has also produced good remissions in acute myeloblastic leukemia.[104] Intermittent therapy in combination with prednisone, cyclophosphamide and vincristine has produced a complete remission rate of 47 percent.[105]

Cytosine arabinoside has been shown to be effective for the treatment of acute lymphoblastic leukemia as well. Children's Cancer Study Group A reported on the effect of cytosine arabinoside given as a rapid intravenous injection to children with acute leukemia who had received prior therapy.[106] It was found that 30 percent of these children achieved a good partial remission. In another study a combination of cytosine arabinoside and prednisone produced an overall complete and partial remission rate of 49 percent in children with acute lymphoblastic leukemia or acute myeloblastic leukemia who had become refractory to conventional chemotherapy.[107] There is an intrathecal preparation of cytosine arabinoside which can be used in children who are refractory to intrathecal methotrexate. Nausea and vomiting occur and can usually be controlled by an antiemetic such as Compazine.®

Immunotherapy

In principle this consists of stimulating or inducing the patient's own immune response (active immunotherapy) or giving him antibodies or immunocompetent cells (passive immunotherapy).[108] Mathé reported thirty children with acute lymphoblastic leukemia who were induced into remission by prednisone alone or in combination with vincristine and daunorubicin. The patients were then given additional intensive chemotherapy in an effort to further reduce the leukemic population of cells. All ten of the children who received no further therapy had relapsed by 130 days. Twenty children further treated at weekly intervals with either innoculations of BCG or pooled allogenic leukemic lymphoblasts pretreated with formalin and irradiated *in vitro,* or a combination of the two, had remissions ranging from fifteen days to more than 1150 days.[109] Of interest is a report from Canada that deaths from leukemia were found to be half as common among BCG-vaccinated children less than fifteen years of age for each of the years 1960–1963 in the province of Quebec.[110]

CURRENT STATUS OF THERAPY FOR ACUTE LYMPHOBLASTIC LEUKEMIA

There is ample evidence, as mentioned before, that children who go into remission survive longer.[111,112] Therefore the immediate aim of treatment is to produce very prolonged remissions. At the present time more prolonged remissions are being sought through the use of (a) new drugs, (b) finding better ways of using the drugs available today, (c) using combinations of drugs and (d) reinduction therapy.

Remission Induction

Here one uses combination chemotherapy. This may be in the form of vincristine and prednisone or 6-mercaptopurine and prednisone. Larger combinations, using vincristine, prednisone and daunorubicin or l-asparaginase have not significantly increased the rate of remission induction.

Intensification–Consolidation Therapy

Once the child is in a complete remission there still is a reservoir of leukemic cells.[113] More intensive chemotherapy at this time is directed at further decreasing this population of cells. This can be done by using one drug such as methotrexate and administering it intensively in five-day courses.[112] One can use combinations of drugs such as methotrexate, 6-mercaptopurine, and cyclophosphamide for this intensification phase.[57]

Central Nervous System Prophylaxis

It has been recognized that many children in bone marrow remission will have a residue of leukemic cells in the central nervous system.[113] An attempt is being made now to prophylactically treat the central nervous system in order to achieve two goals: the first to prevent symptomatic leukemic menengitis and second, and most important, to produce very prolonged remissions. Aur has used intrathecal methotrexate and cranial irradiation with very encouraging results.[57] We now believe all children with acute lymphoblastic leukemia in remission should receive CNS prophylaxis after approximately two months of consolidation chemotherapy. Intrathecal methotrexate is given at a dose of 12 mg/m^2 every four days for a total of six doses. Cranial irradiation is given over a sixteen-day period in a dose of 2400 rods.

Maintenance Therapy

One can give one drug continuously until relapse. Krivit reported on the use of five drugs (methotrexate, vincristine, prednisone, Cytoxan and 6-mercaptopurine) given sequentially or cyclically.[114] Sequentially each drug was given alone until evidence of relapse, at which time the child was placed on the next drug in sequence. In the cyclical regimen each drug was administered for six-week periods in rotation. No difference was found in the median length of remission maintenance on either regimen, both lasting about 17.5 months. In an effort to increase the duration of remission the concept of reinduction therapy was introduced. During the maintenance phase when the child is usually, though not always, on a single drug he is given additional therapy (reinduction) at timed intervals, usually monthly. One injection of vincristine and seven days of prednisone given at monthly intervals is one form of the reinduction therapy. It has been shown that monthly reinduction with vincristine and prednisone increases the time in remission of children being maintained on daily 6-mercaptopurine.[115]

Though immunotherapy is a new and exciting adjunct to the overall treatment of acute leukemia, it is difficult to assess its role at the present time. If the initial promising results are duplicated at other centers, then immunotherapy of some type will undoubtedly become part of the maintenance therapy.

CURRENT STATUS OF THERAPY FOR ACUTE MYELOBLASTIC LEUKEMIA

It is only within the last several years that progress has been made in the treatment of this type of acute leukemia and we are finally seeing an increase in survival.[112] We now have new drugs such as cytosine arabinoside and daunorubicin that are effective for remission induction. Combinations of drugs such as cytosine arabinoside and 6-thioguanine or vincristine, prednisone, Cytoxan and cytosine arabinoside are effective for remission induction and perhaps for maintenance also. New combinations of drugs are now being studied in an effort to obtain higher remission rates.

SUMMARY

There is no question that great progress has been made in the treatment and control of childhood acute leukemia. Certainly our immediate goal of prolonged remissions is encouraging for there are several reported cases of children living five years and longer.[57, 60,112] It is reasonable to believe that the etiology of leukemia will be unravelled in the foreseeable future. We look forward to a future time when we will be able to state that the majority of children with this dread disease are surviving more than five years and many may therefore be on the way to a cure.

REFERENCES

1. Ederer, F., Miller, R.W., and Scotto, J.: United States childhood cancer mortality patterns, 1950-1959. *JAMA, 192*:593-596, 1965.

2. Heath, C.W., and Hasterlik, R.: Leukemia among children in a suburban community. *Am J Med, 34*:796-812, 1963.
3. Meighan, S.S., and Knox, G.: Leukemia in childhood. Epidemiology in Oregon. *Cancer, 18*:811-814, 1965.
4. Ellermann, V., and Bang, O.: Experimentelle leukämie bei hühnern. *Centrabl J Bakt Abt I, 46*:595-609, 1908.
5. Bryan, W.R., Dalton, A., and Rauscher, F.: The viral approach to human leukemia and lymphoma; its current status. *Progr Hematol, 5*: 137-179, 1966.
6. Jarrett, W., Martin, W., Crighton, C. *et al.*: Leukemia in the cat. *Nature (Lond), 202*:566-568, 1964.
7. Dmochowski, L.: Electron microscope studies of leukemia in animals and men. In *Current Research in Leukaemia.* Cambridge, Cambridge University Press, 1965, pp. 23-33.
8. Bayer, M.E., Blumberg, B.S., and Werner, B.: Particles associated with Australia antigen in the sera of patients with leukaemia, Down's syndrome, and hepatitis. *Nature (Lond), 218*:1157-1159, 1968.
9. Blumberg, B., Sutnick, A., and London, W.: Hepatitis and leukaemia; their relation to Australia antigen. *Bull NY Acad Med, 44*:1566-1586, 1968.
10. Temin, H., and Mitutani, S.: RNA-dependent DNA polymerase in virions of Rous sarcoma virus. *Nature (Lond), 226*:1211-1213, 1970.
11. Baltimore, D.: Viral RNA-dependent DNA polymerase. *Nature (Lond), 226*:1209-1211, 1970.
12. Trallo, R., Young, S., and Ting, R.: RNA-dependent DNA polymerase of human acute leukemic cells. *Nature (Lond), 228*:927-929, 1970.
13. Spiegelman, S.: Personal communication.
14. Heath, C.W., and Moloney, W.: Familial leukemia. *N Engl J Med, 272*: 882-887, 1965.
15. Rigby, P., Pratt, P., Rosenlof, R., and Lemon, H.: Genetic relationships in familial leukemia and lymphoma. *Arch Intern Med, 121*:67-70, 1968.
16. McMahon, B., and Levy, M.A.: Prenatal origin of childhood leukemia. Evidence from twins. *N Engl J Med, 270*:1082-1085, 1964.
17. Kamada, N., Okada, K., Ito, T. *et al.*: Chromosomes 21-22 and neutrophil alkaline phosphatase in leukemia. *Lancet, 1*:364, 1968.
18. Khouri, F., Shahid, M.J., and Yenikomshian, S.: Cytogenetic studies in acute leukemia. *Acta Haematol Jap, 40*:192-199, 1968.
19. Holland, W., Doll, R., and Carter, C.: The mortality from leukemia and other cancers among patients with Down's syndrome and among their parents. *Br J Cancer, 16*:177, 1962.
20. Jackson, E., Turner, J., Kauber, M., and Norris, F.: Down's syndrome. Variation of leukemia occurrence in institutionalized populations. *J Chronic Dis, 21*:247-253, 1968.

21. Miller, R.W.: Persons with exceptionally high risk of leukemia. *Cancer Res, 27*:2420-2423, 1967.
22. Zuelzer, W., and Cox, D.E.: Genetic aspects of leukemia. *Semin Hematol, 6*:228-249, 1969.
23. Stewart, A., Webb, J., and Hewitt, D.: Survey of childhood malignancies. *Br Med J, 1*:1495-1508, 1958.
24. Murray, R., Heckel, P., and Hempelmann, L.H.: Leukemia in children exposed to ionizing radiation. *N Engl J Med, 261*:585-588, 1959.
25. Gibson, R.W., Bross, I., Graham, S. *et al.*: Leukemia in children exposed to multiple risk factors. *N Engl J Med, 279*:906-909, 1968.
26. Sang, K.: Superior mediastinal syndrome in a young child. *JAMA, 208*: 1177-1179, 1969.
27. Krakoff, I.H., and Meyer, R.: Prevention of hyperuricemia in leukemia and lymphoma. *JAMA, 193*:1-6, 1965.
28. DeConti, R.C., and Calabresi, P.: Use of allopurinol for prevention and control of hyperuricemia in patients with neoplastic disease. *N Engl J Med, 274*:481-488, 1966.
29. Jordan, G.W.: Serum calcium and phosphorus abnormalities in leukemia. *Am J Med, 41*:381-390, 1966.
30. Zucker, S., Hanes, D.J., Vogler, W., and Eames, R.: Plasma muramidase; a study of methods and clinical applications. *J Lab Clin Med, 75*: 83-92, 1970.
31. Perillie, P.E., Kaplan, S., Lefkowitz, E. *et al.*: Studies of muramidase (lysozyme) in leukemia. *JAMA, 203*:317-322, 1968.
32. Wiernik, P.H., and Serpick, A.: Clinical significance of serum and urinary muramidase activity in leukemia and other hematologic malignancies. *Am J Med, 46*:330-343, 1969.
33. Hardisty, R.M., Speed, D., and Till, M.: Granulocytic leukaemia in childhood. *Br J Haematol, 10*:551-566, 1964.
34. Miller, D.R.: Raised foetal haemoglobin in childhood leukemia. *Br J Haematol, 17*:103-112, 1969.
35. Whitecar, J.P.: Disseminated intravascular coagulation in patients with acute leukemia. *Proc Am Assoc Cancer Res, 12*:46, 1971.
36. Kwan, O., and Gross, S.: The G immunoglobulins in acute leukemia in children. Hematologic and immunologic relationships. *Blood, 33*:198-206, 1969.
37. Lindqvist, K.I., Ragab, A., and Osterland, K.: Paraproteinemia in a child with leukemia. *Blood, 35*:213-221, 1970.
38. Stoop, J., Zegers, B., van der Heiden, C., and Ballieux, R.: Monoclonal gammapathy in a child with leukemia. *Blood, 32*:774-786, 1968.
39. Constantoulakis, M., Phocas, E., and Theodosopoulos, G.: Atypical leukaemia of long duration with monoclonal hypergammaglobulinemia. *J Clin Pathol, 23*:156-160, 1970.
40. Hersh, E., Bodey, G., Nies, B., and Freireich, E.J.: Causes of death in

acute leukemia; A ten-year study of 414 patients from 1954–1963. *JAMA, 193*:105-109, 1965.

41. Viola, M.: Acute leukemia and infection. *JAMA, 201*:923-926, 1967.
42. Bodey, G., Bieckley, M., Sathe, Y.S., and Freireich, E.J.: Quantitative relationships between circulating leukocytes and infection in patients with acute leukemia. *Ann Intern Med, 64*:328-340, 1966.
43. Strauss, R., Paul, B., Jacobs, A. *et al.*: The metabolic and phagocytic activities of leukocytes from children with acute leukemia. *Cancer Res, 30*:480-488, 1970.
44. Senn, H.J., and Holland, J.: Funktionelle beurteilung der infeklabwehr bei leukamien. *Schweiz Med Wochenschr, 100*:308-310, 1970.
45. Murray, J., Haegelin, H.F., Hewitt, W. *et al.*: Opportunistic pulmonary infections. *Ann Intern Med, 65*:566-594, 1966.
46. Hutter, R., and Collins, H.S.: The occurrence of opportunistic fungus infections in a cancer hospital. *Lab Invest, 11*:1035-1045, 1962.
47. Young, R., Vogel, C.L., and De Vita, V.: Aspergillus lobar pneumonia. *JAMA, 208*:1156-1162, 1969.
48. Holland, E., Simone, J.V., and Johnson, W.: Remission fatalities in childhood acute leukemia. *Proc Am Assoc Cancer Res, 11*:38, 1970.
49. DeVita, V., Emmer, M., Levine, A. *et al.*: *Pneumocystis carinii* pneumonia. Successful diagnosis and treatment of two patients with associated malignant processes. *N Engl J Med, 280*:287-290, 1969.
50. Cangir, A., and Sullivan, M.P.: The occurrence of cytomegalovirus infections in childhood leukemia. *JAMA, 195*:616-622, 1966.
51. Dyment, P., Orlando, S.J., Issacs, H., and Wright, H.: The incidence of cytomegaloviruria and postmortem cytomegalic inclusions in children with acute leukemia. *J Pediatr, 72*:533-536, 1968.
52. Freireich, E.J., Thomas, L., Frei, E. *et al.*: A distinctive type of intracerebral hemorrhage associated with "blastic crisis" in patients with leukemia. *Cancer, 13*:146-154, 1960.
53. Fritz, R., Forkner, C.E., Freireich, E.J. *et al.*: The association of fatal intracranial hemorrhage and "blastic crisis" in patients with acute leukemia. *N Engl J Med, 261*:59-64, 1959.
54. Nies, B.A., Thomas, L.B., and Freireich, E.J.: Meningeal leukemia. *Cancer, 18*:546-555, 1965.
55. Evans, A., Gilbert, E.S., and Zandstra, R.: The increasing incidence of central nervous system leukemia in children. *Cancer, 26*:404-409, 1970.
56. Sullivan, M.T., Vietti, T., Fernbach, D. *et al.*: Clinical investigations in the treatment of meningeal leukemia. Radiation therapy regimens vs. conventional intrathecal methotrexate. *Blood, 34*:301-319, 1969.
57. Aur, R., Simone, J., Hustu, H. *et al.*: Central nervous system therapy and combination chemotherapy of childhood lymphocytic leukemia. *Blood, 37*:272-281, 1971.

58. Jampol, M.L., and Ohnysty, J.: Acute leukemia seen as testicular tumor. *NY State J Med, 67*:1903-1906, 1967.
59. Givler, R.L.: Testicular involvement in leukemia and lymphoma. *Cancer, 23*:1290-1295, 1969.
60. Burchenal, J.: Long term survivors in acute leukemia and Burkett's tumor. *Cancer, 21*:595-599, 1968.
61. Silverman, F.N.: The skeletal lesions in leukemia. Clinical and roentgenographic observations in 103 infants and children, with a review of the literature. *Am J Roentgenol, Radium Ther Nucl Med, 59*:819-843, 1948.
62. Hilbish, T., Besse, B., Lusted, L.B. *et al.*: Acute leukemia. Skeletal manifestations in children and adults. *Arch Intern Med, 104*:741-747, 1959.
63. Nies, B.A., Kundel, D.W., Thomas, L., and Freireich, E.J.: Leukopenia, bone pain, and bone necrosis in patients with acute leukemia. *Ann Intern Med, 62*:698-705, 1965.
64. Simmons, C., Hable, T.S., and Singleton, E.: The osseous manifestations of leukemia in children. *Radiol Clin North Am, 6*:115-130, 1968.
65. Reardon, G., and Moloney, W.C.: Chloroma and related myeloblastic neoplasms. *Arch Intern Med, 108*:864-871, 1961.
66. Bluefarb, S.: *Leukemia cutis*. Springfield, Charles C Thomas, 1960, pp. 1-338.
67. Roberts, W., Bodey, G., Westlake, P.: The heart in acute leukemia: A study of 420 autopsy cases. *Am J Cardiol, 21*:388-412, 1968.
68. Sumners, J., Johnson, W., and Ainger, L.E.: Childhood leukemic heart disease. A study of 116 hearts of children dying of leukemia. *Circulation, 40*:575-581, 1969.
69. Freireich, E.J.: Effectiveness of platelet transfusion in leukemia and aplastic anemia. *Transfusion, 6*:50-54, 1966.
70. Schwarzenberg, L., Mathé, G., Amiel, J.L. *et al.*: Study of factors determining the usefulness and complications of leukocyte transfusions. *Am J Med, 43*:206-213, 1967.
71. Zubrod, C.G.: Treatment of the acute leukemias. *Cancer Res, 27*:2557-2560, 1967.
72. Zuelzer, W.: Implications of long term survival in acute stem cell leukemia of childhood treated with composite cyclic therapy. *Blood, 24*:477-494, 1964.
73. Henderson, E.S.: Treatment of acute leukemia. *Ann Intern Med, 69*:628-632, 1968.
74. Pinkel, D.: Five-year follow up of "total therapy" of childhood lymphocytic leukemia. *JAMA, 216*:648-652, 1971.
75. Evans, A., Farber, S., Brunet, S., and Mariano, P.: Vincristine in the treatment of acute leukemia in children. *Cancer, 16*:1302-1306, 1963.
76. Heyn, R., Beatty, E.C., Hammond, D. *et al.*: Vincristine in the treatment of acute leukemia in children. *Pediatrics, 38*:82-91, 1966.

77. Selawry, O.S., and Hananian, J.: Vincristine treatment of cancer in children. *JAMA, 183*:741-746, 1963.
78. Sandler, S.G., Tobin, W., and Henderson, E.S.: Vincristine-induced neuropathy; A clinical study of fifty leukemia patients. *Neurology (Minneap), 19*:367-374, 1969.
79. Farber, S., Diamond, L., Mercer, R.D. *et al.*: Temporary remissions in acute leukemia in children produced by folic acid antagonist 4-aminopteroyl-glutamic acid (aminopterin). *N Engl J Med, 238*:787-793, 1948.
80. Selawry, O.S.: New treatment schedule with improved survival in childhood leukemia. Intermittent parenteral vs. daily oral administration of methotrexate for maintenance of induced remission. *JAMA, 194*: 75-81, 1965.
81. Djerassi, I., Farber, S., Abir, E., and Neikirik, W.: Continuous infusion of methotrexate in children with acute leukemia. *Cancer, 20*:233-242, 1967.
82. Djerassi, I.: Methotrexate infusions and intensive supportive care in the management of children with acute lymphocytic leukemia, Follow-up report. *Cancer Res, 27*:2561-2564, 1967.
83. Clarysse, A., Cathey, W.J., Cartwright, G., and Wintrobe, M.: Pulmonary disease complicating intermittent therapy with methotrexate. *JAMA, 209*:1861-1864, 1969.
84. Moore, D., Carnahan, C.E., Mills, S., and Burgert, E.: *Pneumocystis* carinii pneumonitis complicating leukemia. *Mayo Clin Proc, 44*:162-168, 1969.
85. Colsky, J., Greenspan, E., and Warren, Y.W.: Hepatic fibrosis in children with acute leukemia after therapy with folic acid antagonists. *Arch Pathol, 59*:198-206, 1955.
86. Ragab, A.H., Frech, R.S., and Vietti, T.: Osteoporotic fractures secondary to methotrexate therapy of acute leukemia in remission. *Cancer, 25*:580-585, 1970.
87. Fernbach, J.D., Griffith, K., Haggard, M. *et al.*: Chemotherapy of acute leukemia in childhood; Comparison of cyclophosphamide and mercaptopurine. *N Engl J Med, 275*:451-456, 1966.
88. Rundles, R.W., Wyngaarden, J.B., Hitchings, G. *et al.*: Effects of xanthine oxidase inhibitor on thiopurine metabolism, hyperuricemia and gout. *Trans Assoc Am Physicians, 76*:126-140, 1963.
89. Einhorn, M., and Davidson, I.: Hepatotoxicity of mercaptopurine. *JAMA, 188*:802-806, 1964.
90. McIllvanie, S., and MacCarthy, J.D.: Hepatitis in association with prolonged 6-mercaptopurine therapy. *Blood, 14*:80-90, 1959.
91. Holton, C., Vietti, T., Nora, A.H. *et al.*: Daunomycin and prednisone for induction of remission in advanced leukemia. *N Engl J Med, 280*: 171-174, 1969.

92. Jones, B.: Daunorubicin plus vincristine plus prednisone vs. daunorubicin plus vincristine plus prednisone in resistant childhood leukemia. *Proc Am Assoc Cancer Res, 11*:41, 1970.
93. Bernard, J., Jacquillat, C., Boiron, M. *et al.*: Experimental treatment of acute lymphoblastic and myeloblastic leukemias with a new antibiotic, rubidomycin. *Presse Med, 75*:951-957, 1967.
94. Bornstein, R.S., Theologides, A., and Kennedy, B.J.: Daunorubicin in acute myelogenous leukemia in adults. *JAMA, 207*:1301-1306, 1969.
95. Bonadonna, G., and Monfardini, S.: Cardiac toxicity of daunorubicin. *Lancet, 1*:837, 1969.
96. Broome, J.: Studies on the mechanism of tumor inhibition by l-asparaginase. Effects of the enzyme on asparagine levels in the blood, normal tissues and 6 C3HED lymphomas of mice; differences in asparagine formation and utilization in asparaginase-sensitive and resistant lymphoma cells. *J Exp Med, 127*:1055-1071 1968.
97. Broome, J.: Evidence that the l-asparaginase of guinea pig serum is responsible for its antilymphoma effects; II. lymphoma 6C3HED cells cultured in a medium devoid of l-asparagine lose their susceptibility to the effects of guinea pig serum *in vivo*. *J Exp Med, 118*:121-148, 1963.
98. Tallal, L., Tan, C., Oettgen, H. *et al.*: Asparaginase in 111 children with leukemias and solid tumors. *Proc Am Assoc Cancer Res, 10*:92, 1969.
99. Rausen, A., and Glidewell, O.: l-Asparaginase in advanced childhood leukemia. Comparative trial of drug schedules singly and in combination. *Proc Am Assoc Cancer Res, 11*:66, 1970.
100. Gralnick, H., and Henry, P.H.: l-Asparaginase induced coagulapathy. *Proc Am Assoc Cancer Res, 10*:32, 1969.
101. Schein, P.S., Rakieter, N., Gordon, B.M. *et al.*: The toxicity of *E coli* l-asparaginase. *Cancer Res, 29*:426-434, 1969.
102. Haskell, C., Cavellos, G.P., Leventhal, B. *et al.*: l-Asparaginase toxicity. *Cancer Res, 29*:974-975, 1969.
103. Carey, R.W.: Comparative study of cytosine arabinoside therapy alone and combined with thioguanine, mercaptopurine or daunomycin in acute myelocytic leukemia. *Proc Am Assoc Cancer Res, 11*:15, 1970.
104. Gee, T.S., Yu, K., Augustin, B. *et al.*: Combination therapy of adult acute leukemia with thioguanine and 1-B-D arabinofuranosylcytosine. *Proc Am Assoc Cancer Res, 9*:23, 1968.
105. Whitecar, J.R., Bodey, G., and Freireich, E.J.: Combination chemotherapy (COAP) of adult acute leukemia. *Proc Am Assoc Cancer Res, 11*:83, 1970.
106. Howard, J.P., Alba, V., and Newton, W.: Cytosine arabinoside. Results of a cooperative study in acute childhood leukemia. *Cancer, 21*: 341-345, 1968.

107. Nesbit, M.E., and Hammond, D.: Cytosine arabinoside and prednisone therapy of previously treated acute lymphoblastic and undifferentiated leukemia of childhood. *Proc Am Assoc Cancer Res, 11*:59, 1970.
108. Mathé, G., Schwarzenberg, L., Amiel, J. *et al.*: The role of immunology in the treatment of leukemias and hematosarcomas. *Cancer Res, 27*: 2542-2553, 1967.
109. Mathé, G. ,Amiel, J.L., Schwarzenberg, L. *et al.*: Active immunotherapy for acute lymphoblastic leukemia. *Lancet, 1*:697-699, 1969.
110. Davigon, L., Lemonde, P., Robillard, P., and Frappier, A.: B.C.G. vaccination and leukaemia mortality. *Lancet, 2*:638, 1970.
111. Henderson, E.S.: Treatment of leukemia. *Semin Hemat, 6*:271-319, 1969.
112. Holland, J.F.: Therapy of Acute Leukemia. *International Congress of Hematology* (XIII). Munich, 1970, pp. 58-65.
113. Mathé, G., Schwarzenberg, L., Mery, A.N. *et al.*: Extensive histological and cytological survey of patients with acute leukemia in "complete remission." *Br Med J, 1*:640-642, 1966.
114. Krivit, W., Brubaker, C., Thatcher, L. *et al.*: Maintenance therapy in acute leukemia of childhood; comparison of cyclic vs. sequential methods. *Cancer, 21*:352-356, 1968.
115. Chevalier, L., and Glidewell, O.: Schedule of 6-mercaptopurine and effect of inducer drugs in prolongation of remission maintenance in acute leukemia. *Proc Am Assoc Cancer Res, 8*:10, 1967.

Chapter 2

UNUSUAL FORMS OF CHILDHOOD LEUKEMIA

THOMAS F. NECHELES

OVER 95 percent of all cases of childhood leukemia can be classified as lymphoblastic, myeloblastic or "stem cell" acute leukemias. Only rarely do children present with a form of leukemia which does not fit into one of these categories. However, such unusual cases do occur and may present problems in diagnosis as well as management, especially since they may not respond to the therapeutic regimens found useful in the common forms of childhood acute leukemia.

Leukemia can conceivably arise in any one of the various hematopoietic cell lines and indeed most, if not all, of the possible types have been identified in some cases. However, in children, only a few of the unusual forms are of any clinical significance: chronic granulocytic leukemia, some of the variants of acute myeloblastic leukemia, and monocytic leukemia. Chronic lymphocytic leukemia and malignancies involving the plasma cells have never been unequivocally demonstrated in the pediatric age group and other possible varieties such as basophilic leukemia, megakaryocytic leukemia, and so forth, are so rare, if they even occur, so as not to warrant more than passing mention.

CHRONIC GRANULOCYTIC LEUKEMIA

Chronic granulocytic leukemia (CGL) can be defined as a self-perpetuating proliferative disorder involving the myeloid elements of the bone marrow resulting in a persistently elevated number of mature granulocytes in the peripheral blood, infiltration both into hematopoietic organs, such as the spleen, and nonhematopoietic organ systems, and eventual death. Less than 5 percent of all cases of childhood leukemia fit this definition of chronic granulocytic leukemia.[1] However, despite their morphological similarities, this is not a homogeneous group and two distinct forms of chronic granulocytic leukemia have been recognized in the pediatric age group. These have been classified, by Bloom *et al.*[2] into the juvenile type and adult type. Although similar in histological appearance, these two forms of chronic granulocytic leukemia differ sufficiently (Table 2-1) as to warrant consideration as two distinct entities.

TABLE 2-1
FORMS OF CHILDHOOD CHRONIC GRANULOCYTIC LEUKEMIA

	Juvenile Form	*Adult Form*
Age of maximum incidence (yrs)	1 to 5	10 to 15
Skin rash	Frequent	Rare
Splenomegaly	Moderate	Marked
Suppurative lymphadenitis	Frequent	Rare
Initial white blood cell count	Rarely above 100,000/mm^3	Frequently above 100,000/mm^3
Thrombocytopenia	Usually present	Infrequent
Blast forms in peripheral blood	Frequent	Infrequent
Ph^1 chromosome	Absent	Almost always present
Hemoglobin F levels	Moderately to markedly elevated	Normal
Leukocyte alkaline phosphatase	Normal	Reduced
Response to therapy	Poor	Usually excellent

Modified from Bloom *et al.*[2]

Juvenile Type of CGL

This form of leukemia is typically seen in the first several years of life. The patients often come to the physician's attention because of eczematoid rash usually involving the face. Infection is another frequent initial complaint; skin involvement and suppurative lymphadenitis are probable the most common presenting complaints. The involvement of skin and superficial lymph nodes is of interest in that the most frequent forms of infection in agranulocytosis show similar patterns of involvement. This finding suggests that infants with the juvenile type of CGL may well have functionally deficient granulocytes. In fact, Mauer[3] has compared the clinical presentation of the juvenile type of CGL with that of chronic granulomatous disease of childhood in which the defect of granulocyte function is well known.[4] The appearance of clinical signs of purpura and mucosal bleeding usually serves to draw attention to the hematopoietic system and mitigates against the diagnosis of primary sepsis or inherited disease of the granulocytes. At this point, pallor is a common finding. The physical examination usually reveals hepatosplenomegaly. Lymphadenopathy in the absence of suppurative adenitis is not very remarkable.

Laboratory data at the time of diagnosis usually includes a normocytic, normochromic anemia, thrombocytopenia and leukocytosis. Leukocytosis may be quite marked but it is unusual for the white blood cell count to be above 100,000/mm^3. Other laboratory data helpful at this time is the presence of bizarre myeloid forms in the peripheral blood smear including usually a small number of myeloblasts. The nitro-blue tetrazolium test,[5] used to diagnose chronic granulomatous disease, shows that the granulocytes can reduce the dye and presumably are effective in killing bacteria. Bone marrow examination reveals a hyperplastic marrow with a large number of myeloid precursors at all stages of development. The "leukemic hiatus" often seen in acute myeloblastic leukemia is absent. Erythroid and megakaryocytic precursors are usually decreased, accounting for the anemia and thrombocytopenia. Differentiation from a leukemoid reaction to infection may, at this point, present some difficulty.

Ancillary hematologic studies are often of some help. Of particular interest and of significant aid in establishing the diagnosis is the finding of a marked elevation of fetal hemoglobin concentration in the peripheral blood. Bloom *et al.*[2] quote levels of 15 to 50 percent but other authors have reported levels of 76 percent[6] and levels above 90 percent have been seen.[7] These levels of fetal hemoglobin suggest that the disease process involves the erythroid as well as the myeloid elements of the marrow. The leukocyte alkaline phosphatase activity, in contrast to the adult form of this disease, is usually either in the normal range or is elevated.[8] Chromosome studies are helpful only in differentiating the juvenile type from the adult type of CGL. In contradistinction to the adult type of chronic granulocytic leukemia, chromosome studies in the juvenile type usually reveal only nonspecific changes. The characteristic defect in the G-group chromosomes, the so-called Philadelphia chromosome, is typically lacking.[8a] In fact, the presence of the Ph^1 chromosome mitigates against the diagnosis of the juvenile type of chronic granulocytic leukemia. Chromosome abnormalities, when present, are limited to nonspecific breaks and gaps.

Chemotherapy of the juvenile type of chronic granulocytic leukemia is unsatisfactory. These children usually do not respond to the treatment regimens effective in the adult type of this disease. The various modalities of treatment that have been tried include busulfan, 6-mercaptopurine and cyclophosphamide. None of these appear to be uniformly useful in obtaining a remission, as defined by the return of the bone marrow morphology and peripheral hematologic values to normal. Partial remissions with transitory clinical improvement have been reported but these are usually short lived and the disease pursues a relentless downhill course. The average duration of survival does not appear to have been significantly changed by chemotherapy and is usually measured in terms of months. The use of newer chemotherapeutic agents in this disease has not as yet been reported and the evaluation of such modalities of treatment is limited by the low incidence of suitable cases. However, it appears that a trial of cytosine arabinoside and cyclophosphomide in such cases (analogous to COAP therapy)[9] might well be warranted. Splenectomy has induced prolonged remission in a few cases.[11] It is interesting to note that Weatherall and Brown[10] have suggested that this may be a form of congenital leukemia in which there is a proliferation of a myeloid cell line which has not undergone normal differentiation. Several instances of chronic myeloid leukemia in siblings have also been reported,[11] supporting the possible congenital origin of this disease.

Adult Type of CGL

The adult type of chronic granulocytic leukemia is usually found in the older child, typically towards the end of the first decade of life, but occasional cases of this form of the disease have been seen in infancy as well. In contrast to other childhood forms of leukemia, the onset may be insidious with few or no presenting symptoms. The child may be seen by the physician because of fever, pallor or nonspecific malaise. Occasionally the diagnosis may arise from findings on a routine physical examination. Rarely the child may be referred by the dentist because of prolonged bleeding following a dental extraction. Purpura as one of the major presenting complaints is quite uncommon. Physical examination is noteworthy primarily for the presence of marked hepatosplenomegaly, usually associated with a moderate degree of pallor. Lymphadenopathy is usually inconspicuous. Petechiae and purpura, if present, are minimal.

Laboratory studies usually reveal a normocytic, normochromic anemia with a reticulocytopenia. Thrombocytopenia is uncommon and indeed the platelet count may be elevated. Platelet function may, however, be impaired so that one has clinical evidence of bleeding even in the presence of thrombocytosis. The white blood count is elevated and frequently above 100,000/mm^3 and may be as high as 500,000/mm^3. Examination of the peripheral blood reveals myeloid elements at all stages of maturation ranging from myeloblasts to mature neutrophils. The latter predominate at the initial stages of the disease and immature forms may comprise only a small proportion of the circulating myeloid elements. Various morphological abnormalities of the mature neutrophils may be noted, the pseudo–Pelger-Huet anomaly is probably the most common, but none are of any particular diagnostic significance. Increased numbers of basophils are frequently found and may range as high as 20 percent of the total leukocyte count. The bone marrow is hypercellular with a marked increase in all stages of myeloid elements. The erythroid precursors are usually decreased both on a relative and absolute basis. The megakaryocytes are frequently normal in number although at times an increase may be noted.

A marked decrease in the leukocyte alkaline phosphatase (LAP) activity is considered to be diagnostic of the adult type of chronic granulocytic leukemia,[8] in contrast to the juvenile type. This decrease in LAP activity persists even during periods of clinical and hematologic remission. Increased activity is seen, how-

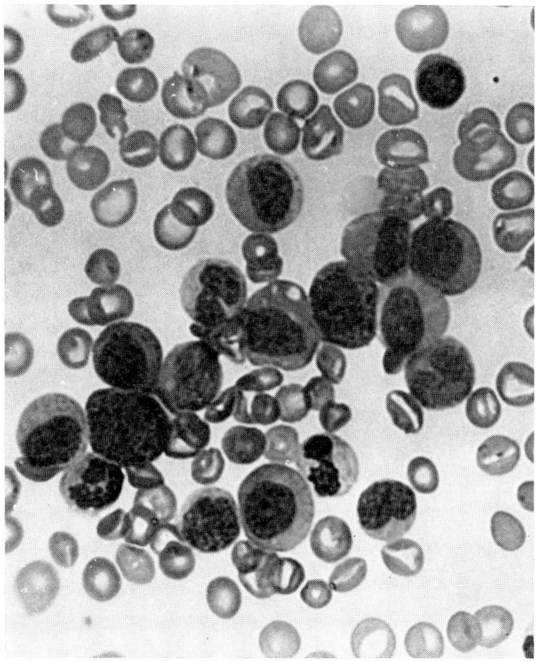

Figure 2-1. Peripheral blood smear in chronic granulocytic leukemia (×40). The majority of leukocytes are myelocytes, metamyelocytes or mature neutrophils, although an occasional promyelocyte can be recognized.

ever, in the face of coexisting infection or chronic inflammatory disease such as ulcerative colitis.[12] Fetal hemoglobin levels are within normal limits.

Chronic granulocytic leukemia is the only human neoplasm in which a specific chromosomal abnormality has been identified in a high percentage of newly diagnosed cases. Depending upon the center reporting and the diagnostic criteria used, 70 to 90 percent[13,14] of all cases of chronic granulocytic leukemia show the specific chromosomal abnormality known as the Philadelphia chromosome (Ph^1). This is a small acrocentric autosome (Fig. 2-2) which lacks the distal portions of its long arms and is usually considered to be a member of the G-22 pair.[15] The Ph^1 chromosome is frequently found in all of the marrow metaphases examined at the time of diagnosis and has been identified in megakaryocytes[16]

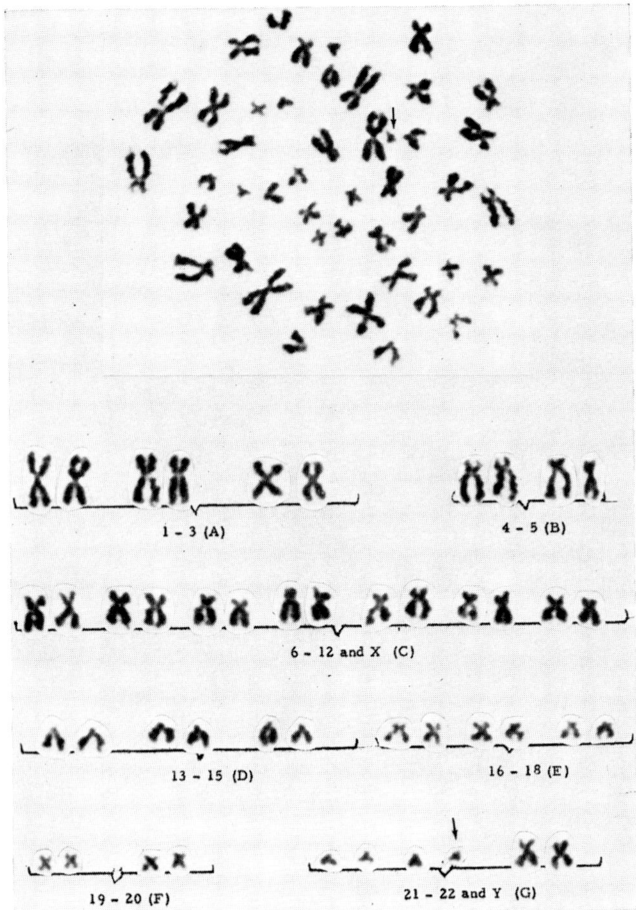

Figure 2-2. A karyotype of a patient with chronic granulocytic leukemia showing a typical Ph^1 chromosome (arrow).

and erythroid precursors[17] as well as cells of the granulocytic series. The anomaly persists in the bone marrow even during clinical and hematological remission, suggesting that current therapy does not begin to eradicate the abnormal (malignant) stem cell line. The Ph^1 chromosome is present only in cells of the myeloid series; it is absent in lymphoid cells and in skin fibroblasts.[18] Its presence is a postzygotic phenomenon as evidenced by its absence in monozygotic twin pairs, one of whom had the disease.[19] The role of the Ph^1 chromosome in the pathogenesis of chronic granulocytic leukemia is still unclear. Although adult cases of chronic granulocytic leukemia which are Ph^1-negative are notoriously unresponsive to therapy,[13] a similar clinical-cytogenetic correlation has not been described in the pediatric literature, possibly because of the limited amount of clinical material.

Treatment of the adult type of chronic granulocytic leukemia is usually relatively uncomplicated, especially in the early stages of this disease. Almost 100 percent of previously untreated patients respond to busulfan.[20] A dose of 0.05 mg/kg/day by mouth leads to prompt control of the white count and reduction of the size of the spleen. Close monitoring of the blood counts, especially platelets, is important and the drug should be discontinued when the white count falls below 15,000/mm^3. Marrow suppression and particularly thrombocytopenia are extremely difficult to manage and should be avoided. Other toxic effects of long-term busulfan therapy have been described and include pulmonary fibrosis[21] and a syndrome suggestive of adrenal cortical insufficiency.[22] Eventually the patient becomes increasingly resistant to busulfan therapy as evidenced by a lack of response in the white blood cell count and increasing splenomegaly. Dibromomannitol[23] and hydroxyurea[24] have been used successfully in some patients who have become resistant to busulfan. Good therapeutic control is much more difficult and unpleasant gastrointestinal side effects are more common with these two drugs. 6-Mercaptopurine in a dose of 2.5 mg/kg/day has also been found useful in some such resistant cases.

Complications which may occur during the course of the disease include local accumulations of leukemic cells in the form of chloromas. These tumor masses frequently produce symptomatology secondary to impingement on neighboring structures. The most striking example is an intradural chloroma leading to spinal cord compression. These local collections may appear even in the face of satisfactory control of the peripheral blood counts and often require local irradiation for relief. Progressive splenomegaly may also pose problems in management since a rapidly enlarging spleen may produce local discomfort, may undergo infarction and subcapsular bleeding with associated clinical symptomatology, and may produce a significant degree of hypersplenism leading to a marked thrombocytopenia and anemia difficult to control with transfusions. Irradiation to the splenic area is usually helpful in the temporary control of the clinical symptomatology. Splenectomy in the late stages of the disease, at a time when the symptoms of hypersplenism become troublesome, carries with it a relatively high risk, especially in the face of the thrombopathy often present in these patients. Early splenectomy, at a time when the disease is under good control, has recently been suggested[20] to avoid these late complications.

Eventually in most patients the disease evolves into a phase morphologically similar to acute myeloblastic leukemia, the so-called blast crises. The presence of large numbers of circulating myeloblasts associated with severe anemia and thrombocytopenia is usually a grave prognostic sign and these patients no longer respond to busulfan or 6-mercaptopurine. Hydroxyurea has been tried for the treatment of the "blast crises" but the results have been disappointing. A combination of vincristine and prednisone produced complete remissions in 25 percent of patients in one series.[25] The combination of cytosine arabinoside and 6-thioguanine has produced remissions in 30 to 50 percent of patients, most of whom were not children. The remissions in both trials were of short duration and the patients usually succumbed soon thereafter. These patients usually die from either hemorrhage or infection.

Survival in chronic granulocytic leukemia, with optimal therapy, is, on the average, thirty-six to forty months from the time of diagnosis.[20] Therapy has done little to prolong survival but has improved the quality of life. There is need for trials of more intensive chemotherapy of CGL as measures to eradicate the Ph^1 chromosome-positive clone of cells, delay the onset of the "blast crises" and improve overall survival.

UNUSUAL VARIANTS OF ACUTE LEUKEMIA

Over 95 percent of all cases of acute leukemia can be classified as lymphoblastic, undifferentiated ("stem cell") or myelocytic.

Only about 3 percent of a large series of children with acute leukemia could be classified as one of the less common variants.[26] Despite the rarity of these forms, they are important because of the unusual clinical problems involved in the recognization, management and treatment of these children.

Promyelocytic Leukemia

Acute promyelocytic leukemia has only recently been recognized as a separate variant of acute leukemia. The predominant cell type is an atypical promyelocyte usually with coarse irregular cytoplasmic granulations. The outstanding clinical characteristic of this disease is the associated hemorrhagic tendency which often overshadows all other manifestations of the leukemic process. The patient usually presents with bleeding manifestations such as purpura, epistaxis or gingival bleeding. Hemorrhage into the central nervous system has occasionally been the first sign of leukemia. In some cases, local infiltrates of leukemic cells without signs of frank bleeding may be the presenting symptom, unilateral exophthalmos in a twelve-month-old girl was one such example.[27] Physical examination usually reveals signs of bleeding but is otherwise frequently unremarkable. Neither lymphadenopathy nor hepatosplenomegaly are characteristic. Anemia and thrombocytopenia are common although the reduction in platelets may be only moderate.

Promyelocytes may or may not be present in the peripheral blood, but they constitute the predominant cell in the bone marrow. These cells are rather large with a primitive nucleus containing nucleoli. The cytoplasm is relatively abundant and light blue in color. The specific feature is the many large coarse irregularly staining cytoplasmic granules. Auer rods may be present and may also be abnormally large. A decrease in plasma fibrinogen level and factor V deficiency are the characteristic features of this disease. Fibrinogen synthesis appears to be normal. Infused fibrinogen disappears rapidly[28] and a consumptive coaguloapthy has been postulated as the basis for the hemorrhagic tendency. Other authors have suggested the presence of a plasmin activator.[29] The breakdown of the abnormal promyelocytes may release activators which in themselves produce the clinical picture of disseminated intravascular coagulation. 6-Amino-caproic acid has had no effect on the hypofibrinogenemia[30] and heparin therapy has been only partially successful.[31] Therapy directed towards the underlying leukemic process has, in general, been discouraging. Most patients survive only a few weeks from the time of diagnosis and less than 10 percent survive over eight months. A recent report suggests that daunomycin may be active in the treatment of this disease in inducing a significant number of clinical and hematologic remissions.[32]

Erythroleukemia

Erythroleukemia, or DiGuglielmo's syndrome, is an uncommon form of leukemia which, in its early stages, involves primarily the erythroid precursors. This is primarily a disease of the older age groups although a number of cases have been reported in the pediatric literature including in the newborn period. The incidence is thought to be about 1 percent of all cases of childhood acute leukemia,[26] depending, of course, on the criteria used to establish the diagnosis. Dameshek and Baldini[33] pointed out the polyphasic aspect of this syndrome which may evolve from a stage of abnormal red cell proliferation, characterized by bizarre megaloblastoid proliferation, through a stage of mixed erythroblastic and myeloblastic proliferation, into an end-stage indistinguishable from acute myeloblastic leukemia.

The initial symptomatology is usually related to the anemia and these children are occasionally diagnosed as megaloblastic anemia of undetermined etiology. Nonspecific symptoms include fever, weight loss and general malaise. Physical examination reveals pallor and splenomegaly, often of a marked degree. Lymphadenoapthy and hepatomegaly are less common. The most striking laboratory finding early in the disease is the severe refractory anemia. Some degree of thrombocytopenia is usually present; leukopenia is more variable and usually mild. Examination of the peripheral smear reveals, in almost all cases, some degree of normoblastemia even in the presence of a reticulocytopenia. The nucleated red cells are usually abnormal in appearance with bizarre nuclei. The mature red cells usually show a marked degree of anisocytosis and poikilocytosis. The morphology of the leukocytes is usually normal in the early stages of the disease although a rare myeloblast may be found.

Bone marrow smears reveal erythroid hyperplasia with bizarre erythroblasts, many with megaloblastoid changes, others with abnormal nuclear forms, and still others with abnormal mitotic figures (Fig. 2-3). Multilobed nuclei are common and the nuclear chromatin pattern may show abnormal clumping. Cytoplasmic

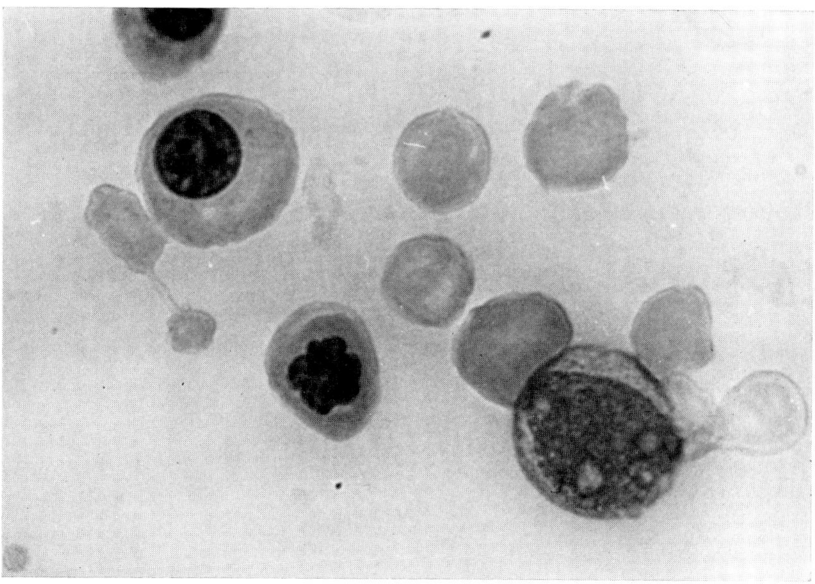

Figure 2-3. Peripheral blood smear in erythroleukemia (×100). Nucleated red cells, one with a bizarre nucleus, and the blast are typical features.

vacuolization is common. Quaglino and Hayhoe[34] have described the presence of PAS-positive material in the abnormal erythroblasts as well as in myeloblasts which may be present (but not in myeloblasts in typical acute myeloblastic leukemia) suggesting that these "blasts" may, in fact, be undifferentiated erythroid precursors. Ringed sideroblasts may also be identified on iron stains of the marrow. Myeloblasts are usually inconspicuous in the early stages of the disease. Associated with the morphological features of disturbed erythroid proliferation are various abnormalities of hemoglobin synthesis.[35]

Chromosomal studies have indicated a number of nonspecific abnormalities including the aneuploidy commonly seen in acute myeloblastic leukemia. The presence of such anomalies is, however, useful in establishing the preleukemic or leukemic nature of the severe refractory anemia. Most cases of DiGuglielmo's syndrome evolve, in a matter of weeks or months, into a picture indistinguishable from acute myeloblastic leukemia. This, plus the fact that the numbers of abnormal erythroid elements can be suppressed by red cell transfusions,[36,37] has led some authors[37] to question the concept of a primary malignancy of the erythroid cell line. The unusual histochemical characteristics of the erythroblasts and myeloblasts in these cases, the associated biochemical abnormalities in hemoglobin synthesis, and the generally poor response to chemotherapy all serve to distinguish erythroleukemia from more typical cases of acute myeloblastic leukemia. Erythroleukemia is one of the myeloproliferative disorders and this disease has been observed in the progression of polycythemia vera[38] and paroxysmal nocturnal hemoglobinuria[39] into acute myeloblastic leukemia. In this context, a malignancy initially involving primarily the erythroid cell line is not unexpected.

In general, the response of erythroleukemia to chemotherapy has been quite poor. In view of the anticipated poor response, judicious therapy with transfusions of whole blood and packed red cells should probably be used as long as anemia is the major clinical problem. Treatment with 6-mercaptopurine, vincristine, prednisone, cyclophosphamide and methotrexate has been unrewarding. The only drug combination which appears to have produced any clinical response, and that only in a limited number of patients, is cytosine arabinoside and 6-thioguanine. The remissions are transitory at best. Survival in erythroleukemia is quite variable in duration but, in general, the median appears to be about six months.

Eosinophilic Leukemia

The causes of eosinophilia in the pediatric age group are so numerous as to almost defy classification. Only rarely, however, does the absolute number of eosinophils rise above 5,000 to 10,000/mm^3. Such cases comprise a group of diseases termed the "hypereosinophilic syndromes" by Hardy and Anderson.[40] Among these syndromes is eosinophilic leukemia. This entity is quite uncommon, occurring in only 0.3% of children with acute leukemia,[26] but its differentiation from other nonmalignant causes of hypereosinophilia may be extremely difficult. Furthermore, an occasional patient with acute myeloblastic leukemia may develop abnormal neutrophils containing large golden granules superimposed on an orange cytoplasmic background. Special histochemical stains and electron microscopy may be required to establish the true neutrophilic nature of such cells.[41] A reactive eosinophilia may also occur in some cases of acute leukemia. Thus, problems in the clinical differentiation between Loeffler's endocarditis, atypical forms of acute myeloblastic leukemia, and eosinophilic leukemia have resulted in a considerable controversy over the characterization, or even the existence, of eosinophilic leukemia.[42] Differentiation of these three clinical entities appears to be of some clinical significance, however, since the optimal therapeutic approach is probably different for each.

The symptomatology in eosinophilic leukemia differs from that seen in other forms of acute leukemia. Malaise, fever, sweats, cough, dyspnea, chest pain, weight loss and pruritus are all frequent presenting complaints. Symptoms referable to heart failure, pulmonary involvement, central nervous system manifestations, rash and fever have all been reported.[43] Not all symptoms are present simultaneously at the onset of the disease but in most instances the majority were seen some time during the course of the illness. Physical examination frequently reveals cardiomegaly with a sinus tachycardia or arrhythmias, or both. Pulmonary findings may include wheezes, rales and other signs of bronchopulmonary disease. Hepatosplenomegaly is usually prominent, lymphadenopathy is noted in only about 50 percent of the reported cases.

Thrombocytopenia and anemia are frequent initial laboratory findings. There is almost always a leukocytosis of 50,000/mm^3 or more. Examination of the peripheral blood smear reveals marked

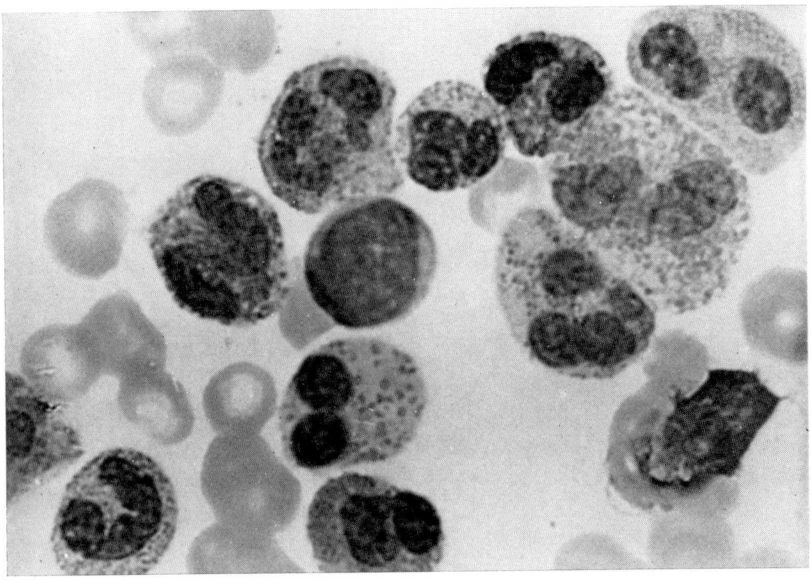

Figure 2-4. Peripheral blood smear in acute eosinophilic leukemia (×100). Abnormalities in the cytoplasmic granules and in the nuclear segmentation are typical features. The cell in the center of the field is a myeloblast.

eosinophilia often with abnormalities of the nuclear chromatin pattern and formation of the granules. In addition, eosinophilic promyelocytes, myelocytes and metamyelocytes are found in at least half of the patients. Myeloblasts are also frequently seen in the blood smear, especially in the later stages of the disease. Bone marrow aspiration or biopsy usually reveals a marked myeloid hyperplasia with an eosinophilia. Occasionally, however, the marrow is fibrotic and only a few nests of myeloblasts can be seen. Chromosomal studies are usually normal although abnormalities have been identified in a few instances.[44,45] The leukocyte alkaline phosphatase activity is normal.

As the disease progresses, increasing numbers of myeloblasts may appear in the peripheral circulation and the morphological appearance may become indistinguishable from acute myelogenous leukemia. The usual course of the disease is characterized by more or less rapid deterioration. Survival is almost always less than one year from diagnosis. An occasional patient will have a transitory response to prednisone with a decrease in eosinophilia, fever and hepatosplenomegaly. More frequently, prednisone proves to be ineffective. Other forms of therapy which have been tried include splenic irradiation, busulfan, nitrogen mustard and cyclophosphamide. None have proved effective. Perhaps the newer agents, cytosine arabinoside or daunomycin, may prove effective in selected cases.

Several aspects of this disease deserve special consideration. Some authors[46] have denied the existence of eosinophilic leukemia as a distinct clinical entity, considering it as a form of Loeffler's endocarditis or related collagen disease. The existence of anemia and thrombocytopenia and the presence of increased numbers of myeloblasts in blood and bone marrow argue strongly for a primary hematologic disorder. Furthermore, the finding at autopsy of widespread organ infiltration by immature eosinophilic precursors as well as undifferentiated myeloblasts argues against a simple allergic or autoimmune disorder and fulfills one of the basic criteria for leukemia—namely, invasion of immature hematopoietic cells into nonhematopoietic tissues. The other noteworthy characteristic of this disease is the atypical spectrum of clinical manifestations. Cardiac, pulmonary and central nervous system involvement contrast markedly with the other forms of leukemia where these particular organ systems are usually not involved, at least in the early stages of the disease. These particular clinical manifestations are probably a consequence of the marked eosinophilia rather than due to the leukemic process per se. Breakdown of excessive numbers of eosinophils with the liberation of granular enzymes may be the cause of endocardial damage, pulmonary infiltration and frequent thrombi seen in both eosinophilic leukemia and Loeffler's endocarditis.[41] Thus, although the clinical symptomatology of eosinophilic leukemia may in some respects be quite similar to that seen in other forms of hypereosinophilia, the etiology and pathogenesis of the latter may be quite different.

Monoblastic Leukemia

True acute monoblastic leukemia comprises about 2 percent of all cases of childhood acute leukemia.[26,47] It shows no predilection for any particular age group and, indeed, has been seen in infancy.[48] The clinical manifestations are similar to that of other forms of acute leukemia except for the unusually high frequency of gingival hypertrophy and ulcerations, findings which were present in almost 50 percent of all patients with this form of leukemia.[49] Signs of a hemorrhagic diathesis are also common at the time of diagnosis. The morphology of the leukemic cell in acute monocytic leukemia is usually somewhat more mature than the typical blasts in other forms of acute leukemia. The monoblast has an irregular nucleus which may appear folded or lobulated and the chromatin material is very finely reticulated. There is an abundant blue-gray cytoplasm which may contain a number of small red granules. Auer rods are occasionally seen.

Two types of "acute monocytic leukemias" have been recognized: the Naegeli type, in which typical myeloblasts are present in addition to the monocytoid forms, and the Schilling type in which the monoblast is the only leukemic cell type present. The Naegeli type is considered to be a form of acute myeloblastic leukemia in which either the monocytoid forms are derived from myeloblasts or are present as a reaction to the myeloblast proliferation. The Schilling type, on the other hand, is considered to be a neoplastic disorder of the monocytes derived from the reticuloendothelial system and at times has been termed "histiocytic leukemia." The differentiation between the Naegeli and Schilling forms is reinforced by examination of the bone marrow; the myelomonocytic variant is characterized by myeloblastic proliferation, whereas the Schilling type is associated with proliferation of immature reticulum cells.

Serum and urinary muramidase levels have been found to be elevated in both the Naegeli and Schilling types.[50] However, when the serum muramidase level is expressed as a ratio in terms of the total leukocyte count, it is significantly elevated in monoblastic leukemia (Schilling) as compared with the myelomonocytic (Naegeli) form.[51] The serum and urinary muramidase levels depend on the cellular content and this is related to the degree of cellular maturation.[52] Thus, "falsely" low levels may be found in patients in whom the monoblasts are extremely undifferentiated.

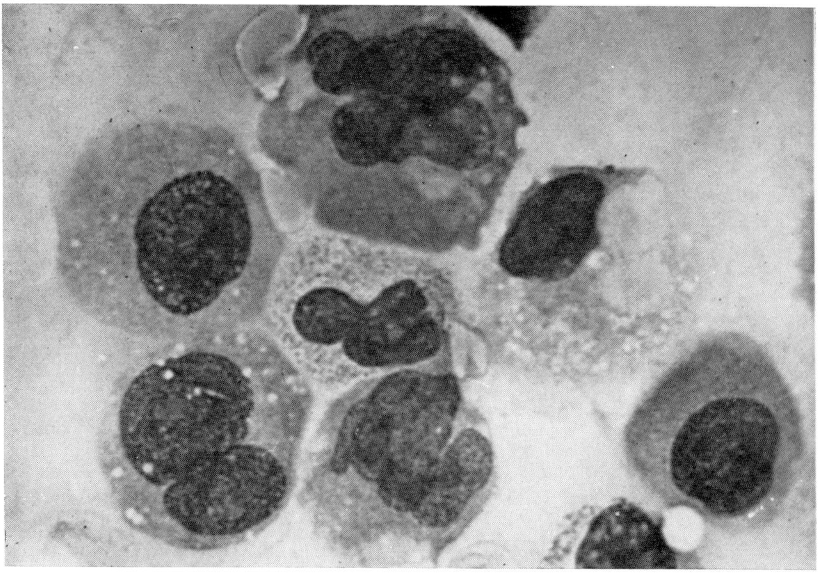

Figure 2-5. Bone marrow aspirate in acute monocytic leukemia (×100). The fine reticulated chromatin pattern and bizarre folding of the nucleus in some of the cells are obvious. Erythrophagocytosis is seen in several of the cells.

Hypofibrinogenopenia has been observed in acute monoblastic leukemia and is frequently associated with a hemorrhagic diathesis out of proportion to the degree of thrombocytopenia. The presence of a circulating fibrinolysis has been observed on occasion.[53] The differentiation of the Schilling or "pure" monoblastic leukemia from the monomyelocytic forms is of some clinical significance since the Naegeli type is similar to myeloblastic leukemia in terms of clinical response to therapy whereas the Schilling type of acute monoblastic leukemia appears, in most cases, to be refractory to all forms of chemotherapy. The median survival from time of diagnosis is about three months and few patients achieve remissions.

Congenital Leukemia

Leukemia appearing at birth or during the first month of life is atypical in a number of respects. Only about one hundred well-documented cases exist in the literature and over 80 percent of these are myeloblastic. Although a few cases have been associated with irradiation *in utero*,[54,55] no antecedent cause has been identified in the majority of instances. Pierce, in a review of forty-five acceptable cases,[56] pointed out the very high incidence of nodular skin lesions in those infants who presented signs of leukemia at birth. These consisted of slightly raised nodules, slate-gray in color, which appeared to arise in the deep layers of the skin and were freely movable over the subcutaneous tissues. Other findings at birth included hepatosplenomegaly and hemorrhagic manifestations including ecchymoses and bleeding into the umbilical stump, bleeding into the mucous membranes and into the gastrointestinal and urinary tracts. Interestingly enough, anemia was usually not present at birth but developed over the next several days. Hyperleukocytosis with counts ranging from 50,000 to over 100,000/mm^3 was a frequent finding with predominance of immature granulocytes. Thrombocytopenia was also very common. Infants in whom leukemia was diagnosed during the first several weeks of life had similar findings but anemia was much more common as a presenting sign. Survival was uniformly short with few infants living longer than two months.

Therapy has, in general, been highly ineffective and has included exchange transfusions to lower the very high white blood cell counts, as well as chemotherapy with vincristine, prednisone, 6-mercaptopurine and methotrexate. In addition, the newer agents, cytosine arabinoside, 6-thioguanine and cyclophosphamide, did not induce a remission when tried in one case. Congenital leukemia must be differentiated from a number of conditions often found in the neonatal period including sepsis, cytomegalic inclusion body disease, congenital syphilis, erythroblastosis fetalis (including incompatabilities in the ABO, subgroup, leukocyte and platelet systems), congenital thrombocytopenic purpura and rare cases of congenital aplastic anemia. Leukemoid reactions in the young infant may be quite bizarre and the differential diagnosis difficult even for the experienced hematologist.

Congenital anomalies are present in a high proportion of patients with congenital leukemia. Approximately 15 percent of the cases in one series[53] were associated with Down's syndrome and it was postulated that the malformations and the leukemia were both due to a common intrauterine event. The diagnosis of leukemia in an infant with Down's syndrome must, however, be made with caution in view of the number of reports[57-60] of transient abnormalities of myelopoiesis typical of acute myeloblastic leukemia, followed by complete recovery and prolonged survival, in some cases without specific therapy. In view of the present lack of effective therapy in this age group, it appears wisest that infants with Down's syndrome and a leukemia-like disease be treated conservatively.

Preleukemic and Paraleukemic States

Leukemia is probably the end result of one or more of a number of different insults to the hematopoietic system. Genetic, viral, immunological and environmental agents all probably play a role in the development of any particular form of leukemia. The role of any given agent is still a matter of speculation and it is impossible to predict with any degree of certainty who will develop leukemia. Even in individuals exposed to heavy doses of radiation, as in the case of the atomic bomb survivors, the development of leukemia can only be measured as a statistical event. Development of leukemia in such individuals is correlated closely with the total amount of irradiation absorbed but still, in a given individual, development of leukemia is apparently a random statistical event. In other words, at a given dose of irradiation, only a certain proportion of individuals will develop the disease. Despite this degree of uncertainty, it is of some interest to identify "preleukemic states"—that is, disease states which can, in a significant number of cases, be expected to evolve into leukemia. A number of such disease states have been identified.

The presence of aneuploidy and apparently random chromosomal anomalies in a significant proportion of cases of acute leukemia is well known. Furthermore, the presence of a specific chromosomal anomaly in chronic granulocytic leukemia has been referred to earlier in this chapter. These anomalies are undoubtedly due either to the leukemic process itself or are the result of the original insult to the hematopoietic tissue, the insult which also resulted in the leukemic process. The development of leukemia in an unexpectedly high proportion of individuals who have definite constitutional chromosomal abnormalities appears to be a different process. An increased incidence of leukemia has been reported in individuals with Down's syndrome,[61,62] Klinefelter's syndrome,[63] trisomy 13-15,[64] and Bloom's syndrome.[65,66] An increased incidence of other prezygotic chromosomal abnormalities has also been reported in children with acute leukemia.[67] These observations suggest that aneuploid cell lines are more susceptible to malignant transformation.

Aplastic anemia is another disorder in which an increased incidence of leukemia is well recognized. Constitutional aplastic anemia of the Fanconi type is associated both with nonspecific chromosomal anomalies, such as breaks, fragmentation and ring formation, and with an increased incidence of acute leukemia.[68] Fibroblasts cultured from individuals with Fanconi's anemia have a greatly increased susceptibility to *in vitro* transformation by the simian vacuolating virus (SV40),[69] suggesting that constitutional chromosomal anomalies are unusually susceptible to the leukemogenic action of oncogenic viruses.[20] Acquired aplastic anemia may also evolve into acute leukemia. In some cases, the leukemic process became quickly evident following a short course of corticosteroids,[70] and it is probable that the initial hypoplastic phase was in reality only one stage in the leukemic process.[71] In other patients, aplastic anemia may persist for a number of years before the leukemic process becomes evident. This appears to be particularly true in the aplasia following benzene intoxication,[72] the leukemic process has occurred up to seven years following apparent recovery. Leukemia has also been seen following aplastic anemia secondary to chloramphenicol.[73] The differentiation between the hypoplastic phase of acute leukemia and the "empty" marrow of aplastic anemia may be difficult at times. The presence of primitive nests of "blasts" in an otherwise hypoplastic marrow may represent early marrow regeneration or, on the other hand, the appearance of leukemic cells in a damaged marrow. Reticulum stains of the bone marrow biopsy is frequently of value of differentiating the two; acute leukemia is frequently associated with an increased deposition of reticulum fibers whereas aplastic anemia rarely is.

Myelofibrosis in childhood[74] is an exceedingly rare disease and is of interest primarily in the correlation with other disease entities. In most cases, the disease, characterized by fibrous replacement of the bone marrow, is secondary to another malignancy. Thus, myelofibrosis in childhood has been described in association with neuroblastoma and lymphoma. These instances might be regarded as secondary myelofibrosis, due perhaps to stimulation of marrow fibrous tissue by the infiltrative disease. In some patients no evidence of an underlying tumor can be found. It is in these patients that one must suspect a preleukemic state. The diagnosis at times may be difficult, especially in the early stages, since small numbers of myeloblasts are seen in uncomplicated, or idiopathic, myelofibrosis. Aggressive antileukemic chemotherapy at this stage is usually unrewarding and conservative management of the anemia appears to be the most useful course. In adults myelofibrosis may persist for years with little change in the clinical picture. The disease appears to be more aggressive in children and the leukemic process, when it becomes overt, responds poorly to chemotherapy.

Block *et al.*[75] originally described a syndrome, found primarily in older individuals, which they termed "preleukemic acute leukemia," characterized by refractory anemia, a persistent monocytosis and a peripheral pancytopenia. This preleukemic phase was usually brief and usually evolves into acute myeloblastic leukemia. A similar preleukemic state has been described in children characterized by leukocytosis, anemia, thrombocytopenia and hepatosplenomegaly associated with the loss of a C-group chromosome.[76-81] In 7 out of the 10 patients described, acute leukemia, usually myeloblastic, appeared after a preleukemic phase of one to four years. Loss of the C-group chromosome may thus predispose to the development of acute leukemia.

Finally, Randall *et al.*[82] described a family in which nine children developed a severe myeloproliferative disorder suggestive of subacute myeloblastic leukemia characterized by hepatosplenomegaly, anemia, leukocytosis and thrombocytopenia. The bone marrow revealed marked granulocytic hyperplasia. The leukocyte alkaline phosphatase was decreased both in affected children and in non-affected family members. Chromosomal karyotypes revealed an increased proportion of aneuploid cells but no consistent defect. The course was variable with early death in three, chronic symptoms in four and apparent complete recovery in two children. This may represent still another manifestation of the myeloproliferative disorders.

REFERENCES

1. Barrett, O., Conrad, M., and Crosby, W.H.: Chronic granulocytic leukemia in childhood. *Am J Med Sci, 240:*587, 1960.
2. Bloom, G.E., Gerald, P.S., and Diamond, L.K.: Chronic myelogenous leukemia in an infant. *Pediatrics, 38:*295, 1966.
3. Mauer, A.M.: Pediatric Hematology. New York, McGraw-Hill, 1969, p. 372.
4. Holmes, B., Quie, P., Windhorst, D., and Good, R.A.: Fatal granulomatous disease of childhood. An inborn abnormality of phagocyte function. *Lancet, 1:*1225, 1966.
5. Baehner, R.L., and Nathan, D.: Leukocyte oxidase: Defective activation in chronic granulomatous disease. *Science, 155:*835, 1967.
6. Ozsoylu, S., and Balci, S.: Fetal hemoglobin in various forms of childhood leukemia. Relation to relapse and remission. *Clin Pediatr, 9:* 152, 1970.
7. Necheles, T.F.: Unpublished data.
8. Rosen, R.B., and Nishiyama, H.: Leukocyte alkaline phosphatase in chronic leukemia of childhood. *Ann NY Acad Sci, 155:*933, 1968.

8a. Reisman, L.E., and Trujillo, J.: Chronic granulocytic leukemia of childhood. *J Pediatr, 62:*710, 1963.

9. Freireich, E.J., Bodey, G.P., Hart, S. *et al.:* Remission induction in adults with acute myelogenous leukemia. *Recent Results in Cancer Research, 30:*85, 1970.
10. Holton, C.P., and Johnson, W.: Chronic myelocytic leukemia in infant siblings. *J Pediatr, 72:*377, 1968.
11. Weatherall, D.J., and Brown, M.J.: Juvenile chronic myeloid leukemia. *Lancet, 1:*526, 1970.
12. Rosen, R.B., and Teplitz, R.: Chronic granulocytic leukemia complicated by ulcerative colitis. *Blood, 26:*148, 1965.
13. Ezdinli, E.Z., Sokal, J.E., Crosswhite, L., and Sandberg, A.: Philadelphia-chromosome-positive and-negative chronic myelocytic leukemia. *Ann Intern Med, 72:*175, 1970.

14. Tough, I.M.: Cytogenetic studies in cases of chronic myeloid leukaemia with a previous history of radiation. *In* Hayhoe, F.G.J. (Ed.): *Current Research in Leukaemia.* Cambridge, The University Press, 1965.
15. Court Brown, W.M., and Tough, I.M.: Cytogenetic studies in chronic myeloid leukemia. *Adv Cancer Res, 7*:351, 1963.
15a. Casperson, T. *et al.:* Identification of the Philadelphia chromosome as a number 22 by quinicrine mustard fluorescence analysis. *Exp Cell Res, 63*:238, 1970.
16. Tough, I.M., Jacobs, P.A., Court Brown, N.M. *et al.:* Cytogenic studies in bone marrow in chronic myeloid leukaemia. *Lancet, 1*:844, 1963.
17. Rastrick, J.M., Fitzgerald, P.H., and Gunz, F.: Direct evidence for the presence of Ph' chromosome in erythroid cells. *Br Med J, 1*:96, 1968.
18. Baikie, A.G., Court Brown, W.M., Buckton, K.E. *et al.:* A possible specific chromosome abnormality in human chronic myeloid leukaemia. *Nature (Lond), 188*:1165, 1960.
19. Goh, K.-O., and Swisher, S.N.: Identical twins and chronic myelocytic leukemia. *Arch Intern Med, 115*:475, 1965.
20. Galton, D., and Spiers, A.: Progress in the leukemias. *Progr Hematol, 7*:343, 1971.
21. Boyles, P.W.: Interstitial pulmonary fibrosis after long-term busulfan therapy. *Clin Med, 76*:11, 1969.
22. Kyle, R.A., Schwartz, R.S., Oliner, H.L., and Dameshek, W.: A syndrome resembling adrenal cortical insufficiency associated with long-term busulfan (Myleran) therapy. *Blood, 18*:497, 1961.
23. Ramaran, C.V., and Israels, M.: Treatment of chronic myeloid leukaemia with dibromannitol. *Lancet, 2*:125, 1969.
24. Kennedy, B.J., and Yarbro, J.W.: Metabolic and therapeutic effects of hydroxyurea in chronic myeloid leukemia. *JAMA, 195*:1038, 1966.
25. Carbone, P., Canellos, G.P., and DeVita, V.: Therapy of the blastic phase of chronic granulocytic leukemia. *Recent Results in Cancer Research, 30*:142, 1970.
26. Fraumeni, J., Manning, M.D., and Mitus, W.: Acute childhood leukemia: Epidemiologic study by cell type. *J Natl Cancer Inst, 46*:461, 1971.
27. Crombie, A.L.: Proptosis in leukemia. *Br J Ophthal, 51*:101, 1967.
28. Didisheim, P., Trombold, J.S., Vanderroot, L., and Mibashan, R.: Acute promyelocytic leukemia with fibrinogen and factor V deficiencies. *Blood, 23*:717, 1964.
29. Cooperberg, A.: Acute promyelocytic leukemia. *J Can Med Assoc, 97*:57, 1967.
30. Ryder, R.: Promyelocytic leukemia and hypofibrinogenemia. *Acta Haematol, 35*:181, 1966.
31. Bentegeat, J., Leger, H., Got, M., *et al.:* Interpretation of histo-pathologic data in the evolution of two promyelocytic acute leukemias with consumption coagulopathy. *Bord Med, 3*:2687, 1970.

32. Armata, J., Wyszkowski, J., and Cyklis, R.: Rubidomycin in blastic phases of acute promyelocytic and myeloblastic leukaemia in children. *Acta Paediatr Scand, 60:*471, 1971.
33. Dameshek, W., and Baldini, M.: The DiGuglielmo syndrome. *Blood, 13:*192, 1958.
34. Quaglino, D., and Hayhoe, F.: Periodic-acid-Schiff positively in erythroblasts with special reference to DiGuglielmo's disease. *Br J Haematol, 6:*26, 1960.
35. Necheles, T.F., and Dameshek, W.: DiGuglielmo syndrome; studies on hemoglobin synthesis. *Blood, 29:*550, 1967.
36. Adamson, J.W., and Finch, C.A.: Erythropoietin and the regulation of erythropoiesis in DiGuglielmo's syndrome. *Blood, 36:*590, 1970.
37. Schwartz, A.D., Zelson, J.H., and Pearson, H.: Acute myelogenous leukemia with compensatory but ineffective erythropoiesis: DiGuglielmo's syndrome. *J Pediat, 77:*653, 1970.
38. Bank, A., Larsen, P.R., and Anderson, H.: DiGuglielmo's syndrome after polycythemia. *N Engl J Med, 275:*489, 1966.
39. Carmel R., Coltman, C., Yatteau, R.F., and Costanzi, J.J.: Association of paroxysmal nocturnal hemoglobinuria with erythroleukemia. *N Engl J Med, 283:*1329, 1970.
40. Hardy, W.R., and Anderson, R.E.: The hypereosinophilic syndromes. *Ann Intern Med, 68:*1220, 1968.
41. Yam, L.T., Li, C.Y., Necheles, T.F., and Katayama, I.: Pseudoeosinophilia, eosinophilic endocarditis and eosinophilic leukemia. *Am J Med,* (In press).
42. Zucker-Franklin, D.: Eosinophilia of unknown etiology: A diagnostic dilemna. *Hosp Practice, 6:*119, March 1971.
43. Benvenisti, D.S., and Ultmann, J.E.: Eosinophilic leukemia. *Ann Intern Med, 71:*731, 1969.
44. Goh, K.O., Swisher, S.A., and Rosenberg, C.N.: Cytogenetic studies in eosinophilic leukemia. *Ann Intern Med, 62:*80, 1965.
45. Gruenwald, H., Kiossoglon, K.A., Mitus, W.J., and Damashek, W.: Philadelphia chromosome in eosinophilic leukemia. *Am J Med, 39:* 1003, 1965.
46. Rickles, F.R., and Miller, D.: Eosinophilic leukemoid reaction. *J Pediatr 80:*418, 1972.
47. Thompson, R.B., and Walker, W.: Fifty cases of acute leukaemia in childhood. *Br Med J, 1:*1165, 1962.
48. Whorton, C.M.: Congenital histiocytic leukemia. *Lab Invest, 9:*199, 1960.
49. Roath, S., Israels, M., and Wilkinson, J.F.: The acute leukaemias. *Q J Med, 33:*257, 1964.
50. Osserman, E.F., and Lawlor, D.P.: Serum and urinarylysozyme (muramidase) in monocytic and monomyelocytic leukemia. *J Exp Med, 124:* 921, 1966.

51. Perillie, P.E., Kaplan, S.S., Lefkowitz, E. *et al.:* Studies on muramidase (lysozyme) in leukemia. *JAMA, 203:*79, 1968.
52. Asamer, H., Schmalzi, F., and Braunsteiner, H.: Immunocytological demonstration of lysozyme (muramidase) in human leukaemic cells. *Br J Haematol, 20:*571, 1971.
53. Boggs, D.R., Wintrobe, M., and Cartwright, G.: The acute leukemias. Analysis of 322 cases and review of the literature. *Medicine (Baltimore), 41:*163, 1962.
54. Cooper, A., and Steinbeck, A.W:. Leukaemia following irradiation in utero. *Br J Radiol, 32:*265, 1959.
55. Schuleri, E., and Magheru, H.: Case of acute granulocytic leukemia in a newborn infant, probably congenital, and caused by repeated exposure of the mother to x-rays during pregnancy. *Arch Anat Pathol (Paris), 19:*25-29, 1971.
56. Pierce, M.I.: Leukemia in the newborn infant. *J Pediatr, 54:*691, 1959.
57. Ross, J.D., Moloney, W., and Desforges, J.F.: Ineffective regulation of granulopoiesis masquerading as congenital leukemia in a mongoloid child. *J Pediatr, 63:*1, 1963.
58. Wegelius, R., Vaananen, I., and Koskela, S.L.: Down's syndrome and transient leukaemia-like disease in a newborn. *Acta Paediatr Scand, 56:*301, 1967.
59. Nagao, T., Lampkin, B.C., and Hug, G.: A neonate with Down's syndrome and transient abnormal myelopoiesis: Serial blood and bone marrow studies. *Blood, 36:*443-447, 1970.
60. Rioux, E., and Leclerc, R.: Congenital acute myelocytic leukemia associated with Down's syndrome. Complete, long-lasting remission after exchange transfusion. *Union Med Can, 100:*951-954, 1971.
61. Krivit, W., and Good, R.A.: Simultaneous occurrence of mongolism and leukemia. *Am J Dis Child, 94:*289, 1957.
62. Wald, N., Borges, W.H., Li, C. *et al.:* Leukaemia associated with mongolism. *Lancet, 1:*1228, 1961.
63. Mamunes, P., Lapidus, P.H., Abbot, J., and Roath, S.: Acute leukaemia and Kleinfilter's syndrome. *Lancet, 2:*26, 1961.
64. Schade, H., Schoeller, L., and Schultz, K.W.: D-trisomie (Putaw-syndrome) mit kongenitaler myeloischer leukaemia. *Med Welt, 50:*2690, 1962.
65. German, J., Archibald, R., and Bloom, D.: Chromosomal breakage in a rare and probably genetically determined syndrome of man. *Science, 148:*506, 1965.
66. Schroeder, T.M., and Kurth, R.: Spontaneous chromosomal breakage and high incidence of leukemia in inherited disease. *Blood, 37:*96, 1971.
67. Borges, W.H., Nicklas, J.W., and Hamm, C.: Prezygotic determinants in acute leukemia. *J Pediatr, 70:*180, 1967.
68. Bloom, G.E., Warner, S., Gerald, P., and Diamond, L.: Chromosome

abnormalities in constitutional aplastic anemia. *N Engl J Med, 274*:8, 1966.

69. Dosik, H., Hsu, L.Y., Todaro, G.J. *et al.*: Leukemia in Fanconi's anemia: Cytogenetic and tumor virus susceptibility studies. *Blood, 36*:341-352, 1970.
70. Melhorn, D.K., Gross, S., and Newman, A.J.: Acute childhood leukemia presenting as aplastic anemia: the response to corticosteroids. *J Pediatr, 77*:647-652, October 1970 .
71. Shahidi, N.T.: Leukemia presenting as aplastic anemia. *J Pediatr, 78*:549, 1971.
72. Forni, A., and Moreo, L.: Cytogenetic studies in a case of benzene leukaemia. *Eur J Cancer, 3*:251, 1967.
73. Brauer, M.J., and Dameshek, W.: Hypoplastic anemia and myeloblastic leukemia following chloramphenicol therapy. *N Engl J Med, 277*: 1003, 1967.
74. Say, B., and Berkel, I.: Idiopathic myelofibrosis in an infant. *J Pediatr, 64*:580, 1964.
75. Block, M., Jacobson, L., and Bethard, W.F.: Preleukemic acute human leukemia. *JAMA, 152*:1018, 1953.
76. Freireich, E.J., Whang, J., Tjio, J.H. *et al.*: Refractory anemia, granulocytic hyperplasia of bone marrow, and a missing chromosome in marrow cells. A new clinical syndrome(?). *Clin Res, 12*:284, 1964.
77. McClure, P.D., Thaler, M.M., and Conen, P.E.: Chronic erythroleukemia with chromosome mosaicism. *Arch Intern Med, 115*:697, 1965.
78. Jackson, J.R., and Higgins, L.: Group C monosomy in myelofibrosis with myeloid metaplasia. *Arch Intern Med, 119*:403, 1967.
79. Tuesdale, J.M., Worth, A.J., and Corey, M.: A missing C chromosome in the bone marrow cells of three children with myeloproliferative disease. *Cancer, 25*:1468, 1970.
80. Polak, J., and Zizka, J.: Myeloproliferative disease in a child with monosomia of a C group chromosome. *Acta Paediatr Scand, 59*:591, 1970.
81. Humbert, J.R., Hathaway, W.E., Robinson, A. *et al.*: Pre-leukemia in children with a missing bone marrow C chromosome and a myeloproliferative disorder. *Br J Haematol, 21*:205, 1971.
82. Randall, D.L., Reignam, C.W., Githens, J.H., and Robinson, A.: Familial myeloproliferative disease. *Am J Dis Child, 110*:479, 1965.

Chapter 3

THE LYMPHOSARCOMAS

CARL POCHEDLY

SINCE LYMPHOSARCOMAS comprise only 5 percent of childhood neoplasms, few large series of cases have been reported.[1-6] The general term "lymphosarcoma" is used to include all primary malignant tumors of lymphoid origin, except Hodgkin's disease, showing no evidence of leukemia in the peripheral blood or in the bone marrow at the time of diagnosis. The three main types of lymphosarcoma are small cell lymphosarcoma, reticulum cell lymphosarcoma and giant follicle lymphosarcoma. Burkitt's lymphoma is probably also a member of this group.[7-10]

The *etiology* of the lymphosarcomas is obscure, but oncogenic viruses and immunological abnormalities may be important factors. There are tumors of cattle, dogs and cats which are indistinguishable histologically from human lymphosarcomas.[11-14] Virus particles have been observed in bovine lymphomas.[15] The lymphosarcoma in African children described by Burkitt gives epidemiological evidence of being caused by a transmissable oncogenic virus.[16-19] Recent reports showed that Epstein-Barr virus (EBV) is etiologically related to infectious mononucleosis, but the possibility persists that the virus might be involved under rare conditions also in the genesis of Burkitt's lymphoma and other malignancies of the lymphoreticular system. Although the virus is rarely detectable directly in Burkitt tumor biopsies, it emerges with a high degree of frequency in cultures derived therefrom.[20] African patients with Burkitt's lymphomas were found regularly to possess antibodies to EBV, generally in high titers.[20,21] Patients with clinically and morphologically identical tumors have been identified in several countries, and at least two patients who have lived all their lives in the western hemisphere have had no detectable antibody to EBV in serum samples studied by several investigators. Thus, the EBV data in "American Burkitt's" is in marked contrast to the African data.[22]

Dameshek suggested that lymphosarcomas are immunoproliferative disorders.[19] Lymphoid tissue is constantly changing, being subject to the bombardment of antigens derived from both self and the external environment. New clones of immunologically competent cells may develop from previously uncommitted lymphocytes. Possibly a lymphosarcoma represents neoplastic overgrowth of one of these clones. This clone may not be overwhelmed by the body's defenses but may be tolerated by the body as part of its own tissues. Under these circumstances, such an abnormal or "wild" clone might continuously replicate itself, eventually forming a tumor. Such a neoplasm may thus be the end result of an immunoproliferative response which has for some reason "gone wrong."[19,23] Clinically, lymphosarcomas are not uncommonly associated with immunologic disease.[24] It is also possible that oncogenic viruses and immunologic abnormalities may *interact* in giving rise to abnormal lymphoid proliferation.[25]

A possible lymphoma-producing effect of diphenylhydantoin (Dilantin®) has been suggested.[26-29] A number of children and adults receiving diphenylhydantoin for prevention of convulsions have developed marked adenopathy and splenomegaly (pseudolymphoma) which regressed on discontinuance of the drug. But in one case a fatal malignant lymphoma ensued.[27]

CLINICAL PICTURE

Lymphosarcomas originate within and outside of lymph nodes wherever lymphoid tissue is present. Lymphoid tissue is scattered widely throughout the body. Even the bone marrow, for example, contains small foci of lymphoid cells. Large collections of lymphoid cells are found in lymph nodes, spleen, thymus, tonsils and Peyer's patches of the small intestine. Since lymphosarcoma may be present in any of these foci, a large variety of clinical manifestations may result. Overgrowth of malignant cells results in destruction of the normal architecture of lymphoid tissue and infiltration of surrounding tissues and organs. At the time of diagnosis the disease may be limited to a single focus or to a region, or it may be generalized with constitutional symptoms and signs. Symptoms and signs originate in the area of primary involvement or from the areas invaded by direct extension from affected lymph nodes. The symptoms may cover a wide spectrum, depending on the location and effects of the infiltrating or enlarging neoplastic tissue. Thus, lymphosarcoma may simulate almost any disease.[30]

No organ is immune to involvement by the lymphosarcomas, but the major presenting signs in nearly two-thirds of children with this disease is painless peripheral lymphadenopathy. These nodes, particularly the cervical, axillary and inguinal nodes, are the site most commonly involved first. Next in order of frequency are retroperitoneal and mesenteric nodes. The intestinal wall (especially the ileum), the liver or the spleen may be primarily involved (Figs. 3-1 and 3-2). Many patients present with mediastinal lymph node enlargement. The tumor may also involve bone[31,32] (Fig. 3-3), skin and special organs such as prostate, testes[33] and central nervous system.[1] Lymphosarcomas may also involve the pericardium and myocardium and cause cardiac temponade or pericardial constriction.[3,34,35] Pleural effusion may result from involvement of the pleura (Fig. 3-4). Compression of the superior vena cava and trachea, with dyspnea, cyanosis, venous engorgement and edema of the upper half of the body, is a serious complication.[36]

The stomach, small intestine or colon may be primary sites involved.[37] Gastric lesions most often consist of a diffuse infiltration that may be recognized on barium x-ray examination of the stomach because of the presence of exaggerated or stiffened rugae and diminished peristalsis. The most frequent site of disease in the small bowel is the terminal ileum, where the lesion may produce bleeding, intussusception (Fig. 3-5) or intestinal obstruction.[38-40] In rare cases primary lymphosarcoma of the upper small intestine may present with steatorrhea.[41,42] Renal involvement, which is often not recognized clinically, occurs in about half of patients with lymphosarcomas.[43] Involvement of the nasopharynx and tonsillar areas (Waldeyer's ring) occasionally occurs.[44,45] Lesions of the nervous system and skeleton occurs more frequently in reticulum cell lymphosarcoma than in small cell lymphosarcoma.[46,47]

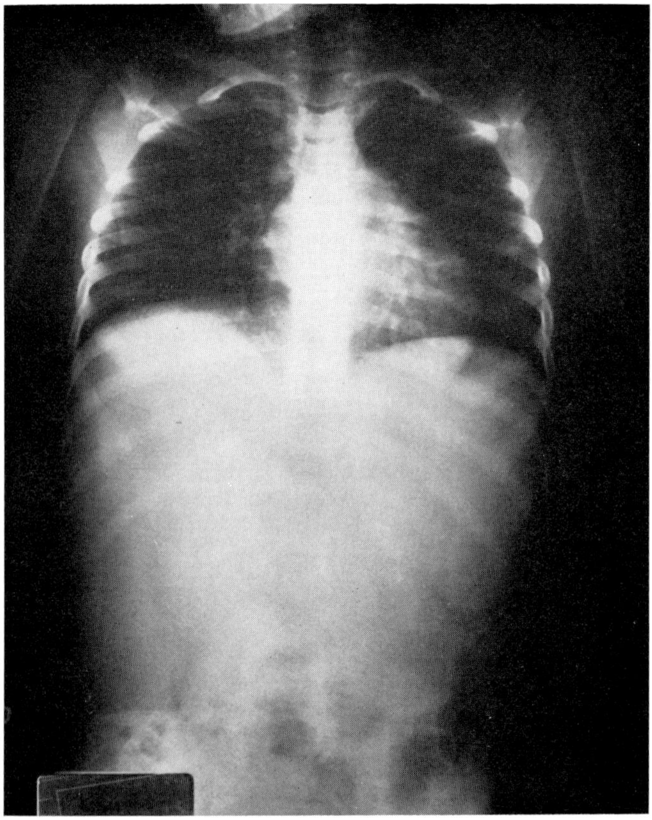

Figure 3-1. Marked enlargement of liver and spleen and mediastinal lymphadenopathy due to reticulum cell lymphosarcoma. Complete remission occurred on chemotherapy. (Courtesy of Dr. John McGovern.)

The lymphosarcomas must be distinguished from other diseases that may produce similar clinical manifestations. Infectious mononucleosis, tuberculosis, brucellosis and disseminated lupus erythematosis may present problems in differential diagnosis.[46]

The *course* of a child with lymphosarcoma can be acute, recurrent or chronic. Some patients fail to respond from the outset to all known methods of treatment, and the disease may pursue an unremitting course to death within a few months or even weeks. In others, the disease is recurrent and requires constant if

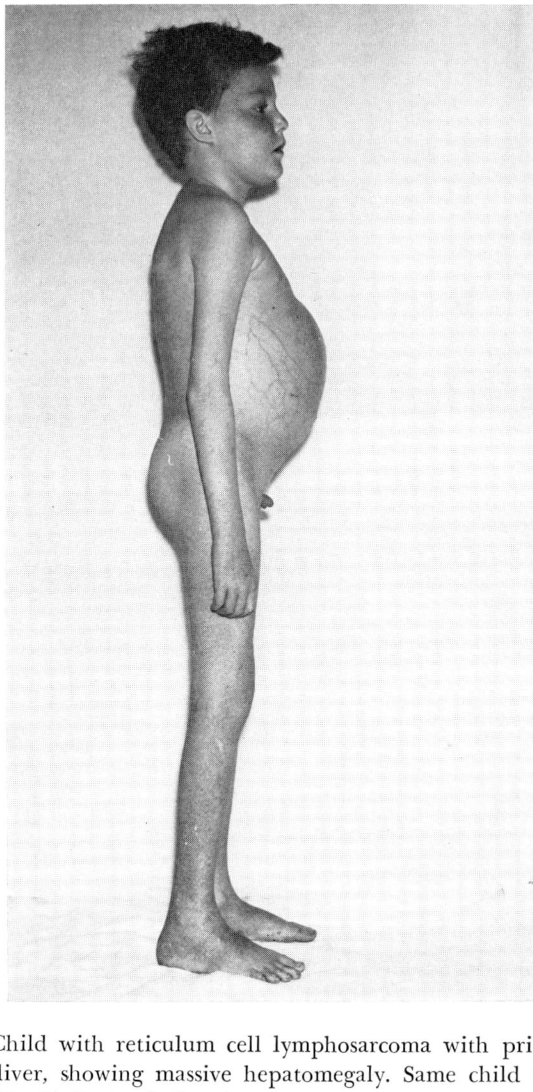

Figure 3-2. Child with reticulum cell lymphosarcoma with primary localization to the liver, showing massive hepatomegaly. Same child as Figure 3-1. (Courtesy of Dr. Philip McCaffrey.)

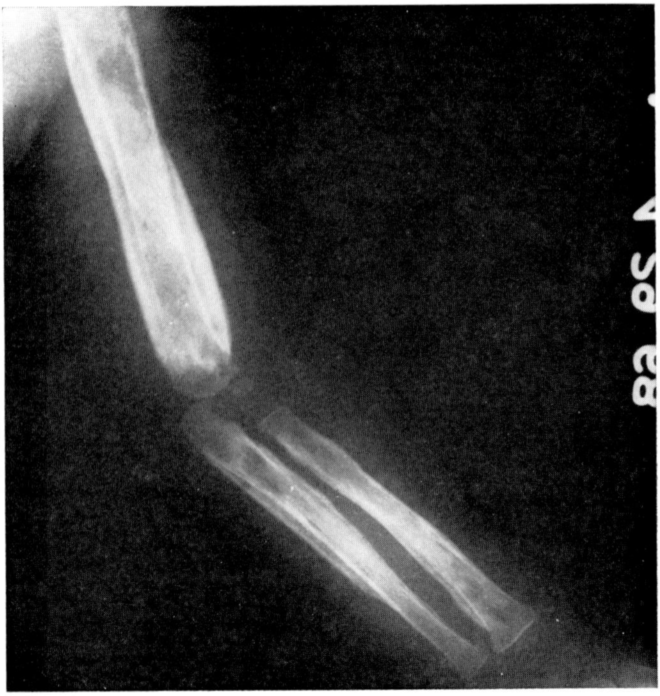

Figure 3-3. Arm of a two-year-old child with reticulum cell sarcoma with primary bone involvement. There are irregular osteolytic areas, coarsening of the bony architecture and periosteal cloaking. Similar lesions were present in the opposite arm and in both legs. These lesions largely disappeared with chemotherapy, but the condition later converted to acute leukemia.

not continuous treatment. In many cases, however, particularly those of giant follicle lymphosarcoma, the disease is chronic and presents few therapeutic problems for the greater part of its course. This type of disease responds well to treatment and may remain inactive for long periods.[48]

Lymphosarcoma in *children* differs in certain respects from the adult disease. The incidence is lower in childhood and boys are affected more than twice as often as girls.[3] Presentation of lymphosarcoma as an intra-abdominal tumor is twice as frequent in children compared with adults. Transformation of lymphosarcoma to leukemia is much more common in children. Extranodal sites

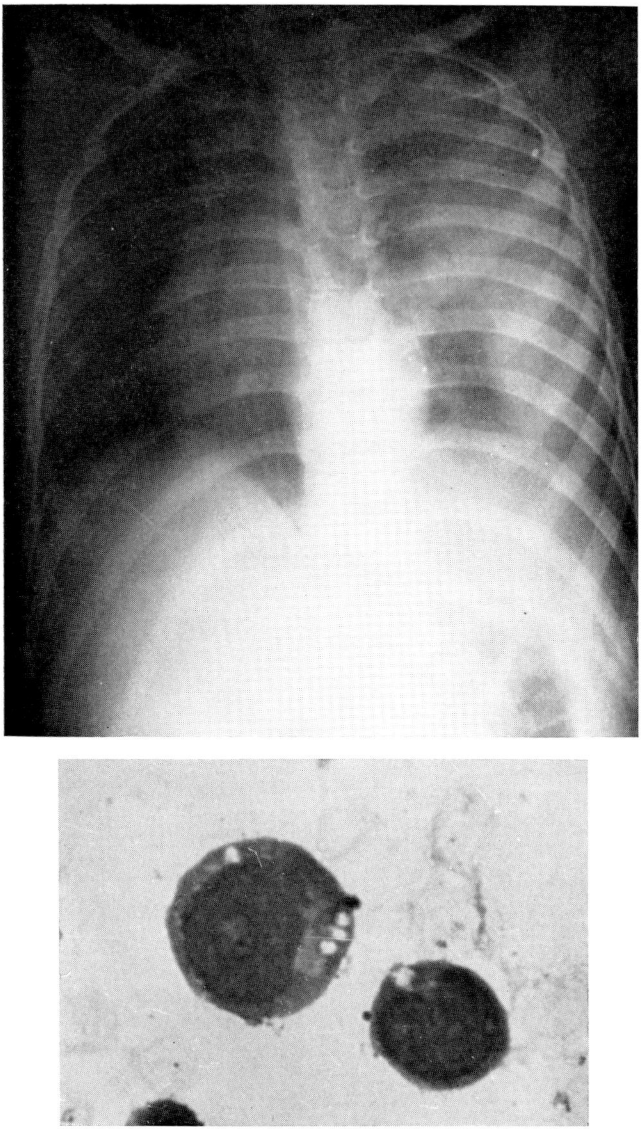

Figure 3-4. *(Top)* Marked left-sided pleural effusion and tracheal deviation in a child with primary abdominal lymphosarcoma. *(Bottom)* Cells resembling lymphoblasts found in sediment of pleural fluid (Wright's stain).

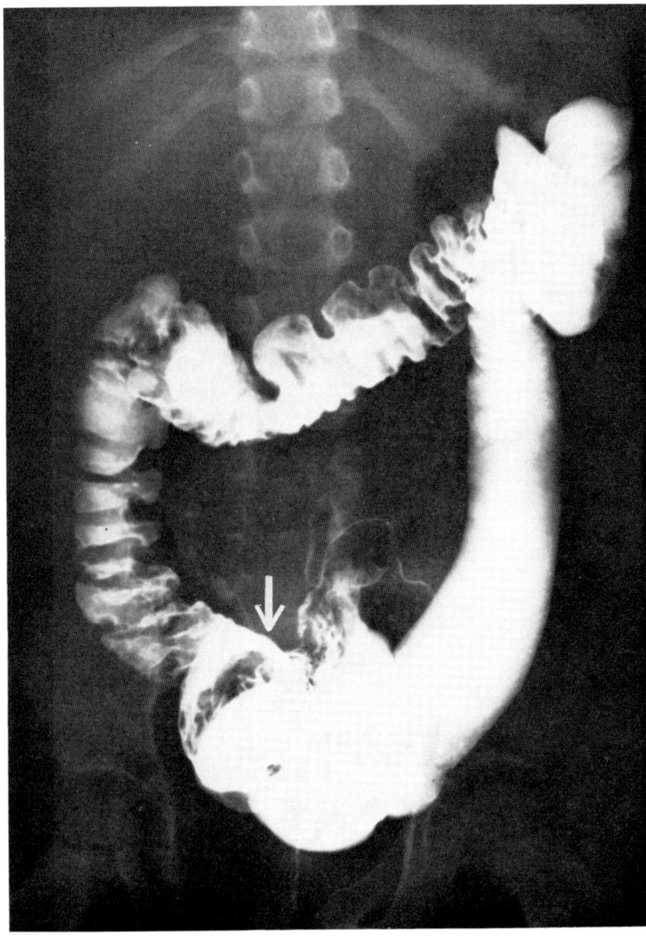

Figure 3-5. Postevacuation x-ray following barium enema showing ileocecal intussusception (arrow) in a five-year-old boy. Enlarged lymph nodes removed at surgery contained lymphosarcoma. (Courtesy of Dr. Allen Steinhardt.)

are primary foci of the disease more frequently in children than in adults. This is most evident in the reticulum cell type which may occur in tonsils, bone, liver or intestine. Intussusception is more frequently seen in children. Symptomatic obstruction of the superior vena cava is about four times more frequent in the younger age group. In contrast primary gastric lesions are rarely seen in childhood.[3] lymphosarcomas in children do not usually respond as well to therapy as the histologically similar disease in adults and clinically are much more aggressive than the adult form of the disease.

STAGING

Determining the anatomic extent of the disease, clinical staging (Table 3-1), is probably the most important factor in planning treatment and estimating prognosis in the child with lymphosarcoma. The staging of lymphosarcomas is also important for analysis of survival data. Certain clinical and laboratory studies are necessary for accurate staging (Table 3-2). Chest x-rays may reveal hilar or other chest involvement. If mediastinal adenopathy is suspected, tomography should be done. In addition, the thoracolumbar spine and pelvis should be x-rayed for evidence of bony metastasis. Intravenous pyelography is included as part of the work-up to reveal the presence of retroperitoneal lymphosarcoma. Lymphangiography may also be indicated.[49]

TABLE 3-1
ANATOMICAL AND CLINICAL CRITERIA FOR STAGING OF LYMPHOSARCOMAS*

Stage O. A single nodule has developed and its removal for biopsy represents, as far as can be detected, excision of all lymphomatous disease.

Stage I. Disease is localized to a single node or to contiguous structures without systemic symptoms.

Stage II. Disease limited by the diaphragm to the upper or lower half of the body, but present in more than a single site

A. Without systemic symptoms
B. With systemic symptoms (fever, anemia, weight loss)

Stage III. Disease above and below the diaphragm

A. Without systemic symptoms
B. With systemic symptoms

Stage IV. Disease demonstrated in any of the following areas: bone marrow (cytology), bone lesions by x-ray, pulmonary parenchymal lesions, more than one cutaneous or subcutaneous lesion, gastrointestinal tract when considered secondary, and hepatic lesions.

*Acute Leukemia Group B.

TABLE 3-2
STUDIES NEEDED FOR ACCURATE STAGING OF LYMPHOSARCOMAS

1. History, with careful attention to systemic symptoms (fatigue, fever, weight loss)
2. Physical examination, with special attention to lymph node enlargement and hepatosplenomegaly
3. Complete blood count, platelet count, reticulocyte count, red cell sedimentation rate and urinalysis
4. Posteroanterior and lateral chest x-ray films (whole lung tomograms if hilar lymphadenopathy is present)
5. Liver function tests, especially alkaline phosphatase, SGOT, bilirubin and LDH. Also determine total serum protein, protein electrophoresis and blood uric acid
6. X-ray of skull and long bones
7. Intravenous pyelogram
8. Bone marrow examination, preferably with needle biopsy technic
9. Biopsy of lymph nodes, preferably several nodes
10. Liver biopsy (if indicated)
11. Inferior vena cavagram (if indicated)
12. Lymphoangiogram (if indicated)
13. Exploratory laparatomy (if indicated)

Bone marrow aspiration is performed both to assess the general morphologic state of the hematopoietic system and to rule out occult leukemia. Histological sections of the aspirated marrow should also be examined.[50] If the aspirated specimen is unsatisfactory, needle biopsy (using a Conrad-Crosby or Turkel needle) should be done (Fig. 3-6). There is seldom evidence of bone marrow invasion by lymphosarcoma until late in the course. Liver function tests, especially alkaline phosphatase, SGOT and LDH may lead to the discovery of lymphomatous liver involvement. If the liver is enlarged or if more than one of the liver function tests are abnormal, liver biopsy should be done. Laparotomy, with splenectomy, liver biopsy and para-aortic lymph node biopsy, may be indicated when intra-abdominal involvement is suspected and cannot be proven by other methods. In fact laparotomy may be recommended in all cases that are not obviously stage IV. Such precise staging is necessary to exclude the presence of disseminated disease before recommending extended field radiation therapy.[51]

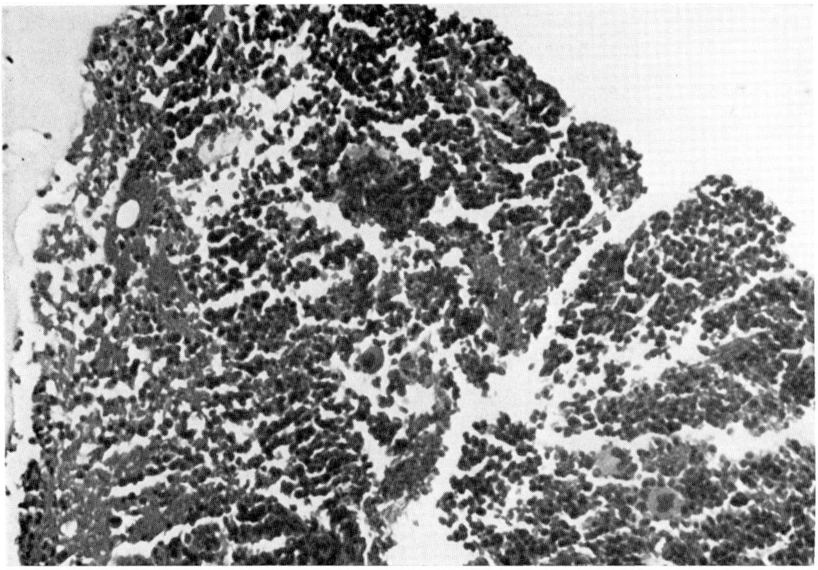

Figure 3-6. Section of bone marrow from a child with disseminated reticulum cell lymphosarcoma, obtained by Conrad-Crosby needle biopsy. Lacunar cartilage is shown on the left. The marrow is diffusely infiltrated by neoplastic cells, which were identifiable on higher magnification.

Laboratory Findings

Anemia may be present at time of initial diagnosis in children with stage IV disease. Refractory hypochronic anemia may also occur with less extensive lymphomatous disease.[52,53] When bone marrow involvement occurs thrombocytopenia is often present. Hemolytic anemia of the autoimmune type occasionally occurs and is usually accompanied by a positive direct Coombs' test.[24] When there is hepatic involvement, the liver function tests and liver enzymes are abnormal. The lactic acid dehydrogenase level is increased in presence of any malignant neoplasm.[54] Increased chromosomal breakage may be found by karyotype analysis of tumor cells. Skin tests for delayed hypersensitivity may show a defect in cellular immunity and the immunoglobulins may be deficient.[55] Low levels of IgM are present in untreated children with Burkitt's lymphoma.[56]

Serum proteins show a variety of nonspecific abnormalities including hypoalbuminemia, elevation of alpha- and beta-globulins and either an increase or a decrease in gamma-globulins. The occurrence of "myeloma-type" protein is not rare. The erythrocyte sedimentation rate is a good measure of lymphosarcoma activity; it probably reflects changes in the serum proteins and seems to be more sensitive than the electrophoretic pattern.[54] Serum lipoproteins may also be abnormal.[57] Hyperuricemia is common in all the malignant lymphomas and all patients with stage III or stage IV disease should be tested for it.

In order to estimate the prognosis for the patient with lymphosarcoma and to plan treatment it is important to know the extent of involvement. When only the physical examination is relied on for an examination of the abdomen, considerable disease can be present in the retroperitoneal nodes and not be detected. The use of techniques that opacify the ureters (intravenous pyelogram), the vena cava (inferior vena cavagram) and the abdominal lymph nodes (lymphangiogram) are the most reliable indirect methods at present available for this. Lymphangiography probably reveals more disease than inferior vena cavagraphy does, but it is technically more difficult to perform, especially in small children. Lymphangiography has shown that nearly half of patients with Hodgkin's disease classed as stage I or stage II by the usual methods of examination are in reality stage III.[46,58]

Visualization of the retroperitoneal lymph nodes by lymphangiography (Fig. 3-7) often provides valuable information, but it should be done only when fully indicated. Oil embolization of lungs, liver and other organs, allergic reactions to iodine and cellulitis at the site of cutdown can occur.[54,59] Indications for lymphangiography are stage I disease involving only cervical or axillary nodes and stage II disease in which node involvement is supradiaphragmatic. No useful purpose is served by lymphangiography if the intravenous pyelogram shows ureteral distortion, if inguinal or iliac nodes are involved or if clear evidence of stage III or stage IV disease is present. However, lymphangiography often gives false negative findings. Thus, lymphangiograms may not detect disease in retroperitoneal or para-aortic nodes in nearly

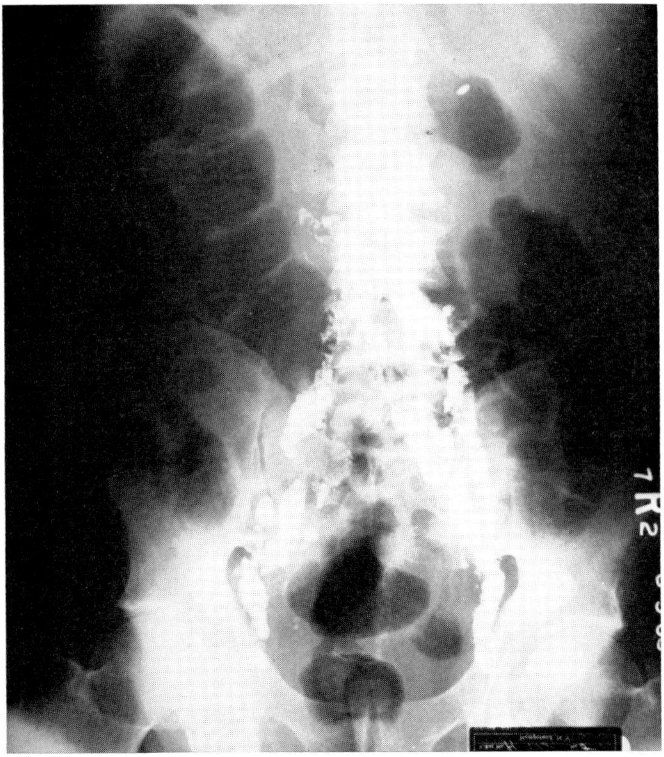

Figure 3-7. Lymphoangiogram showing marked enlargement of iliac and femoral lymph nodes in a patient with lymphosarcoma. (Courtesy of Dr. J. J. LaVine.)

one-third of patients in whom the results of this test were compared to the actual biopsy of the nodes on laparotomy. It now appears that laparotomy with splenectomy should be done in the staging of all patients with lymphosarcoma, except those who are obviously stage IV.

HISTOLOGICAL DIAGNOSIS

The presence of a lymphosarcoma is suggested by the clinical manifestations, but the definite diagnosis can be made only by biopsy. The histopathological approach to precise classification of lymphosarcomas has been frustrated by the fact that these tumors are morphologically labile, not static, and many intermediate stages and cytological variations from the main three types may be observed.[60] Lymphosarcomas arise from lymphoid cells, from reticuloendothelial cells, or their derivatives. The tumor may arise from these cells in any stage of their development. Thus, a lymphosarcoma may be composed mainly of small, adult lymphocytes, large primitive cells or any intermediate stage of development. Transitions from one pattern to another are found as frequently as one searches for them. These transitions are often seen in the same lymph node if one studies sections from all parts of it.[61]

Although a specific diagnosis can usually be made by the histologic study of involved tissue, at times the pathologist may have difficulty in identifying the disease from biopsy. Different nodes from the same patient have been diagnosed as different types of lymphosarcoma, and changes considered to be characteristic of Hodgkin's disease, reticulum cell lymphosarcoma and giant follicle lymphosarcoma have been observed in one and the same lymph node. In patients with lymphosarcoma, biopsies repeated after intervals of time often reveal a histological diagnosis different from the initial one. This histological lability has led to the suggestion that the whole lymphoma group is but a single neoplastic entity that has a number of variants.[46,61]

Histological appearance does not predict with much degree of certainty the clinical course, extent of involvement or the prognosis of these diseases. These tumors do not exist as clear-cut clinical entities, and many intermediate histological variations occur. There have been repeated efforts to classify lymphosarcomas into subdivisions based on histological appearance and probable cell of origin, but no completely satisfactory classification has achieved widespread acceptance.[3] It is desirable for purposes of study to classify these tumors as accurately as possible according to their histological appearance, but minute histopathological subdivisions are probably of little clinical importance.

In *small cell* lymphosarcoma, the predominant cell type is similar to the mature lymphocyte. This type is found in about 60 percent of children with lymphosarcoma (Fig. 3-8). *Reticulum*

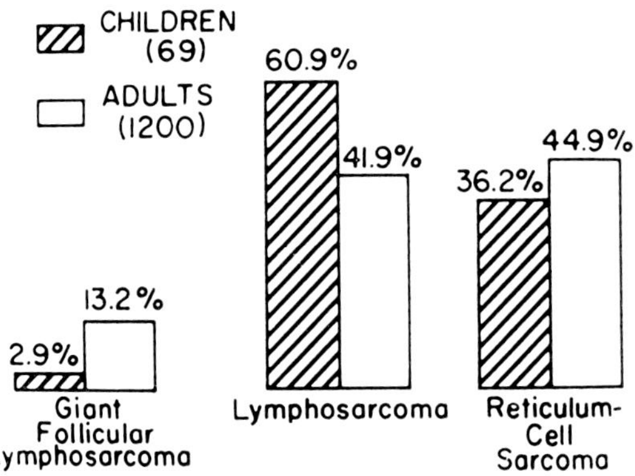

Figure 3-8. Histological types of 1269 cases of lymphosarcoma. Incidence of the types in children and adults are compared. (Courtesy of Dr. S. Rosenberg.)[3]

cell lymphosarcoma is found in about 35 percent. The cells in this case are one and a half times larger than lymphocytes and are variable in shape. Of all the malignant lymphomas, this type is most likely to occur in an extranodal primary site. Reticulum cell lymphosarcoma is the most undifferentiated type, is more highly malignant and invasive, and metastasizes more readily than small cell lymphosarcoma.[3]

Giant follicle lymphosarcoma shows the presence of numerous large follicles or germinal centers. Transitions of this histologic pattern to one of the other two types is often seen, and in borderline cases the separation of this group from the less differentiated forms may be vague. The condition ultimately becomes malignant, although long periods may elapse before clinical signs of malignancy are apparent.[62] When, in the later stages, the condition becomes malignant, repeat biopsy will show that the histological appearance has evolved into that characteristic of another type of lymphosarcoma.[63] The giant follicle type is found in less than 5 percent of children with lymphosarcomas but may occur even in early childhood.[63,64] A nodular sclerotic type of lymphosarcoma is associated with improved prognosis.[65] The frequency of the various histological types of lymphosarcoma in children is shown in

Figure 3-7. Similar data have been obtained from epidemiological surveys.[66]

LEUKEMIC TRANSFORMATION

Leukemic transformation is the term applied to those situations in which there is no evidence of leukemia at the time of the initial diagnosis of lymphosarcoma as determined by peripheral blood and bone marrow examinations, but in which a typical leukemic picture subsequently develops. Such leukemic transformation occurs in 30 to 40 percent of children with lymphosarcomas.[1,67] Occurrence of leukemic transformation in lymphosarcoma does not appear to be related to histologic type of lymphosarcoma or primary site of involvement.[67] A child whose lymphosarcoma is converting to leukemia shows pallor, petechiae, hemorrhages and hepatosplenomegaly. Early signs of leukemic transformation include increase in percentage of lymphocytes in the blood smear, presence of immature myeloid cells, decrease in platelet count, and splenomegaly. The bone marrow picture of these children may change to that for leukemia with surprising suddenness.[67] Lymphosarcomas in children undergo leukemic transformation about twice as frequently as in adults. The resulting leukemia is predominantly an acute lymphoblastic type in children, while adults commonly convert to chronic lymphocytic leukemia.[68] It is very unusual for patients with reticulum cell lymphosarcoma to convert to acute leukemia.[69,70] Burkitt's lymphoma, a type of childhood lymphosarcoma, also may convert to a picture of acute leukemia.[7,10,71,72]

The appearance of a leukemic picture in a child with a lymphosarcoma is an ominous sign: a potentially curable disease thereby acquires a fatal prognosis. In leukemic transformations spontaneous remissions are rare.[73] When leukemic transformation occurs, the therapy is changed to that for acute childhood leukemia. The leukemic phase of lymphosarcoma does not respond to chemotherapy as well as "simple" acute leukemia. The average duration of survival of these children is much shorter than that of children with acute leukemia.

THERAPY

The occasional long-term survival of children with localized lymphosarcoma provides reason for optimism. It is wrong to consider all lymphosarcomas to be merely the solid tumor phase of acute leukemia, since localized tumors may occasionally be cured.[3] Furthermore, children with disseminated disease may be maintained in remission for prolonged periods. It is important to establish a diagnosis histologically before treatment is started. Decision regarding the type and amount of treatment must be based on a careful evaluation and staging of the individual patient, taking into consideration the general condition of the patient as well as the type, extent and location of the disease.

Surgery

Since lymphosarcomas are sometimes unifocal in origin, surgical excision gives hope of cure. Occasionally children are found to have isolated involvement of the small bowel or spleen. In these patients the entire lesion may be removed at the time of biopsy. When there is hypersplenism and splenomegaly, splenectomy may be indicated.[74]

X-ray Therapy

Postoperative radiation to the tumor bed should be given at a dose of 3000 to 5000 rads.[46,75] The higher dose is given to the reticulum cell type. Chemotherapy may also be given since intra-abdominal lymphosarcomas are often not unifocal. Patients with disease limited to two contiguous node-bearing areas without evidence of bone marrow or visceral involvement (stage II) are treated with radiotherapy delivering 4000 to 5000 rads to the tumor at a rate of 1000 rads per week.[76-78] A generous margin of normal tissue should be included in the radiation fields, and regional normal lymph nodes may be radiated as well.[79-81] Kaplan is using total nodal irradiation in stage II and stage III disease. Chemotherapy may also be given. Children whose disease is classified as stage III or stage IV are given radiation directed at the involved areas plus chemotherapy.

Chemotherapy

When the disease is disseminated, systemic therapy with antineoplastic drugs is indicated. Control of anemia, specific antibiotic therapy for infections and prevention of hyperuricemia also are needed.[48] Hyperuricemia due to increased tumor cell breakdown before or during treatment may cause renal damage. Therefore, liberal fluid intake and allopurinol (Zyloprim®) should be given, at a dose of 10 mg/kg/day in three divided doses.[82] Serum uric acid determinations should be done on the day after therapy and every other day for about seven days, until it is certain that an acute uric acid overload will not occur. White blood cell and platelet counts should be performed twice weekly until recovery from toxicity occurs, usually within three weeks. Antineoplastic drugs are toxic to all cells, and the aim in chemotherapy is to establish the best possible balance between therapeutic effect and undesirable toxic side effects.

Once treatment has been started with a particular antineoplastic drug, it should be given an adequate trial. This means, generally, that the patient should be observed for at least four to six weeks to see whether he benefits from the drug. During that time some estimate must be made as to whether the treatment is successful. A simple method of evaluation is to observe a tumor that can be measured. This may be an enlarged lymph node, a palpable subcutaneous tumor or a tumor visible by x-ray, such as lung lesion. Measurements should be taken before treatment starts and then at intervals as treatment progresses. Preferably the measurements should be taken in two directions. A 50 percent or greater decrease in tumor size can be called an objective response or remission. To note simply that the patient feels better or that perhaps the drug has slowed the tumor's rate of growth are inadequate criteria of successful therapy.[83] If there has been an objective response to a drug, then it is reasonable to give it for maintenance therapy or to give repeat courses of the drug. The same drug should be used until progression of the tumor is noted while the patient is still on the drug. When progression occurs, a different agent is tried, and the same clinical evaluations are made.[83]

In the previously untreated patient, therapy is designed initially to induce a remission, *remission induction,* followed by the second phase, *remission maintenance.* The drugs of choice for inducing remission in a previously untreated child with evidence of disseminated lymphosarcoma is a combination of vincristine (Oncovin) and cyclophosphamide (Cytoxan®).[84,85] Many dosage schedules and regimens using these two drugs have been tried. In general, vincristine is given intravenously weekly at a dose of 1.5 to 2.0 mg/m^2. Cyclophosphamide is given orally at a dose of 3 to 5 mg/kg. daily. Courses of fourteen days each using these two drugs can be given, allowing one to two weeks between courses. Prednisone 2 mg/kg/day should also be given during the induction period. Corticosteroids exert a lympholytic effect on malignant lymphoid tumors. In addition, the immunosupressant action of these drugs is useful when there is hemolytic anemia or when there is massive breakdown of tumor and release of antigenic products during x-ray therapy or chemotherapy.[86,87] If the child achieves a remission, this may be maintained with courses of vincristine and cyclophosphamide given every four to six weeks. Maintenance therapy with oral cyclophosphamide, 2.5 mg/kg, may be given as a daily dose after recovery from toxicity associated with induction. The dose should be adjusted to maintain minimal leukopenia. Patients can also be maintained on intermittent cyclophosphamide, 15 mg/kg weekly, given intravenously.[76]

Drugs that may induce remission in children with lymphosarcomas who have become refractory to the drugs already mentioned include BCNU (1, 3-bis, 2-chlorethyl-1-nitrosourea),[88] cytosine arabinoside,[89,90] methotrexate, chlorambucil,[91] nitrogen mustard, actinomycin D, procarbazine (Matulane®),[92,93] daunomycin[94] and streptonigran.[95] 1-Asparaginase may occasionally produce marked regression of these tumors.[96-98] Combination chemotherapy with the MOPP regimen (mustard, Oncovin, prednisone and procarbazine) has given encouraging results in trials on patients with disseminated lymphomas.[81,99,100] MOPP may be given as initial therapy when there is extensive disease. When conversion to acute leukemia occurs, the therapy is changed to that for leukemia.[101]

In addition to evaluating the therapeutic effects of the drug, the signs and symptoms of drug toxicity must be carefully followed. Bone marrow depression, in particular, is dose-limiting. It is often necessary to modify drug dosage, since nearly all antineoplastic agents are effective only at levels at which there is toxicity. Because of the toxicity of these agents, it is important to stop a drug when it becomes no longer effective. Blood counts should be obtained twice a week as a guide to adjusting drug dosage.[75] Carefully planned therapy, precise evaluation of response and exact adjustment of dosage to avoid serious toxic effects may give the child considerable benefit.[75] However the results of present modalities of therapy are unsatisfactory. New approaches, as through manipulation of tumor immunology, may offer new hope for prolonged survival or cure of these tumors.[56,102,103] Thus, a virus-induced lymphosarcoma of chickens can now be prevented by a live vaccine.[104]

With our present therapeutic armamentarium we often eventually reach the point where definitive medicine has failed. Our objective then is palliation. The proper management of the terminal phase of the disease requires skillful use of analgesics and sedatives, and control of infection, hemorrhage and anemia.[105]

PROGNOSIS

It is difficult to gain an accurate picture of the prognosis in the lymphosarcomas because of the different histological and clinical classifications that have been used. Also, aggressive combined use of x-ray therapy, surgery and chemotherapy have not been employed long enough to enable one to fully assess their beneficial effects. The survival curve of sixty-nine children with lymphosarcoma is shown in Figure 3-9. When the involved lymph nodes are peripheral, such as in the neck, axillae or groin, the prognosis and response to treatment tend to be good. Alternatively, when the involved nodes are central, as in the mediastinum or retroperitoneal area, the prognosis tends to be poor and the response to treatment is also poor.[86] Hepatic involvement is, in general, a sign of advanced progressive lymphosarcoma and bodes a poor prognosis. On the other hand, the frequent induction of permanent remissions by chemotherapy in children with Burkitt's lymphoma is reason for optimism.[10,99,106,107]

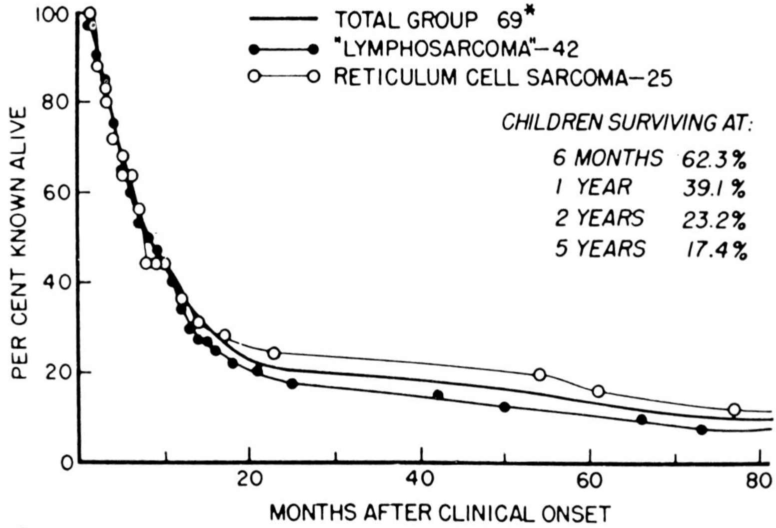

Figure 3-9. Survival curve of sixty-nine children with lymphosarcoma. (Courtesy of Dr. S. Rosenberg.)[3] Many of the currently used chemotherapeutic agents were not available when these data were collected.

REFERENCES

1. Jones, B., and Klingberg, W.: Lymphosarcoma in children. *J Pediatr, 63*:11-20, 1963.
2. Baily, R., Burgert, E., and Dahlin, D.: Malignant lyphomas in children. *Pediatrics, 28*:985-992, 1961.
3. Rosenberg, S. *et al.*: Lymphosarcoma in childhood. *N Engl J Med, 259*: 505-512, 1958.
4. Charache, H.: Lymphosarcoma in infancy and childhood. *Am J Roentgenol Radium Ther Nucl Med, 76*:594-598, 1956.
5. Borella, L.: Reticulum cell sarcoma in children. *Cancer, 17*:26-33, 1963.
6. Varaguth, P., and Candardjis, P.: Prognosis and treatment of reticulum cell sarcoma. *Schweiz Med Wochenschr, 93*:862-866, 1963.
7. Wright, D.: Burkitt's tumor and childhood lymphosarcoma. *Clin Pediatr, 6*:116-123, 1967.
8. Fagundes, L., Oliveira, R., and Amaral, R.: Childhood lymphosarcoma in the state of Rio Grande do Sul, Brazil; report of 20 cases histologically similar to Burkitt's tumor. *Cancer, 22*:1283-1291, 1968.
9. Dorfman, R.: Childhood lymphosarcoma in St. Louis, Missouri, clinically and histologically resembling Burkitt's tumor. *Cancer, 18*:418-430, 1965.

10. Ziegler, J., Wright, D., and Kyalwazi, S.: Differential diagnosis of Burkitt's lymphoma of the face and jaws. *Cancer, 27*:503-514, 1971.
11. Smith, H.: Malignant lyphomas in animals. *Am J Clin Pathol, 38*:75-81, 1962.
12. Marshak, R. *et al.*: Observations on a Heifer with cutaneous lymphosarcoma. *Cancer, 19*:724-728, 1966.
13. Hatziolas, B. *et al.*: Bovine lymphosarcoma; The effect of inoculations on newborn calves and mice—first year of observations. *Am J Vet Res, 27*:489-493, 1966.
14. Squire, R.: Feline lyphoma. *Cancer, 19*:447-451, 1966.
15. Rauscher, F., Carrese, L., and Baker, C.: Survey of viral oncology with particular reference to lymphomas. *Cancer Res, 26*:1176-1184, 1966.
16. Burkitt, D., and Wright, D.: Geographical and tribal distribution of the African lymphoma in Uganda. *Br Med J, 1*:569-573, 1966.
17. Burkitt, D.: Viral etiology of Burkitt's lymphoma; an alternative hypothesis to a vectored host. *J Natl Cancer Inst, 42*:19-28, 1969.
18. Glemser, B.: *Man Against Cancer*. New York, Funk & Wagnalls, 1969, pp. 4-23, 145-163.
19. Dameshek, W., and Gunz, R.: *Leukemia* (2nd ed.). New York, Grune & Stratton, 1964, pp. 403-423.
20. Henle, G., Henle, W., Clifford, P. *et al.*: Antibodies to Epstein-Barr virus in Burkitt's lymphoma and control groups. *J Natl Cancer Inst, 43*: 1147-1157, 1969.
21. Einhorn, N., Klein, G., and Clifford, P.: Increase in antibody titer against the EBV-associated membrane antigen complex in Burkitt's lymphoma and nasopharyngeal carcinoma after local irradiation. *Cancer, 26*:1013-1021, 1970.
22. Levine, P.: Wanted: Case reports of Burkitt's lymphoma in the U.S. *Med Times, 99*:124-126, Feb. 1971.
23. Cooper, M., Peterson, R., Gabriesen, A., and Good, R.: Lymphoid malignancy and development, differentiation, and function of the lymphoreticular system. *Cancer Res, 26*:1165-1169, 1966.
24. Miller, D.: The association of immune disease and malignant lymphomas. *Ann Intern Med, 66*:507-521, 1967.
25. Schwartz, R., and Schwartz, J.: Malignant lymphoproliferative diseases; interactions between immunological abnormalities and oncogenic viruses. *Ann Rev Med, 19*:269-282, 1968.
26. Hyman, G., and Sommers, S.: The development of Hodgkin's disease and lymphoma during anticonvulsant therapy. *Blood, 28*:416-427, 1966.
27. Gams, R., Neal, J., and Conrad, F.: Hydantoin-induced pseudo-lymphoma. *Ann Intern Med, 69*:557-568, 1968.
28. Choorivathanavanich, P., Wallace, E., and Scaglione, P.: Pseudolyphoma induced by diphenylhydantoin. *J Pediatr, 76*:621-623, 1970.

29. Gams, R.: Pseudolymphoma induced by diphenylhydantoin. *J Pediatr, 77*:1100-1101, 1970.
30. Whitfield, C.: The patient with lymphoma. *GP, 38*:78-88, 1968.
31. Medill, E.: Primary reticulum-cell sarcoma of bone. *J Fac Radiol, 8*: 102-117, 1956.
32. Pochedly, C., and Waldman, A.M.: Reticulum cell sarcoma in a child with primary bony involvement. *J Pediatr Surg.* (In press.)
33. Kiely, J., Massey, B., Harrison, E., and Utz, D.: Lymphoma of the testis. *Cancer, 26*:847-852, 1970.
34. Javier, B., Yount, W., Crosby, D., and Hall, T.: Cardiac metastasis in lymphoma and leukemia. *Dis Chest, 52*:481-484, 1967.
35. Terry, L., and Kligerman, M.: Pericardial and myocardial involvement by lymphomas and leukemia. *Cancer, 25*:1003-1008, 1970.
36. D'Angio, G., Mitus, M., and Evans, A.: The superior mediastinal syndrome in children with cancer. *Am J Roentgenol, 93*:537-544, 1965.
37. Ehrlich, A., Stalder, G., Geller, W., and Sherlock, P.: Gastrointestinal manifestations of malignant lymphoma. *Gastroenterology, 54*:1115-1121, 1968.
38. Frazer, J.: Malignant lyphomas of the gastrointestinal tract. *Surg Gynecol Obstet, 108*:182-190, 1959.
39. Mestel, A.: Lymphosarcoma of the small intestine in infancy and childhood. *Ann Surg, 149*:87-94, 1959.
40. Berry, C., and Kieling, J.: Gastrointestinal lymphoma in childhood. *J Clin Pathol, 23*:459-463, 1970.
41. Austad, W., Carnes, J., Gough, K. *et al.*: Steatorrhea and malignant lymphoma. *Am J Dig Dis, 12*:475-490, 1967.
42. Nasr, K., Hoghighi, P., Baldshandeh, K., and Hoghshevas, M.: Primary lymphoma of the upper small intestine. *Gut, 11*:673-678, 1970.
43. Richmond, J., Sherman, R., Diamond, H., and Craver, L.: Renal lesions associated with malignant lymphomas. *Am J Med, 32*:184-192, 1962.
44. Wang, C.: Malignant lymphoma of Waldeyer's ring. *Radiology, 92*: 1335-1339, 1969.
45. Al-Saleem, T., Harwick, R., Robbins, R., and Blady, J.: Malignant lymphomas of the pharynx. *Cancer, 26*:1383-1387, 1970.
46. Leavell, B., and Thorup, O.: *Fundamentals of Clinical Hematology.* Philadelphia, W.B. Saunders Company, 1966, pp. 445-474.
47. Gendelman, S., Rizzo, F., and Mones, R.: Central nervous system complications of leukemic conversion of the lymphomas. *Cancer, 24*:676-682, 1969.
48. Cridland, M. *et al.: Management of generalized lymphosarcomatous disease. Med J Aust, 2*:195-201, 1968.
49. Gasquet, C. *et al.*: Lymphangiography in malignant disease of childhood. *Am J Roentgenol, 103*:1-12, 1968.
50. Liao, K.: The superiority of histologic sections of aspirated bone marrow in malignant lymphomas. *Cancer, 27*:618-628, 1971.

51. Glatstein, E., Guersney, J., Rosenberg, S., and Kaplan, H.: The value of laparotomy and splenectomy in the staging of Hodgkin's disease. *Cancer, 24*:709-718, 1969.
52. Cline, M., and Berlin, N.: Anemia in Hodgkin's disease. *Cancer, 16*: 526-530, 1963.
53. Maron, B., and Shahidi, N.: Refractory hypochromic anemia in malignant lymphoma. *J Pediatr, 77*:93-97, 1970.
54. Gellhorn, A.: A new look at lymphomas. *Postgrad Med, 43*:136-141, 1968.
55. Freeman, A., Sinks, L., and Cohen, M.: Lymphosarcoma in siblings, associated with cytogenetic abnormalities, immune deficiency, and abnormal erythropoiesis. *J Pediatr, 77*:996-1003, 1970.
56. Ziegler, J., Cohen, M., Morrow, R. *et al.*: Immunologic studies in Burkitt's lymphoma. *Cancer, 25*:734-739, 1970.
57. Barclay, M. *et al.*: Serum lipoproteins in children with cancer. *Clin Chim Acta, 24*:225-231, 1969.
58. Lee, B. *et al.*: Evaluation of lymphangiography, inferior vena cavography, and intravenous pyelogram in clinical staging and management of Hodgkin's disease and lymphosarcoma. *N Engl J Med, 271*: 327-337, 1964.
59. Kusik, H., and Panning, W.: A simple, practical technic of lymphography. *Radiology, 88*:576-583, 1967.
60. Lukes, R.: The pathologic picture of the malignant lymphomas. In Zarofonetis, C. (Ed.): *International Conference on Leukemia-Lymphoma.* Philadelphia, Lea & Febiger, 1968, pp. 333-356.
61. Miale, J.: *Laboratory Medicine; Hematology,* 3rd ed. St. Louis, C.V. Mosby Company, 1967, pp. 939-945.
62. Fiat, D. *et al.*: Giant follicular lymph node disease. *Am J Med, 39*:252-259, 1965.
63. Marsden, H., and Steward, J. :*Tumors in Children.* New York, Springer-Verlag, 1968, pp. 63-85.
64. Kotte, S., and Kotte, W.: Das Grossfollikular Lymphoblastom (Brill-Symmers-Syndrom) in Indesalter. *Arch Kinderheilkd, 175*:302-306, 1967.
65. Millett, Y., Bennett, M., Jelliffe, A., and Farrer-Brown, G.: Nodular sclerotic lymphosarcoma. *Br J Cancer, 23*:683-692, 1969.
66. Anderson, R., Ishida, K., Li, Y. *et al.*:Geographic aspects of malignant lymphoma and multiple myeloma. *Am J Pathol, 61*:85-98, 1970.
67. Sullivan, M.: Leukemic transformation in lymphosarcoma in childhood. *Pediatrics, 29*:589-599, 1962.
68. Zeffren, J., and Ultman, J.: Reticulum cell sarcoma terminating as acute leukemia. *Blood, 15*:277-284, 1960.
69. Kelemen, E.: *Pathophysiology and Therapy of Human Blood Diseases.* New York, Pergamon Press, 1969, pp. 448-456.
70. Lowenbraun, S., Sutherland, J., Feldman, M. and Serpcik, A.: Trans-

formation of reticulum cell sarcoma to acute leukemia. *Cancer, 27:* 579-585, 1971.

71. Clift, R., Wright, D., and Clifford, P.: Leukemia in Burkitt's lymphoma. *Blood, 22:*243-248, 1963.
72. Ten Seldam, R., Cooke, R., and Atkinson, L.: Childhood lymphoma in the territories of Papua and New Guinea. *Cancer, 19:*437-446, 1966.
73. Han, T., and Sokal, J.: Spontaneous remission of leukemic lympho-proliferative disease. *Cancer, 27:*586-595, 1971.
74. Hyatt, D., Skarin, A., Moloney, W., and Wilson, R.: Splenectomy for lymphosarcoma. *Surg Gynec Obstet, 131:*928-932, 1970.
75. Devita, V., and Carbone, P.: *Lymphosarcoma.* In Conn, R. (Ed.): *Current Therapy.* Philadelphia, W.B. Saunders Company, 1968, pp. 265-268.
76. Evans, E., and D'Angio, G.: In Gellis, S., and Kagen, B. (Eds.): *Current Pediatric Therapy.* Philadelphia, W.B. Saunders Company, 1968, pp. 402-404.
77. Easson, E.: Radiotherapy for malignant lymphomas. *Ann Rev Med, 17:* 179-196, 1966.
78. Sagerman, R., Wolff, J., Sitarz, A., and Luke, K.-H.: Radiation therapy for lymphoma in children. *Radiology, 86:*1096-1099, 1966.
79. Parker, R.: "Radical" radiotherapy of lymphosarcomas. *Radiol Clin North Am, 6:*71-82, 1968.
80. Rosenberg, S., and Kaplan, H.: Hodgkin's disease and other malignant lymphomas. *Calif Med, 113:*23-38, October 1970.
81. Ultmann, J.: Current status; the management of lymphoma. *Semin Hematol, 7:*441-459, 1970.
82. Krakoff, I., and Murphy, M.L.: Hyperuricemia in neoplastic diseases of children. *Pediatrics, 41:*52-56, 1968.
83. Brunk, S.: Treatment of lymphomas with antineoplastic agents. *J Iowa Med Soc, 58:*1038-1041, 1968.
84. Carbone, P., and Spurr, C.: Management of patients with malignant lymphoma; a comparative study with cyclophosphamide and vinca alkaloids. *Cancer Res, 28:*811-822, 1968.
85. Hoogstraten, B. *et al.:* Combination chemotherapy of lymphosarcoma and reticulum cell sarcoma. *Blood, 33:*370-378, 1969.
86. White, L.: Treatment of tumors of the hematopoietic system. *Mod Treat, 3:*706-723, July 1966.
87. Kofman, S. *et al.*: Role of corticosteroids in treatment of malignant lymphomas. *Cancer, 15:*338-345, 1962.
88. Lessner, H. *et al.:* B.C.N.U.; effects on advanced Hodgkin's disease and other neoplasia. *Cancer, 22:*451-456, 1968.
89. Howard, J., Albo, V., and Newton, W.: Cytosine arabinoside; results of a cooperative study in acute childhood leukemia. *Cancer, 21:*341-345, 1968.

90. Talley, R. *et al.*: Clinical pharmacology and human antitumor activity of cytosine arabinoside. *Cancer, 20:*809-816, 1967.
91. Ezdinli, E., and Stutzman, L.: Chlorambucil therapy for lymphosarcomas and chronic lymphocytic leukemia. *JAMA, 191:*444-450, 1965.
92. Billmeier, G., and Holton, C.: Procarbazine hydrochloride in childhood cancer. *J Pediatr, 75:*892-895, 1969.
93. Stolinsky, D., Solomon, J., Pugh, R. *et al.*: Clinical experience with procarbzine in Hodgkin's disease, reticulum cell sarcoma, and lymphosarcoma. *Cancer, 26:*984-990, 1970.
94. Tan, C. *et al.*: Daunomycin, an antitumor antibiotic in the treatment of neoplastic disease. *Cancer, 20:*333-353, 1967.
95. Rivers, S., Whittington, R., and Medrick, T.: Methyl ester of streptonigrin in treatment of lylmphoma. *Cancer Chemother Rep.* No. 46, 1965, pp. 17-21.
96. Murphy, M.L.: In Shirkey, H. (Ed.): *Pediatric Therapy.* St. Louis, C.V. Mosby Company, 1968, pp. 941-969.
97. Tallal, L. *et al.: E. coli* I-asparagenase in the treatment of leukemia and solid tumors in 131 children. *Cancer, 25:*306-320, 1970.
98. Haskell, C. *et al.:* I-Asparagenase; therapeutic and toxic effects in patients with neoplastic disease. *N Engl J Med, 281:*1028-1934, 1969.
99. Burchenal, J.: Chemotherapy for leukemia and lymphoma. *Postgrad Med, 48:*164-168, Nov. 1970.
100. Frei, E. :The curative tratment of lymphoma. *Calif Med, 113:*47, 1970.
101. Jones, B. *et al.*: Chemotherapy of the leukemic transformation of lymphosarcoma. *J Pediat, 70:*442-448, 1967.
102. Law, L.: Studies on the significance of tumor antigens in induction and repression of neoplastic diseases. *Cancer Res, 29:*1-21, 1969.
103. Mathé, G. *et al.*: Acative immunotherapy for acute lymphoblastic leukemia. *Lancet, 1:*697-699, 1969.
104. Okozaki, W., Purchase, H., and Burmester, B.: Protection against Marek's disease by vaccination with a herpes-virus of turkeys. *Avian Dis, 14:*413-429, 1970.
105. Carter, R.: Palliation of childhood cancer. In Hickey, R. (Ed.): *Palliative Care of the Cancer Patient.* Boston, Little, Brown & Company, 1967, pp. 459-482.
106. Burkitt, D.: Long-term remissions following one- and two-dose chemotherapy for African lymphoma. *Cancer, 20:*756-759, 1967.
107. Burchenal, J.: In Zarafonetis, C. (Ed.): *International Conference on Leukemia-Lymphoma.* Philadelphia, Lea & Febiger, 1968, pp.469-474.

Chapter 4

HODGKIN'S DISEASE

Thomas F. Necheles

Hodgkin's disease is a neoplasm of the lymphoid tissues characterized by a mixed proliferation of both lymphoid and reticulum elements. A prominent feature is the characteristic multinucleated giant cell, the Reed-Sternberg cell. However, this cell may only reflect disordered lymphohistiocytic proliferation.[1] This disease is usually considered to arise in a unicentric fashion, spreading to adjacent and then distant lymphoid areas and ultimately into parenchymatous tissues. The clinical manifestations are protean and may range from a completely asymptomatic state to a severe toxic state associated with fever, anorexia, weight loss and signs of localized organ involvement or compression, or both.

The etiology of Hodgkin's disease is unknown. Although an infectious origin is strongly suggested by many of the clinical manifestations (such as fever, anorexia, weight loss, etcetera) no definite agent has been identified. Regional[2] and temporal clustering also support an infectious etiology. Recently evidence for the existence of viral agents has been reported[3] but have not, as yet, been confirmed in a larger series of patients. The etiologic role of EB virus, herpes simplex and cytomegalic virus appears to have been ruled out.[4] Epidemiological studies[5] suggest a sharp increase in incidence at age ten to twelve years, particularly in children born during late summer, again suggesting a role for environmental factors. The marked predominance of males presenting with Hodgkin's disease before puberty[6] also suggests the role of a sex-linked factor in the disease as manifested in childhood.

The role of immunological factors in etiology of Hodgkin's disease is suggested by several lines of evidence. The finding of an increased incidence of specific human transplantation antigens[7,8] suggests either a genetic predisposition linked, in some way, to the

HLA loci or possibly a viral etiology. Hodgkin's disease has also been reported in patients with congenital lymphopenic agammaglobulinemia, congenital sex-linked agammaglobulinemia, ataxic telangiectasia, the Wiscott-Aldrich syndrome and, most recently, the Chediak-Higashi syndrome.[9] The association of Hodgkin's disease with these various immunological and leukocyte functional abnormalities is much higher than might be anticipated on the basis of chance alone and is suggestive of an altered host response as one of the determinants in the development of this disease. Furthermore, the peculiar histological characteristics of the Hodgkin's lesion, with the abundant infiltrate of lymphocytes, eosinophils, histiocytes and connective tissue elements suggests an ineffective (?) host response to antigenic stimuli provided by the Reed-Sternberg cell. The lymphocytic depletion associated with progressive late-stage disease is also reminiscent of chronic graft-versus-host disease.[10] Despite all of these studies and numerous speculations, very little is known of the underlying etiological bases of Hodgkin's disease.

Two out of six of Thomas Hodgkin's original patients were children.[11] Similarly, five out of six of Dorothy Reed's patients, used as the basis for the definitive delineation of the Reed-Sternberg cell and the associated cellular environment, were also children.[12] Hodgkin's disease in the pediatric age group has, therefore, been recognized since the earliest descriptions of the disease. It probably represents the least common form of lymphoma in childhood and the incidence in the United States, as calculated from death certificates during the years 1960–1964, is only 1.23 per million population.[13] No definite cases have been identified below the age of three. The rate rises progressively during the first decade of life with a marked preponderance of males.[13]

At puberty the rate suddenly increases and the age ratio changes to that seen in most adult series—that is, almost equal incidence in males and females. The geographical distribution of Hodgkin's disease within the United States also differs for the juvenile versus the adult form. Thus, whereas the adult form of Hodgkin's disease is relatively uncommon in the West South Central States, the incidence of the juvenile form is closer to the national norm.[13] The differences in incidence, sex ratio and geographical distribution have led to the suggestion that there are two different diseases, morphologically similar but distinct in terms of etiology and clinical manifestations; one form is possibly due to an infectious etiology and occurring in the younger population seems to be distinct from that seen in the older age group.[14]

The histopathology of Hodgkin's disease has been the subject of considerable controversy. Although the Reed-Sternberg cell (Fig. 4-1) remains an important diagnostic criterion, and indeed the diagnosis of Hodgkin's disease is untenable in the absence of this cell, it is not sufficient evidence in itself to establish the diagnosis. The cell must be identified within a typical environment. This is particularly important since cells similar, if not identical, to classical Reed-Sternberg cells have been identified in the lymph nodes of patients with typical infectious mononucleosis,[15] as well as a number of other disease states characterized by intense histiocytic proliferation.[1] Variations in the cellular environment within

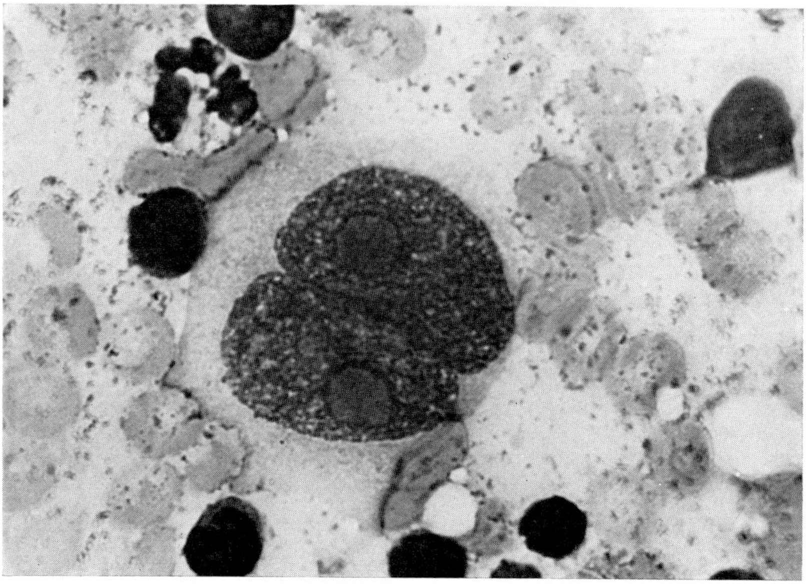

Figure 4-1. A typical Reed-Sternberg cell as seen on a touch imprint of a lymph node. The typical binucleated cell (mirror image) with large nucleoli is seen. (Courtesy of Dr. L. Yam.)

which the Reed-Sternberg cell has been identified have been classified in a number of ways. The currently accepted classification, originally proposed by Lukes and Butler,[16,17] divides Hodgkin's disease into four distinct categories: (a) lymphocytic predominance, (b) nodular sclerosis, (c) mixed cell type and (d) lymphocytic depletion. Typical sections of these histological categories are shown in Figure 4-2.

In adults, at least, the modified Lukes-Butler histological classification has a marked relationship to ultimate survival. Patients who have the lymphocytic predominance type of Hodgkin's disease at the time of original diagnosis have a markedly better survival than those whose biopsies show lymphocytic depletion.[18] In addition, the nodular sclerosis type, which is quite frequent in young females, shows predilection for presentation as a mediastinal mass and is associated with relatively long survival despite continued manifestations of the disease.[19] Frequently the histopathology of Hodgkin's disease tends to merge with the other lymphoproliferative disorders. Thus, it is sometimes difficult to distinguish this entity from lymphoma at one end of the spectrum and reticulum cell sarcoma at the other end. This interrelationship is outlined in Figure 4-3 and Table 4-1. Histological evidence of vascular invasion has recently[20,21] been shown to be of prognostic significance. Vascular invasion was found in about 5 percent of all patients with apparently localized disease and was associated with decreased disease-free intervals following therapy as well as more extensive disease at laparotomy. Five of six such patients had visceral involvement within twelve months.

CLINICAL MANIFESTATIONS

As mentioned above, the presenting manifestations of Hodgkin's disease are protean in character. Many children present as asymptomatic cervical lymphadenopathy which on biopsy proves to be Hodgkin's disease. Other children present with symptoms of persistent cough and a mediastinal mass is found on chest x-ray (Fig. 4-4). Still other children present with diffuse lymphadenopathy, fever and anorexia, a clinical picture strongly suggestive of sepsis. In all of these patients, the diagnosis is established only by biopsy of the appropriate lymph nodes. If the disease appears to be limited to the chest, mediastinal nodes are most likely to be affected, whereas if the disease is present in the cervical region, the largest node is most likely affected. This is an important point since the tendency is usually to sample the most readily accessible rather than most prominent node.

While many patients with lymphadenopathy are completely asymptomatic, occasionally the position of the enlarged node causes symptoms due to compression of surrounding structures. Mediastinal lymphadenopathy can lead to two serious complications: superior vena caval compression and tracheobronchial obstruction. Airway obstruction at times may be quite severe and cause marked respiratory distress with dyspnea and cyanosis. Overaggressive radiation therapy may lead to local edema and further obstruction. One can either use nitrogen mustard as the initial therapy since this agent presumably leads to less local edema or alternatively, one can start with relatively low-dose irradiation coupled with the administration of corticosteroids (2 mg/kg prednisone/day) used for their anti-inflammatory effect. Compression of the superior vena cava leads to cyanosis, venous engorgement and edema of the upper half of the body. Again therapy can consist of either local irradiation or chemotherapy although a combination of the two appears to be safest and yields the best results.[22]

Retroperitoneal lymphadenopathy may, at times, be of sufficient magnitude to cause ureteral compression and hydronephrosis. This is frequently asymptomatic and is recognized only on intravenous pyelogram during the diagnostic work-up (see below). Therapy is similar to that used above. Occasionally Hodgkin's disease may present with neurological symptoms consistent with a lesion compressing the spinal cord. This most commonly occurs in the cervical or thoracic regions. The incidence of cord compression is in the range of 3 to 8 percent. The symptoms are back pain, weakness and superficial sensory loss just below the level of compression. Sphincter difficulties and paraplegia are late results of untreated lesions. The myelogram is the most useful portion of the diagnostic work-up. Therapy with radiation may be

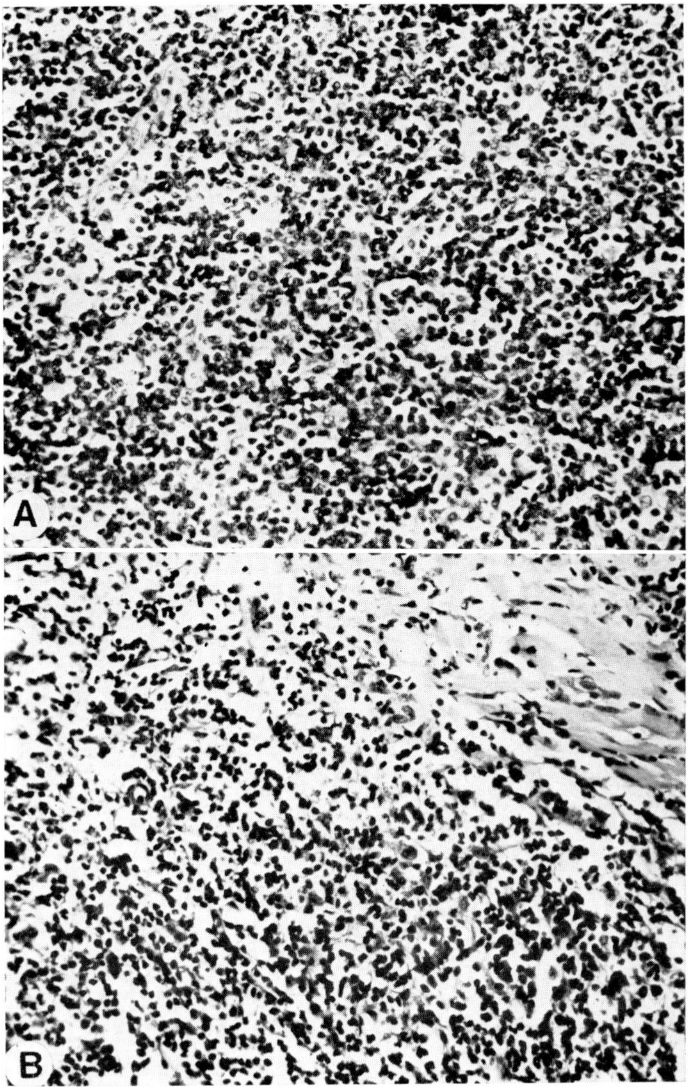

Figure 4-2. Histological section illustrating the various types of Hodgkin's disease as defined by the modified Lukes-Butler classification: (A) Lymphocyte predominance, (B) nodular sclerosis, (C) mixed cell type and (D) lymphocyte depletion. (Courtesy of the Department of Pathology, Tufts University School of Medicine.)

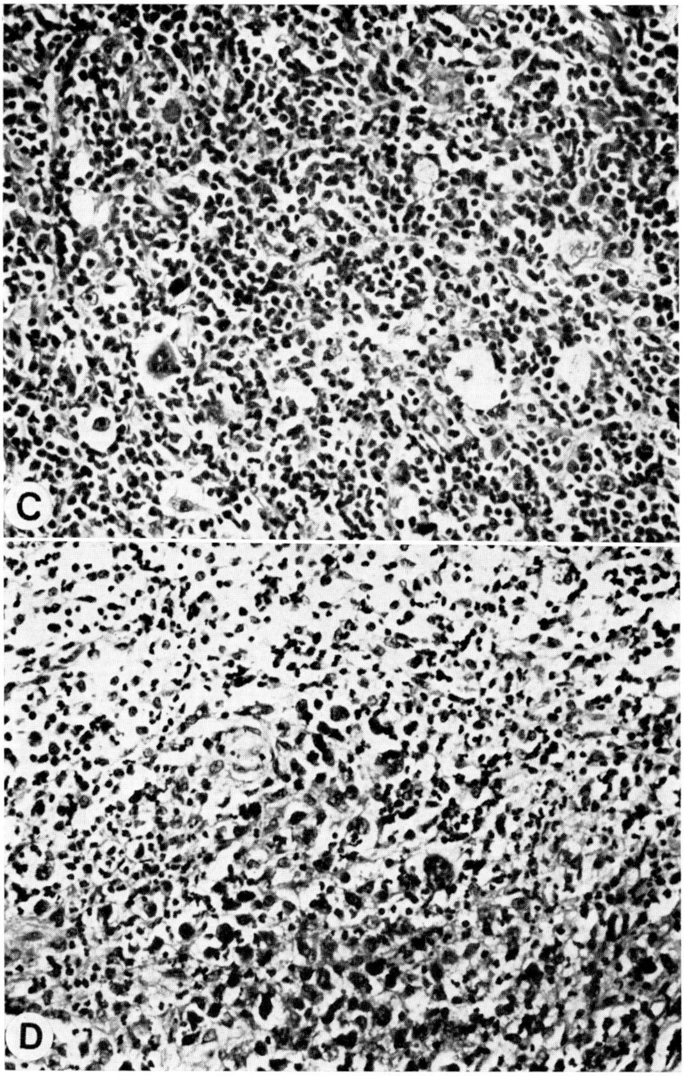

sufficient to control the symptoms but laminectomy with local decompression is usually necessary to restore maximum neurological function. Postoperative radiotherapy is given as early as possible.[23,24] Hodgkin's disease may also involve the lymph nodes of the

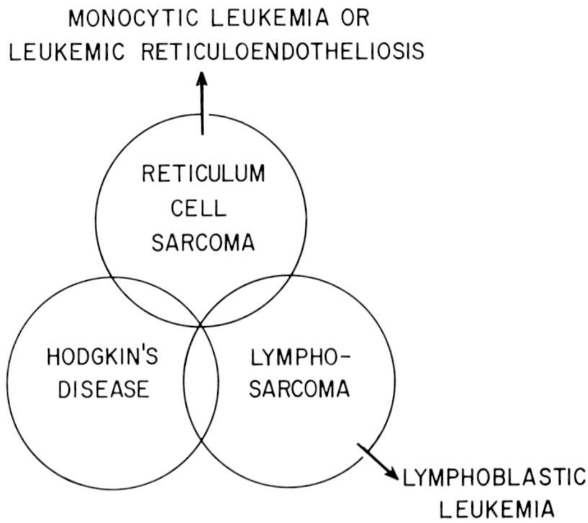

Figure 4-3. Interrelationship of the histologic picture in the various forms of lymphoma. This diagram is based on morphological evidence and may or may not be correlated with the etiological basis of these various entities.

gastrointestinal tract[25] leading to local obstructive phenomena. This may be associated with obstruction of the lymphatic drainage of the intestine and, on occasion, with a malabsorption syndrome. Symptomatology varies with the level of the lesion and the degree of obstruction. Infiltration and obstruction of the lumen of the intestines are uncommon. Hemorrhage and perforation may

TABLE 4-1
CORRELATION OF HISTOPATHOLOGICAL CLASSIFICATION WITH CLINICAL BEHAVIOR

I. *Stable or slowly progressive*
Hodgkin's disease—lymphocytic predominance
Lymphoma—well differentiated
Nodular lymphoma
II. *Moderately progressive*
Hodgkin's disease—nodular sclerosis
Hodgkin's disease—mixed cellularity
Lymphoma—poorly differentiated
III. *Rapidly progressive*
Hodgkin's disease—lymphocytic depletion
Reticulum cell sarcoma

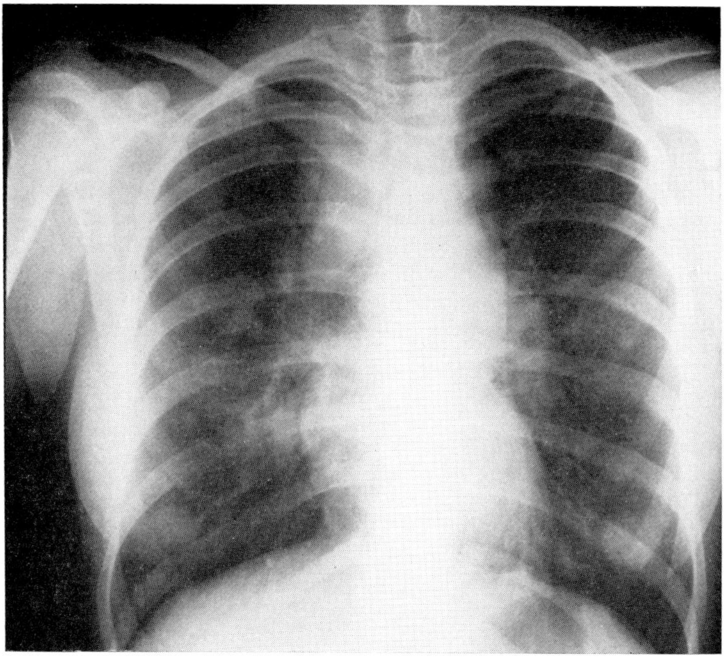

Figure 4-4. A mediastinal mass in the chest of a four-year-old girl. The presenting complaints were cough and fever. Biopsy demonstrated the presence of Hodgkin's disease. (Courtesy of Dr. D. Darling.)

complicate management,[26] especially with radiation therapy. If the disease appears to be localized to a limited segment, surgical resection may aid in long-term therapy.

Symptoms of extranodal involvement by Hodgkin's disease are associated with a poor prognosis (see below for staging). Organs frequently involved include the lung, liver, kidney and bone. Hodgkin's disease of the lung can be of three varieties: local extension from mediastinal nodes, parenchymal involvement independent of adjacent adenopathy, and involvement of the pleura. Local extension probably does not carry with it the poor prognosis that does primary involvement within the parenchymal tissue. In the latter, the x-ray appearance may be either of discrete nodules within the substance of the lung or of a finely reticulated pattern probably due to diffuse involvement of intrapulmonary bronchovascular lymphatics (Fig. 4-5). Local masses may cause compression of secondary bronchi with secondary infection and cavitation. Tuberculosis must, however, also be considered in these patients. Pleural involvement frequently leads to effusion, although the latter may be also secondary to venous obstruction due to massive mediastinal adenopathy. Distinction between the two causes of effusion is important in therapy and may, at times, be difficult. Pleural biopsy is occasionally of help.

Hepatic involvement is very difficult to diagnose without a biopsy and even then may be missed.[27] Most, if not all, parameters of liver function are of little use in the asymptomatic patient. Even hepatomegaly may exist in the absence of histological evidence of intrahepatic Hodgkin's disease in about one-third of biopsied patients. Jaundice sometimes develops and, when present, is almost certainly due to intrahepatic obstruction of portal tracts. Extrahepatic obstruction by nodes is less common. Jaundice may occasionally be secondary to a Coombs' positive hemolytic anemia. Direct invasion of the kidneys[28] must be rare but renal complications secondary to distant disease have been reported with increasing frequency. Thus, a reversible nephrotic syndrome has been ascribed to compression of the inferior vena cava,[29] to amyloidosis,[30] and secondary to distant lymphadenopathy.[31] In the latter patients, the nephrosis improved when the distant nodes responded to irradiation. Tumor-host immunological mechanisms may have played a role in the development of renal symptomatology in these patients.

Invasion of the bones may occur either by local extension from neighboring involved lymph nodes or by distant, presumably hematogenous spread. Local pain is frequently the presenting symptom and may be present for a considerable period of time before changes can be noted on x-ray. Isotopic bone scans, using strontium or gallium, are frequently helpful in localizing lesions in the absence of diagnostic x-ray changes.[32] Bony lesions are said to occur in 10 to 15 percent of all patients[33] and may be quite widespread. The lesions may be either osteolytic or osteoblastic or, as usually is seen, a mixture of the two. Lesions are frequently found in the vertebrae (Fig. 4-6), pelvis, ribs and, less commonly,

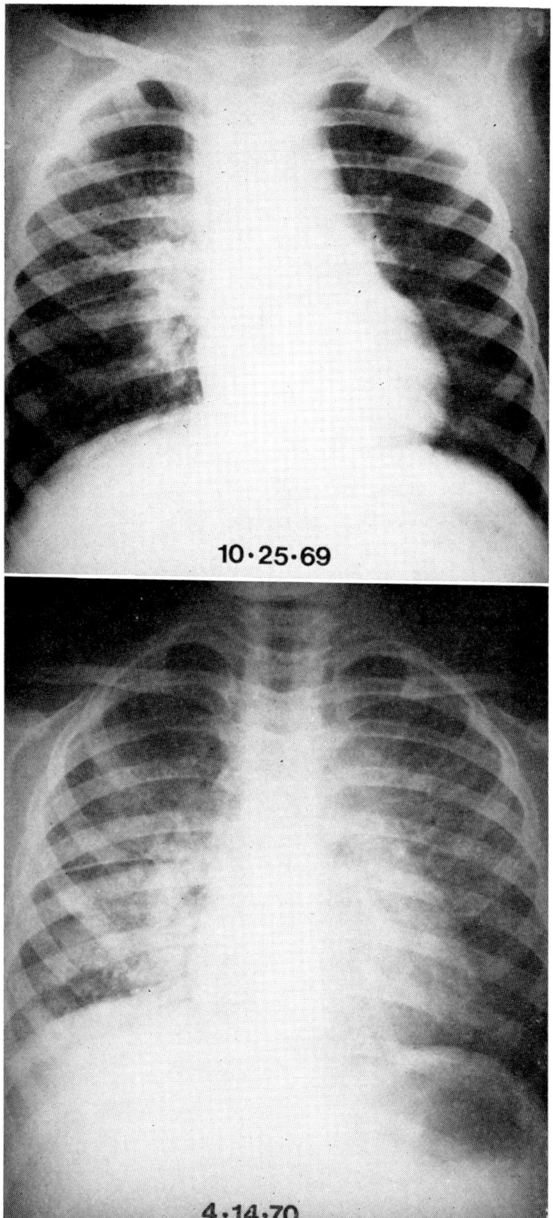

Figure 4-5. Diffuse intrapulmonary involvement by Hodgkin's disease. This pattern represents extension of the disease along bronchovascular lymphatics as was demonstrated by pulmonary biopsy in this patient. (Courtesy of Dr. D. Darling.)

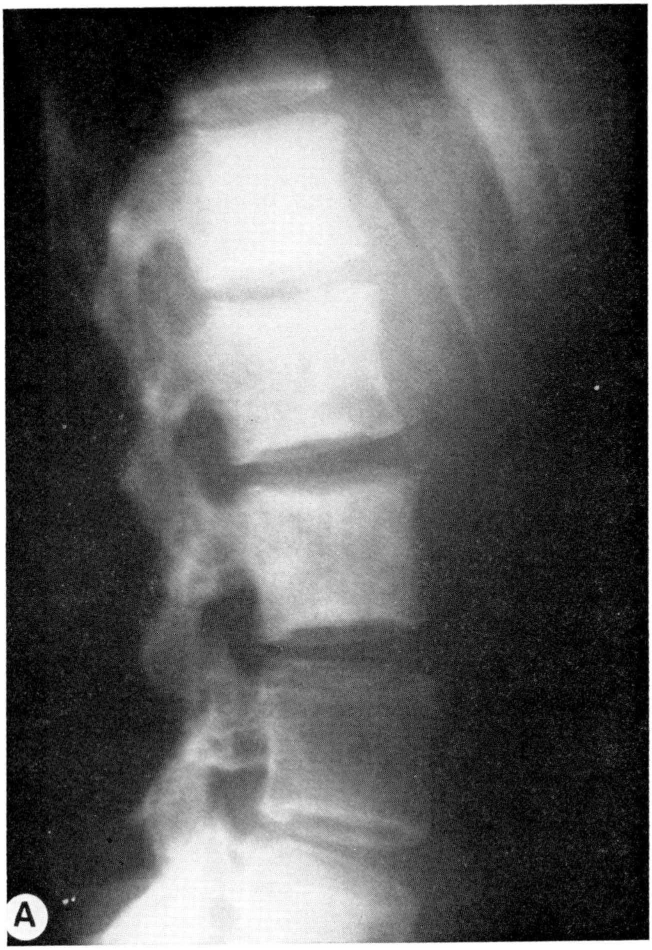

Figure 4-6. An osteoblastic lesion of the lumbar vertebrae. *(Left)* Lateral view. *(Right)* Anteroposterior view. (Courtesy of Dr. D. Darling.)

in the long bones. They are rarely found in the calvarium. Pathological fractures appear to be uncommon, especially if the lesions are treated early with local irradiation. Compression fractures of the vertebrae may, however, be the presenting sign of disease in the spine. The presence of bony lesions, except where due to local spread from mediastinal or retroperitoneal nodes, is associ-

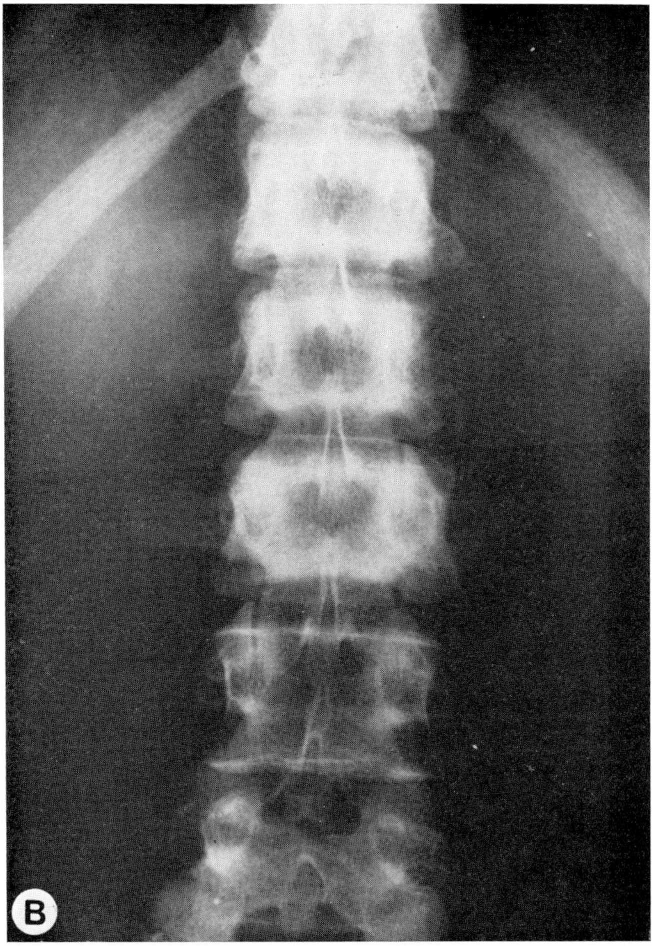

ated with an extremely poor prognosis; 50 percent of such patients are dead within two years. Infiltration of the skin by Hodgkin's disease usually takes the form of discrete nontender nodules which may be either colorless or pigmented. Usually such nodules are thought to represent diffuse or generalized disease. Such infiltrates are also thought to represent retrograde seeding through blocked lymphatics.[34] They frequently appear to be associated with regional node involvement.

In addition to the symptoms referable to lymphadenopathy or organ invasion, systemic symptoms of Hodgkin's disease include fever, night sweats, pruritus and weight loss. The presence of such systemic symptoms often is indicative of widespread disease, frequently of the upper retroperitoneal lymph nodes. Fever in Hodgkin's disease is frequently part of the malignant process and unrelated to the presence of any infectious organisms. This cannot, however, be taken for granted and each febrile episode deserves a careful evaluation. Classically, the fever which occurs in 30 to 50 percent of patients is said to be of the Pel-Ebstein type in which alternate febrile and afebrile episodes last for a few days to a week or longer. Such a pattern is actually relatively uncommon and any type of fever pattern may be noted. Although the cause of the fever is not well understood, two mechanisms have been suggested: (a) the fever is a reflection of the host reaction to cellular spill into the blood and/or (b) the release of a specific polypeptide into the blood, probably by the tumor or granulocytes.[35]

Generalized pruritus may precede the onset of other symptomatology in Hodgkin's disease. It is encountered in about 10 percent of the cases and the underlying cause is unknown. The pruritus, which can be quite bothersome, usually responds to therapy of the generalized disease. It is interesting to note that this symptom is rare in children under ten years. About 15 to 20 percent of the patients with Hodgkin's disease develop severe pain at the site of local active disease on the ingestion of alcohol.[36] This may occur even after the intravenous administration of medications containing alcohol (such as BCNU). In older teenagers and in adults this has, on occasion, been the presenting sign of disease or, more frequently, indicative of a new lesion. The mechanism of this process is unknown.

LABORATORY FINDINGS

Laboratory data is frequently of very little help in the evaluation of patients with Hodgkin's disease, especially in the early stages. Often there is no anemia but as the disease becomes widespread, a normocytic, normochronic anemia may appear. This has frequently been ascribed to bone marrow invasion but the exact mechanism is unknown. Impaired mobilization of iron has also been suggested as the cause. Occasionally, especially in advanced disease, the anemia may be but one aspect of frank hypersplenism. A Coombs' positive hemolytic anemia has also been reported on occasion.[37] The leukocyte count may be normal, increased or reduced. Active disease is frequently associated with granulocytosis but this is not invariably true. Widespread disease, particularly with infiltration of the bone marrow, may be associated with leukopenia and, more consistently, with lymphopenia. Although frequently mentioned, marked eosinophilia and monocytosis are found only in a minority of patients. The platelet count is frequently normal except in cases complicated by hypersplenism or bone marrow invasion. Although the blood sedimentation rate is often used as an index of activity of the disease, elevated values are more directly correlated with the stage of the disease irrespective of state of remission or relapse.[38] If the patient has an elevated blood sedimentation rate at the onset of his disease and it remits when the disease is treated, recurrent elevations are frequently associated with recurrence of active disease.

Bone marrow aspiration is usually of little diagnostic value in Hodgkin's disease. One may see a hypercellular marrow with a generalized increase in myeloid, megakaryocytic and histiocytic elements. A moderate eosinophilia may also be noted. Occasionally, multinucleated cells may be noted but usually, in an aspirated specimen, the positive identification of Reed-Sternberg cells is impossible. Because the identification of bone marrow infiltration is so important in the staging of Hodgkin's disease (and, hence, in therapy), bone marrow biopsy is now advocated in all cases where definite bone lesions are not identified by x-ray. Even the biopsy technique, however, failed to identify over 10 percent of patients who had marrow involvement proven at autopsy.[39]

A number of abnormalities in the serum chemistries of patients with Hodgkin's disease have been reported at one time or another. None of these have been found to be specific either for activity of the disease or for specific organ involvement. Hypercalcemia is often found with widespread bone disease and must be considered when the latter is present. Elevated blood calcium levels are, however, occasionally found in the absence of evidence of bone disease and may be a reflection of a parathyroid-like action of the tumor. Hyperuricemia may be a consequence of aggressive therapy and must be prevented by the use of antiuricemic agents (such as allopurinol). An elevated serum alkaline phosphatase level has been correlated with the stage of the disease and the presence of fever, but not with liver or bone involvement.[40] Even measurement of the organ-specific isozymes did not improve the specificity of the determination. Increase in the leukocyte alkaline phosphatase was also at one time thought to correlate with the presence of active disease but more recently Jaffe and Bishop[38] have reported that a significant number of children may have abnormal values even when in clinical remission. None of the usual liver function tests, including transaminase levels and BSP retention, have been found to correlate with hepatic involvement.[27] Serum ceruloplasmin, transferrin, hydroxyproline and trace metal levels have all at one time or another been thought to reflect the activity of the disease. None, however, have shown consistent correlation with clinical status.

The immunological aspects of Hodgkin's disease have recently received considerable attention. This aspect of the disease process is of particular interest in view of the numerous infectious complications which patients with widespread Hodgkin's disease experience. Thus, herpes zoster, fungal disease and tuberculosis are frequently seen in patients with advanced stages of Hodgkin's disease, even those who have received no radiation or chemotherapy. In addition, one of the few documented instances of a bone marrow transplant with persistent chimera in other than identical twins prior to the era of HLA-typing occurred in a patient with advanced Hodgkin's disease.[41] This clinical observation has been reflected in delayed skin homograft rejection[42] and has been identified as a defect in cellular immunity. Thus Brown *et al.*[43] showed that delayed hypersensitivity in patients with well-localized disease (stage I) was normal whereas a significant decrease in skin sensitivity to various antigens or to sensitization by DNCB was found in patients with more extensive disease. A reduction in lymphocyte blast transformation in response to phytohemagglutinin stimulation was also noted by several groups[43,44] and was thought to indicate a functional defect in the immunological reactivity of the circulating lymphocytes. Recent studies[45] have questioned the relationship of PHA-induced lymphocyte stimulation to immunological competence or clinical status in Hodgkin's disease; indeed, in a series of eleven untreated patients, with apparently localized disease, several showed decreased PHA-induced lymphocyte transformation as well as decreased leukocyte interferon production in response to *in vitro* viral infection.[46] Thus, the defect in cellular immunity may not be as directly related to the extent of disease as was originally thought.

However, a decreasing immunological responsiveness may have some prognostic value; Sokal and Aungst[47] have correlated the response to BCG vaccination to median survival in patients with advanced Hodgkin's disease. The conversion of the tuberculin skin test following BCG vaccination given during remission was found to be a good prognostic sign; 23 of 24 who converted had a median survival of over thirty months whereas failure to convert was associated with rapidly progressive disease. Various other immunological abnormalities have also been reported in Hodgkin's disease. The occurrence of a Coombs' positive hemolytic anemia in the occasional patient has already been alluded to. An occasional patient may also exhibit what appears to be a monoclonal macroglobulinemia[48]; the significance of this is not known. In advanced Hodgkin's disease greatly increased levels of gamma-globulin are frequently found; this appears to be nonspecific. Finally, a recent preliminary observation[49] of a tumor-specific antigen in two patients with Hodgkin's disease may be quite significant, not only in relating the defect in delayed hypersensitivity to the progression of the disease but also in designing new modalities of therapy.

STAGING

Once the definitive diagnosis of Hodgkin's disease has been established by lymph node biopsy, it becomes important to evaluate the extent of the disease. Survival in Hodgkin's disease appears to be directly related to the extent of the disease process at the time of diagnosis. Improvements in survival achieved in recent years are a reflection not only of more aggressive therapy but also of improved techniques for the evaluation of the patient. The relatively poor survival in children as compared to that achieved in adults is quite possibly a reflection of less aggressive attempts to determine the extent of the disease and thus, in many cases, inadequate therapy to areas of occult disease. The currently accepted schema for the clinical staging of Hodgkin's disease, as outlined in Table 4-2, is a recent modification of that agreed upon at the 1965 Conference on Hodgkin's disease held at Rye, New York.[50-52]

The complete evaluation of the patient should include[53] care-

TABLE 4-2
STAGING OF HODGKIN'S DISEASE

Stage I	— Hodgkin's disease present only in a single anatomic region of lymph nodes
Stage I_E	— Hodgkin's disease present only in a localized extralymphatic anatomic region (stomach, thyroid, etc.)
Stage II	— Two or more lymph node regions involved on one side of the diaphragm
Stage II_E	— One or more lymph node regions plus a localized extralymphatic region present on one side of the diaphragm
Stage III	— Involvement of lymph node regions on both sides of the diaphragm
Stage III_S	— Involvement of lymph node regions, including the spleen, on both sides of the diaphragm
Stage IV	— Diffuse involvement of one or more extralymphatic organs or tissues with or without associated lymph node involvement. (A single focus of liver or bone marrow involvement must be considered as diffuse disease.)

Systemic Symptoms: A: no symptomatology; *B:* constitutional symptoms including fever, night sweats, and significant weight loss (greater than 10 percent over past six months)

Complete staging notation includes clinical staging (CS) and pathological stage (PS). Clinical staging includes data obtained from initial biopsy, history and physical examination, routine and special x-rays, laboratory studies and special studies such as isotopic scans. Pathological staging includes laparotomy with biopsies, splenectomy, thoracotomy, as well as any additional biopsies. A patient staged by clinical studies to be stage IIA is noted as CS IIA. If he then undergoes laparotomy and is found to have involvement of the spleen, his classification is then noted as CS IIA PS III_SA.

ful history and physical examination, a complete blood count, chest x-ray and skeletal survey, intravenous pyelogram, bone marrow examination (to include a biopsy), assessment of liver and renal function, and documentation of cutaneous anergy if possible. Ultmann and others have also advocated the use of lower extremity lymphangiogram to delineate involvement of retroperitoneal lymph nodes. However, lymphangiograms are quite difficult to perform in children; in one series[54] only about 50 percent of the attempts resulted in satisfactory studies. An example of a lymphangiogram demonstrating active disease in the hypogastric and iliac lymph nodes is shown in Figure 4-7. The use of the inferior vena cavagram has been advocated as an alternative procedure to visualize the retroperitoneal nodes[55] but, in general, has not proven to be very sensitive. Various problems were encountered in

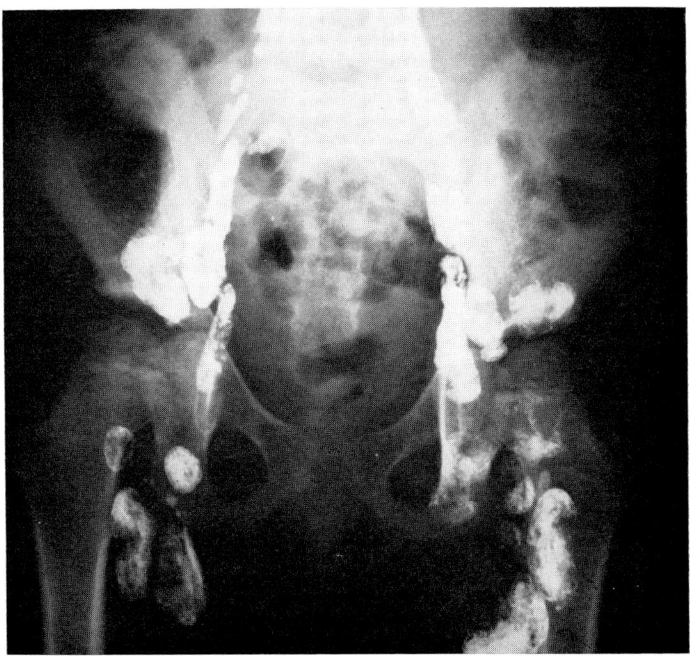

Figure 4-7. A lymphangiogram in a child with Hodgkin's disease. The femoral and iliac nodes not only are enlarged but also demonstrate typical filling defects suggestive (but not absolutely diagnostic) of nodal replacement by tumor. (Courtesy of Dr. D. Darling.)

the clinical staging of Hodgkin's disease as outlined above. Delineation of retroperitoneal and para-aortic nodal involvement was often found to be inaccurate, the biochemical evaluation of liver function was variable and in many cases did not correlate with the clinical course of the disease.[27] In addition, the presence of an enlarged spleen, which often radically changes the stage of the disease if truly secondary to tumor involvement, was frequently difficult to evaluate.

In view of these problems, several centers[56-59] undertook to include an exploratory laparotomy as part of the initial work-up of the patient who had a clinical classification of stage I, II or III. The operative findings were correlated with the clinical staging as determined by routine clinical staging. The results from several large series have been reviewed by Ultmann[56] and Kadin *et al.*[57] The procedure includes biopsy of retroperitoneal nodes (especially those considered suspicious by palpation or on lymphangiogram), liver wedge biopsy, and splenectomy including the removal of perisplenic lymph nodes. The data collected from several such series[75] are tabulated in Table 4-3. The histological diagnoses differed from the preoperative clinical evaluation in 30 percent of the specimens. The lymphangiogram gave misleading results 20 percent of the time and unsuspected splenic involvement was present in over one-third of the patients. Preoperative evaluation of the liver was particularly misleading; only 8 out of 61 patients thought to have clinical evidence of hepatic involvement were found to have evidence of Hodgkin's disease on open biopsy. On the other hand, only 5 out of 126 patients were found to have unsuspected hepatic involvement. Since histological demonstration of hepatic involvement is an ominous finding and represents one of the major contraindications to curative radiotherapy,[60] these findings are of particular pertinence in the evaluation of patients.

Percutaneous needle biopsy has been found to be a relatively insensitive technique for the demonstration of hepatic involvement, yielding false negatives in 10 percent or more patients who later have positive findings on open wedge biopsy.[27,61] An additional advantage of laparotomy is the observation that if in the adults, the weight of the surgically removed spleen is above 400 gm, the liver is involved in 75 percent of the patients. In summary, laparotomy with splenectomy and liver biopsy led to a change in the preoperative evaluation of the extent of the disease in about one-third of all instances.

The role of exploratory laparotomy and splenectomy in the evaluation of unselected patients with Hodgkin's disease has recently been challenged on the grounds that the findings will only rarely change the extent of therapy and radiation to the normal non-enlarged spleen in the adult is quite safe.[62] However, the routine use of x-ray therapy to the spleen in the pediatric age group, except in patients with unequivocal stage IV disease, is warranted for two reasons: First, radiation of the spleen in the child without damage to either the lung or the kidney is technically much more difficult than in the average adult. Secondly, lymphangiography in the pediatric age group is a very difficult and unsatisfactory procedure. Out of three pediatric patients who recently underwent staging laparotomy with splenectomy at our institution, one was found to have unsuspected isolated splenic involvement and consequently was shifted from stage IA to stage IIIA. Isolated involvement of the spleen in the absence of Hodgkin's disease elsewhere in the abdomen is suggestive of hematogenous spread[20,63] which in itself has important implications for therapy. Finally, removal of the spleen at the time of initial work-up may well be of some value in the long-term care of the patient. Thus, by splenectomy one prevents development of subsequent hypersplenism and secondly increases the patient's tolerance to the myelosuppressive effect of radiation and/or chemotherapy.[64]

THERAPY

Radiation plays a primary role in the definitive treatment of Hodgkin's disease. It was demonstrated by a number of authors[65] that, in the early stages at least, Hodgkin's disease spreads by orderly extension to neighboring groups of lymph nodes. This finding led to the concept of curative radiotherapy using extended field prophylactic radiation. Furthermore, Kaplan,[66] Fuller *et al.*,[67] Nobler[68] and others[69,70] have all pointed out that the recurrence rate in lymph node areas treated with irradiation is inversely related to the dose of radiation delivered. The existence of a tumoricidal dose for Hodgkin's disease has been demonstrated (in adults) and a recurrence rate of less than 5 percent can be anticipated in areas treated with 3,500 to 4,000 rads.[66] The longer the relapse-free interval following radiation, the lower the probability of local recurrence.[71] In children, only 1 out of 12 patients treated with tumoricidal doses of radiation had evidence of recurrence within the irradiated field.[72]

At present, three types of radiotherapy are in use for the treatment of localized disease: local high-dose irradiation to involved area, extended field irradiation to include contiguous lymph node areas, and total nodal irradiation to include all of the major lymphatic chains in the torso. Two special types of extended fields have also been employed: mantle irradiation which is designed to include all of the lymph node bearing areas above the diaphragm and the "inverted-Y" field which includes the nodal areas in the abdomen (Fig. 4-8). Long-term experience with the more aggressive forms of radiotherapy is still quite limited, especially in the pediatric age range. However, the data presented by Jenkins *et al.*[72] and Teillet and Schweisguth[73] suggests that extended field irradiation substantially reduces the number of recurrences in patients with stage I and IIA disease. Presently available data in adults suggests such therapy may result in five-year relapse-free survival rates of over 80 percent.[68-70] For patients with IIB (and possibly IIIA) disease, total nodal irradiation may result in five-year relapse-free rates of 60 percent or higher.[10] A possible exception may be those patients who have the nodular sclerosis type of Hodgkin's disease where a definite advantage for total nodal irradiation has not been observed.[74] In more extensive disease, stages IIIB and IV, the role of radiotherapy is to control local manifestations and is used in conjunction with chemotherapy.

Extended field or total nodal radiotherapy is not without its hazards. Complications include hypothyroidism, radiation pneumonitis[75] and radiation pericarditis.[76] The incidence of complications varies from 5 to 10 percent of cases.[56] Probably the most fre-

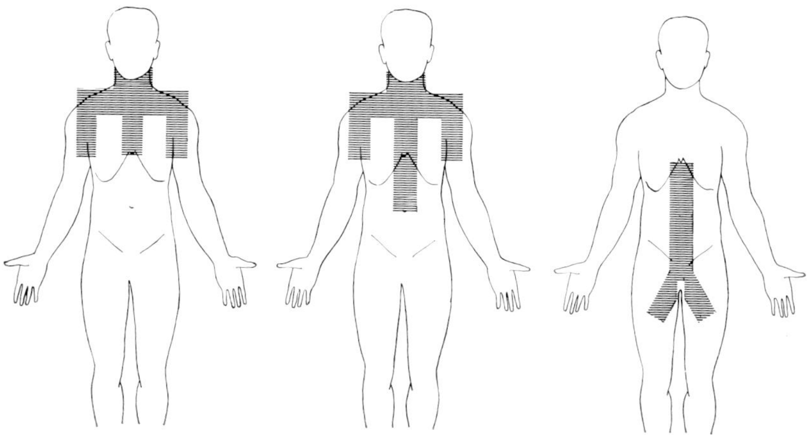

Figure 4-8. Various types of treatment fields in current use in the radiotherapy of Hodgkin's disease: *(a)* mantle field which is designed to include all of the lymph node areas above the diaphragm; *(b)* a modified mantle which has been extended to cover the upper abdominal nodes; and *(c)* an "inverted-Y" field which includes the para-aortic nodes as well as those in the iliac, inguinal and femoral chains. Total nodal irradiation is a combination of a and c, care being taken to avoid overlap at the point where the two fields meet. If splenectomy has not been carried out, the para-aortic field is extended to include the spleen, care being taken to avoid the left lower lung and the left kidney. Otherwise, the current practice is to include the splenic pedicle in the field.

quent significant complication is bone marrow depression which may at times be severe enough to force an interruption in radiation therapy. Decreased bone marrow reserve may persist for a year or more and may limit tolerance to subsequent chemotherapy.[77]

Chemotherapy is generally given to patients who either (a) have relapsed following maximal radiotherapy or (b) have widespread disease. Recently chemotherapy has also been combined with radiotherapy in the definitive therapy of patients who have evidence of hematogenous spread (that is, isolated extension to the spleen). Chemotherapeutic agents which have received adequate clinical trials include nitrogen mustard,[78] vincristine,[79] vinblastine (intravenously),[80] vinblastine sulfate (orally),[81] chlorambucil,[82] cyclophosphamide,[83] procorbazine,[84] BCNU[85] and prednisone.[86] In the past, patients deemed suitable candidates for chemotherapy were given a course of nitrogen mustard (0.4 mg/kg IV in two to four divided doses). This was usually sufficient to induce a clinical remission and the patient was maintained on either no therapy or on chlorambucil (0.2 mg/kg/day) until relapse. Remission induction was again attempted with nitrogen mustard which was repeated until the patient evidenced resistance. Vincristine, vinblastine, procarbazine, cyclophosphamide and prednisone were given singly and sequentially for each relapse. The remissions, in general, tended to be of relatively short duration and often incomplete although at least one patient with stage IIB disease has been reported to have a five-year disease-free survival following a single course of nitrogen mustard.[87]

More recently, combination chemotherapy utilizing vincristine, nitrogen mustard, procarbazine and prednisone (MOPP) has been introduced in the initial therapy of advanced Hodgkin's disease (Table 4-3). These drugs were given in cyclic fashion for six months after which the patients were followed until relapse. Limiting toxicity was bone marrow depression. Roughly 80 percent of the patients achieved a complete remission with a median

TABLE 4-3

Preoperative Assessment	*No.*	*Biopsy Positive*	*Biopsy Negative*	*% False*
Negative LAG	77	10	67	13
Equivocal LAG	29	7	22	
Positive LAG	54	38	16	30
Spleen				
Clinically negative	125	44	17	35
Clinically positive	42	25	18	43
Liver				
Clinically negative	126	5	121	4
Clinically positive	61	8	53	87

duration of over twenty-nine months.[88] Out of the first one hundred patients treated with MOPP, there have been only two drug-related deaths, both secondary to massive tumor necrosis. Recently, MOPP has been compared, in a randomized study, with single agent induction and remission maintenance.[89] Both the response rate and the duration of remissions were greater using combination chemotherapy. Combination chemotherapy has also been evaluated[90] in patients who had received previous therapy, either radiotherapy, chemotherapy, or both; complete remissions were achieved in 70 percent of the patients with unmaintained remissions of up to twenty-four months. The major dose-limiting toxicity was leukopenia and this appeared to be related to the extent of prior radiotherapy. There are no reports of the efficacy of combination chemotherapy in the pediatric age group. Unpublished data from Acute Leukemia Group B includes twenty-nine patients (stage III and IV) in the pediatric age group (4 to 15 years) who were treated with one of several forms of intensive combination chemotherapy. The overall response rate was 86 percent with 52 percent achieving complete remission. The median duration of response was over three hundred days, with 70 percent still in remission twenty-nine to over five hundred days after initiation of therapy. The overall response in this group of children is at least as good as in a similar group of adult patients.

Finally, a few groups[91,92] have started to explore a combination of cyclic chemotherapy with extended field radiotherapy for stage III and IV disease. In an interesting study from France,[91] chemotherapy was given first, followed by radiotherapy which was given in two stages separated by an interval of three to six weeks. Eighty percent complete remissions were obtained with a median duration of thirty months for stage III and eighteen months for stage IV. We have tried a similar combination in a few pediatric patients who tolerated the procedure relatively well; bone marrow depression following drug therapy was the major toxic effect. It is, however, too early to evaluate long-term results.

The optimum therapy for Hodgkin's disease, especially in the pediatric age group, is still a subject of discussion. Total nodal irradiation, as advocated by several groups for localized Hodgkin's disease, will undoubtedly lead to decreased growth. On the other hand, localized irradiation, as so often has been used in the treatment of children, has not proven as effective as extended field irradiation. Certain recommendations for therapy in this age range thus appear justified. Localized disease (stage I or II) should be treated with extended field radiotherapy, either of the modified mantle (Fig. 4-8,b) or "inverted-Y" (Fig. 4-8,c) type. In this scheme, the mantle field of irradiation is extended to include the upper abdominal and retroperitoneal nodes, nodes which are difficult to visualize either by lymphangiogram or at laparotomy. Disease which extends across the diaphragm (stage III and possibly stage IIB) should be treated with total nodal irradiation. In addition, stage III disease, when associated with systemic symptoms, should be treated with combination chemotherapy (MOPP). Finally, generalized disease (stage IV) should be treated with combination chemotherapy with local tumoricidal radiotherapy to troublesome lesions. These recommendations are summarized in Table 4-4.

PROGNOSIS

In adults localized Hodgkin's disease appears to be a potentially curable disease with five-year disease-free survival rates of over 80 percent and significant survival at ten years. Even more extensive disease has an appreciable five-year disease-free survival rate; total nodal irradiation has resulted in 70 percent prolonged remissions in stage IIIA. It is anticipated that improvements in staging, particularly through the use of laparotomy and splenectomy, will lead to further improvements in this survival by revealing loci of occult abdominal disease. Clinical staging is not the sole determinant of survival in Hodgkin's disease; histological classification of the lesion also plays an important determinant role. Patients with lymphocyte-depletion type of Hodgkin's disease at the time of initial diagnosis have, in general, a much poorer prognosis than those with the lymphocyte-predominance type. The factors which underlie the specific type of histological reaction in Hodgkin's disease are not understood but may play an important role in overall prognosis.

TABLE 4-4
THERAPY OF HODGKIN'S DISEASE

Stages I and II

1. Establish diagnosis by lymph node biopsy
2. Explatory laparotomy with lymph node biopsies, liver, biopsy, and splenectomy
3. Modified mantle irradiation (see Fig. 4-8)
4. Observe

Stage III

1. Establish diagnosis by lymph node biopsy
2. Exploratory laparatomy with lymph node biopsies, liver, biospy, and splenectomy
3. Total nodal irradiation
4. MOPP (for stage IIIB)
5. Observe

Stage IV

1. Establish diagnosis by lymph node biopsy
2. MOPP
3. Palliative irradiation as necessary
4. Observe

Combination Chemotherapy (MOPP)

Vincristine	1.5 mg/M^2 once a week (no more than 2 mg per dose)
Nitrogen mustard	6 mg/M^2 once a week
Procarbazine	100 mg/M^2 p.o. daily
Prednisone	40 mg/M^2 p.o. daily

This is to be given in two-week courses with a two-week interval of rest for a total of six courses. The prednisone is to be given on alternate courses only. Complete blood counts must be obtained at weekly intervals. Allopurinol should be used for hyperuricemia. The dose of nitrogen mustarl and procarbazine is to be reduced for leukopenia and/or thrombocytopenia.

In contrast to the long-term survival data in adults, children with Hodgkin's disease tend, on the whole, to do less well. Survival data on sixty children derived from the recent literature[19,93] and from our own experience is summarized in Figure 4-9. For all stages of the disease, the five-year survival is significantly poorer than that seen in adults. Somewhat better experience has recently been reported from France by Teillet and Schweisguth,[73] and even here the five-year survival for stages II through IV was appreciably less than that seen in adults. The histology of Hodgkin's disease in children is not appreciably different from that seen in

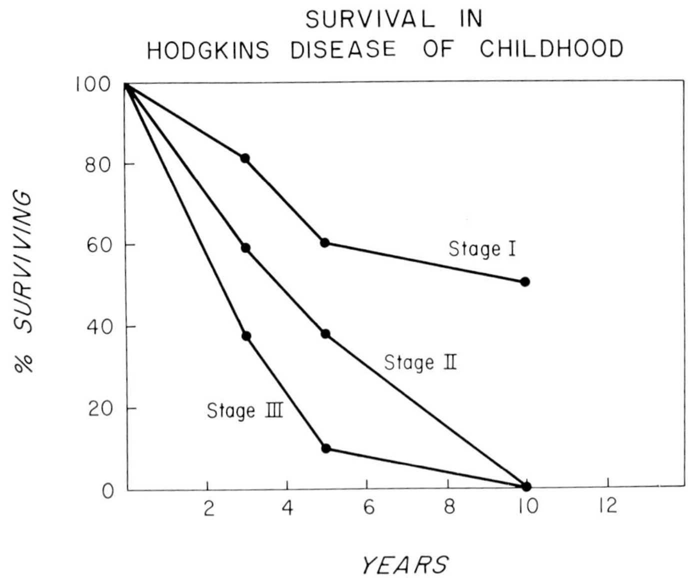

Figure 4-9. Five-year survival data in Hodgkin's disease occurring in the pediatric age range. The curves are based on the reports of Butler[19] and Strum and Rappaport[93] as well as on our own data.

adults. However, Strum and Rappaport[93] have commented upon a predominance of mature lymphocytes noted in most cases, a finding which may have some relevance in terms of host response. The relatively poor prognosis in childhood is, therefore, not because these series are weighted with patients of the lymphocyte-depletion type of disease.

Undue delay in diagnosis is probably one of the major factors contributing to the poor prognosis; the duration of the interval between onset of symptoms and time of diagnosis is inversely related to the length of survival.[73] In the French series, 11 out of 13 patients who were diagnosed within one year of the onset of symptoms were alive five to eight years later; only 2 out of 19 patients who were diagnosed one to four years after the first symptoms were noted were alive; the majority had died within five years of diagnosis. Furthermore, the longer the interval to time of diagnosis, the greater the proportion of stage III cases. Many of these patients were initially misdiagnosed as having cervical lymphadenopathy of infectious origin. The lesson appears obvious: persistent lymphadenopathy in childhood mandates a biopsy. The interval of "watchful waiting" probably should not extend more than six weeks. Only by more aggressive diagnosis, as well as aggressive staging and therapy can we hope to improve long-term survival in childhood Hodgkin's disease.

Prolonged survival does not necessarily mean total eradication of disease. Strum and Rappaport,[94] in a study of individuals dying ten years or more after the diagnosis of Hodgkin's disease, found a significant number who, while the cause of death was unrelated to the previous malignancy, showed evidence of persistent foci of Hodgkin's disease. The authors conclude that in some patients "clinical cure may in fact represent a state of equilibrium in which the host has come to terms with his disease." This is particularly pertinent in view of the recent report[49] of a tumor-specific antigen present in two patients with Hodgkin's disease. One might speculate that if the tumor mass is sufficiently reduced in volume, host immunological mechanisms may serve to control the remaining tumor tissue. On the other hand, deterioration of host immunological mechanisms, as is seen in some patients, will allow rapid progression of the tumor. The clinical utilization of such data may provide entirely new avenues of therapy in Hodgkin's disease.

Finally, there have been a number of reports[95-98] of acute myelocytic leukemia occurring in patients with Hodgkin's disease of long duration. Radiation therapy must be considered as a major causative factor, but the role of alkylating agents as well as genetic or possibly immunologic factors must also be considered.

REFERENCES

1. Strum, S.B., Park, J.K., and Rappaport, H.: Observations of cells resembling Sternberg-Reed cells in conditions other than Hodgkin's disease. *Cancer, 26:*176, 1970.
2. Vianna, N.J., Greenwald, P., and Davies, J.: Extended epidemic of Hodgkin's disease in high school students. *Lancet, 1:*1209, 1971.
3. Eisinger, M., Fox, S., deHarven, E. *et al.*: Virus-like agents from patients with Hodgkin's disease. *Nature (Lond), 223:*104, 1971.

4. Goldman, J.M., and Aisenberg, A.: Incidence of antibody to EB virus, herpes simplex, and cytomegalic virus in Hodgkin's disease. *Cancer, 26*:327, 1970.
5. Miller, R.W.: Mortality in childhood Hodgkin's disease. *JAMA, 198*: 1216, 1966.
6. Evans, H.E., and Nyhan, W.: Hodgkin's disease in children. *Bull Johns Hopkins Hosp, 114*:237, 1964.
7. Forbes, J.F., and Morris, P.M.: Leukocyte antigens in Hodgkin's disease. *Lancet, 1*:849, 1970.
8. Osoba, D., and Falk, J.A.: HL-A antigens in Hodgkin's disease. *Clin Res, 19*:494, 1971.
9. Tan, C., Etcubanas, E., Lieberman, P. *et al.*: Chediak-Higashi syndrome in a child with Hodgkin's disease. *Amer J Dis Child, 121*:135, 1971.
10. Kaplan, H.S.: On the natural history, treatment, and prognosis of Hodgkin's disease. *Harvey Lect, 64*:215, 1968-69.
11. Hodgkin, T.: On some morbid appearances of the absorbent glands and spleen. *Med Chir Soc Trans, 17*:68, 1832.
12. Reed, D.: On the pathological changes in Hodgkin's disease with special reference to its relation to tuberculosis. *Johns Hopkins Hosp Rep*, 10, Nos. 3, 4 and 5, 1902.
13. Fraumeni, J.F., and Li, F.: Hodgkin's disease in childhood; an epidemiologic study. *J Natl Cancer Inst, 42*:681, 1969.
14. Newell, G.R., Cole, S., Miettinen, O.S., and MacMahon, B.: Age differences in the histology of Hodgkin's disease. *J Natl Cancer Inst, 45*: 311, 1970.
15. Lukes, R.J., Tindle, B., and Parker, J.W.: Reed-Sternberg-like cells in infectious mononucleosis. *Lancet, 2*:1003, 1969.
16. Lukes, R.J., and Butler, J.: The pathology and nomenclature of Hodgkin's disease. *Cancer Res, 26*:1063, 1966.
17. Lukes, R., Craver, L.F., Hall, T. *et al.*: Report of the nomenclature committee. *Cancer Res, 26*:1311, 1966.
18. Keller, A., Kaplan, H.S., Lukes, J., and Rappaport, H.: Correlation of histopathology with other prognostic indicators in Hodgkin's disease. *Cancer, 22*:487, 1968.
19. Butler, J.: Hodgkin's disease in children. In *Neoplasia in Childhood.* Chicago, Year Book Medical Publishers, 1969, p. 267.
20. Rappaport, H., and Strum, S.B.: Vascular invasion in Hodgkin's disease; its incidence and relationship to the spread of the disease. *Cancer, 25*:1302, 1970.
21. Strum, S.: Vascular invasion; relationship to histologic type and prognosis. *Symposium on Hodgkin's Disease.* St. Louis, 1971.
22. D'Angio, G., Mitus, A., and Evans, A.E.: The superior mediastinal syndrome in children with cancer. *Am J Roentgenal, 93*:537, 1965.

23. Mullins, G., Flynn, J., El-Mahdi, A.M. *et al.*: Malignant lymphoma of the spinal epidural space. *Ann Intern Med, 74:*416-423, 1971.
24. Silverberg, I.J., and Jacobs, E.: Treatment of spinal cord compression in Hodgkin's disease. *Cancer, 27:*308, 1971.
25. Sternlier, P., Mills, M., and Bollamy, J.: Hodgkin's disease of the small bowel. *Am J Med, 31:*304, 1961.
26. Conger, J.D., Castell, D., and Jacoby, W.: Hodgkin's disease of the jejunum; perforation during radiation therapy. *Arch Intern Med, 121:* 174, 1968.
27. Bagley, C.M., Roth, J., Thomas, L., and DeVita, V.: Clinicopathologic correlations of liver biopsies in Hodgkin's disease. *Clin Res, 19:*489, 1971.
28. Steele, T.H., Presant, C.A., and Serpick, A.: A reversible concentrating defect in predominantly unilateral renal Hodgkin's disease. *Am J Med, 48:*375, 1970.
29. Piessens, W.F., and Zeicher, M.: Hodgkin's disease causing a reversible nephrotic syndrome by compression of the inferior vena cava. *Cancer, 25:*880, 1970.
30. Aach, R., and Kissane, J.: Hodgkin's disease complicated by thrombocytopenia and nephrotic syndrome (CPC). *Am J Med, 51:*109, 1971.
31. Plager, J., and Stutzman, L.: Acute nephrotic syndrome as a manifestation of active Hodgkin's disease. *Am J Med, 50:*56, 1971.
32. Harbert, J.C., and Ashburn, W.: Radiostrontium bone scanning in Hodgkin's disease. *Cancer, 22:*58, 1968.
33. Horan, F.T.: Bone involvement in Hodgkin's disease; a survey of 201 cases. *Br J Surg, 56:*277, 1969.
34. Benninghoff, D.J., Medina, A., Alexander, L., and Camiel, M.: The mode of spread of Hodgkin's disease to the skin. *Cancer, 26:*1135, 1970.
35. Sokal, J., and Shimaoka, K.: Pyrogen in the urine of febrile patients with Hodgkin's disease. *Nature (Lond), 215:*1183, 1967.
36. James, A.: Hodgkin's disease with and without alcohol-induced pain. *Q J Med, 29:*47, 1960.
37. Kyle, R., Kiely, J.M., and Stickney, J.: Acquired hemolytic anemia in chronic lymphocytic leukemia and in the lymphomas. *Arch Intern Med, 104:*61, 1959.
38. Jaffe, N., and Bishop, Y.: The serum iron level, hematocrit, sedimentation rate, and leukocyte alkaline phosphatase level in pediatric patients with Hodgkin's disease. *Cancer, 26:*332, 1970.
39. Webb, D.I., Ubogy, G., and Silver, R.T.: Importance of bone marrow biopsy in the clinical staging of Hodgkin's disease. *Cancer, 26:*313, 1970.
40. Aisenberg, A.C., Kaplan, M., Rieder, S., and Goldman, J.M.: Serum alka-

line phosphatase at the onset of Hodgkin's disease. *Cancer, 26:*318, 1970.
41. Mitus, W.J.: Personal communication, 1971.
42. Kelly, W., Good, R.A., and Varco, R.L.: Anergy and skin homograft survival in Hodgkin's disease. *Surg Gynec Obstet, 107:*565, 1958.
43. Brown, R.S., Haynes, H.A., Foley, H. *et al.*: Hodgkin's disease; immunologic, clinical, and histologic features of 50 untreated patients. *Ann Intern Med, 67:*291, 1967.
44. Jackson, S.M., Garrett, J., and Craig, A.: Lymphocyte transformation during the clinical course of Hodgkin's disease. *Cancer, 25:*843, 1970.
45. Han, T., and Sokal, J.: Lymphocyte response to phytohemagglutinin in Hodgkin's disease. *Am J Med, 48:*728, 1970.
46. Pidot, A., and McIntyre, O.R.: *In vitro* leukocyte interferon production as a test of immune function in patients with Hodgkin's disease. *Clin Res, 19:*495, 1971.
47. Sokal, J.E., and Aungst, C.: Response to BCG vaccination and survival in advanced Hodgkin's disease. *Cancer, 24:*128, 1969.
48. Moore, D., Migliore, P.J., Shullenberger, C.C., and Alexanian, R.: Monoclonal macroglobulinemia in malignant lymphoma. *Ann Intern Med, 72:*43-47, 1970.
49. Order, S., Porter, M., and Hellman, S.: Hodgkin's disease; evidence for a tumor--associated antigen. *N Engl J Med, 285:*471, 1971.
50. Rosenberg, S.: Report of the committee on the staging of Hodgkin's disease. *Cancer Res, 26:*1310, 1966.
51. Rosenberg, S.A.: The clinical evaluation and staging of patients with malignant lymphoma. In Ultmann, J.E., Griem, M.L., Kirsten, W.H., and Wissler, R.W. (Eds.): *Current Concepts in the Management of Lymphoma and Leukemia. Recent Results in Cancer Research.* New York, Springer-Verlag, 1971.
52. Kaplan, H.: Progress and perspectives in staging. *Symposium on Hodgkin's Disease.* St. Louis, 1971.
53. Ultmann, J.E.: Clinical features and diagnosis of Hodgkin's disease. *Cancer, 19:*297, 1966.
54. Grossman, H., Winchester, P., Bragg, D. *et al.*: Roentgenographic changes in childhood Hodgkin's disease. *Am J Roentgenol, 108:*354, 1970.
55. Lee, B.J., Nelson, J.H., and Schwarz, G.: Evaluation of lymphangiography, inferior vena cavography and intravenous pyelography in the clinical staging and management of Hodgkin's disease. *N Engl J Med, 271:*327, 1964.
56. Ultmann, J.E.: Current status; the management of lymphomas. *Semin Hematol, 7:*441, 1970.
57. Kadin, M.E., Glatstein, E., and Dorfman, R.: Clinicopathologic studies

of 117 untreated patients subjected to laparotomy for the staging of Hodgkin's disease. *Cancer, 27*:1277, 1971.

58. Lowenbraun, S., Ramsey, H., Sutherland, J., and Serpick, A.: Diagnostic laparotomy and splenectomy for staging Hodgkin's disease. *Ann Intern Med, 72*:655-663, 1970.
59. Brunk, S., Gulesserian, H.P., Hass, A., and Givler, R.: Exploratory laparotomy and splenectomy in staging lymphomas. *Clin Res, 18*:470, 1970.
60. Glatstein, E., Guernsey, J., Rosenberg, S., and Kaplan, H.: The value of laparotomy and splenectomy in the staging of Hodgkin's disease. *Cancer, 24*:709, 1969.
61. Lokich, J., and Moloney, W.: Staging Hodgkin's disease; a critical appraisal of laparotomy. *Clin Res, 18*:685, 1970.
62. Johnson, R.: Is staging laparotomy routinely indicated in Hodgkin's disease? *Ann Intern Med, 75*:459-462, 1971.
63. Bouroncle, B.: Sternberg-Reed cells in the peripheral blood of patients with Hodgkin's disease. *Blood, 27*:544, 1966.
64. Lowenbraun, S., Ramsey, H.E., and Serpick, A.: Splenectomy in Hodgkin's disease for splenomegaly, cytopenias and intolerance to myelosuppressive chemotherapy. *Am J Med, 50*:49, 1971.
65. Rosenberg, S., and Kaplan, H.S.: Evidence for orderly progression in the spread of Hodgkin's disease. *Cancer Res, 26*:1225, 1966.
66. Kaplan, H.S.: Evidence for a tumoricidal dose level in the radiotherapy of Hodgkin's disease. *Cancer Res, 26*:1221, 1966.
67. Fuller, L., Jung, B., Shullenberger, C., and Butler, J.: Radiotherapeutic management of localized Hodgkin's disease involving the mediastinum. *Br J Radiol, 40*:913, 1967.
68. Nobler, M.: Curative radiotherapy in the malignant lymphomas. *Cancer, 22*:752, 1968.
69. Prosnitz, L., Hellman, S., Von Essen, C.F., and Kligerman, M.: The clinical course of Hodgkin's disease and other malignant lymphomas treated with radical radiation therapy. *Am J Roentgenol, 105*:618, 1969.
70. Musshoff, K., and Boutis, L.: Therapy results in Hodgkin's disease; Freiburg, 1948–1966. *Cancer, 22*:1100, 1968.
71. Kaplan, H.S.: Prognostic significance of the relapse-free interval after radotherapy in Hodgkin's disease. *Cancer, 22*:1131, 1968.
72. Jenkins, R., Peters, M.V., and Darte, J.: Hodgkin's disease in children. *Am J Roentgenol, 100*:222, 1967.
73. Teillet, F., and Schweisguth, O.: Hodgkin's disease in children. *Clin Pediatr, 8*:698, 1969.
74. Johnson, R.E., Thomas, L., and Chretien, P.: Correlation between clinico-histologic staging and extranodal relapse in Hodgkin's disease. *Cancer, 25*:1071, 1970.

75. Moss, W., and Brand, W.: *Therapeutic Radiology*. St. Louis, C.V. Mosby Company, 1969, p. 219.
76. Stewart, J., Cohn, K., Fajardo, L. *et al.*: Radiation-induced heart disease; a study of twenty-five patients. *Radiology, 89:*302, 1967.
77. Curran, R., and Johnson, R.: Tolerance to chemotherapy after prior irradiation for Hodgkin's disease. *Ann Intern Med, 72:*505-509, 1970.
78. Wintrobe, M., Cartwright, G., Fessas, P. *et al.*: Chemotherapy of leukemia, Hodgkin's disease and related disorders. *Ann Intern Med, 41:* 447, 1954.
79. Selawry, O., Holland, J., and Wolman, I.J.: Effect of vincristine on malignant solid tumors in children. *Cancer Chemother Rep, 52:*497, 1968.
80. Wright, T.L., Hurley, J., Korst, D. *et al.*: Vinblastine in neoplastic disease. *Cancer Res, 23:*169, 1963.
81. Wilson, H.E., and Louis, J.: The response of Hodgkin's disease to treatment with oral vinblastine sulfate. *Ann Intern Med, 67:*303, 1967.
82. Lacher, M.J., and Durant, J.R.: Combined vinblastine and chlorambucil therapy of Hodgkin's disease. *Ann Intern Med, 62:*468, 1965.
83. Jacobs, E.M., Peters, F.C., Luce, J.K. *et al.*: Mechlorethamine and cyclophosphamide in the treatment of Hodgkin's disease and the lymphomas. *JAMA, 203:* 392, 1968.
84. Stolinsky, D.C., Soloman, J., Pugh, R.P. *et al.*: Clinical experience with procarbazine in Hodgkin's disease, reticulum cell sarcoma, and lymphosarcoma. *Cancer, 26:*984, 1970.
85. Young, R., DeVita, V., Serpick, A., and Canellos, G.: Treatment of advanced Hodgkin's disease with BCNU. *N Engl J Med, 285:*475, 1971.
86. Hall, T.C., Choi, O., Abadi, A., and Krant, M.: Highdose corticoid therapy in Hodgkin's disease and other lymphomas. *Ann Intern Med, 66:*1144, 1967.
87. Kiely, J., and Harrison, E.: Long-term remission in Hodgkin's disease after nitrogen mustard therapy. *Cancer, 26:*800, 1970.
88. DeVita, V., Serpick, A., and Carbone, P.: Combination chemotherapy in the treatment of advanced Hodgkin's disease. *Ann Intern Med, 73:* 881, 1970.
89. Brook, J., and Goeka, E.: Comparison of single agent with combination therapy in Hodgkin's disease. *Clin Res, 19:*189, 1971.
90. Lowenbraun, S., DeVita, V.T., and Serpick, A.: Combination chemotherapy with nitrogen mustard, vincristine, procarbazine and prednisone in previously treated patients with Hodgkin's disease. *Blood, 36:* 704, 1970.
91. Amiel, J., Schlienger, M., Langier, A. *et al.*: Treatment of disseminated or generalized Hodgkin's disease (stages III and IV) by combined chemotherapy, occasional splenectomy and supplemental radiotherapy. *Nouv Rev Franc Hemat, 10:*597, 1970.

92. Bull, J.M., deKiewiet, J., Rosenberg, S., and Kaplan, H.: Cyclic chemotherapy (MOPP) combined with extended field radiotherapy for Hodgkin's disease. *Clin Res, 18:*189, 1970.
93. Strum, S.B., and Rappaport, H.: Hodgkin's disease in the first decade of life. *Pediatrics, 46:*748, 1970.
94. Strum, S.B., and Rappaport, H.: The persistence of Hodgkin's disease in long-term survivors. *Am J Med, 51:*222, 1971.
95. Ezdinli, E., Sokal, J., Aungst, C. *et al.*: Myeloid leukemia in Hodgkin's disease; chromosomal abnormalities. *Ann Intern Med, 71:*1097, 1969.
96. Newman, D., Maldonado, J., Harrison, E. *et al.*: Myelomonocytic leukemia in Hodgkin's disease. *Cancer, 25:*128, 1970.
97. Osta, S., Wells, M., Viamonte, M., and Harkness, D.: Hodgkin's disease terminating in acute leukemia. *Cancer, 26:*795, 1970.
98. Steinberg, M., Geary, C.G., and Crosby, W.: Acute granulocytic leukemia complicating Hodgkin's disease. *Arch Intern Med, 125:*496, 1970.

Chapter 5

WILMS' TUMOR

CARL POCHEDLY

RECENT CLINICAL, biochemical and histopathological findings in children with Wilms' tumor have caused this common neoplasm to acquire additional features to distinguish it from other childhood malignancies. Wilms' tumor is unique in its response to chemotherapy,[1,2] in its relationship with certain congenital anomalies, in its benign nature when occurring during the newborn period, and in some of its biochemical manifestations. These new findings relating to tumor biology are added to the classical features of the physical examination, x-ray studies and histopathology which have long been used to diagnose Wilms' tumors and to detect recurrences of tumor postoperatively. It would be useful to review briefly the classical clinical features of Wilms' tumor and to integrate these with the new findings.

CLINICAL FEATURES

There are no symptoms of a Wilms' tumor in its early stages. Accidental discovery of an abdominal mass is the usual factor that causes the child to be brought for study. Pain is not a prominent early symptom, but the age group affected is usually the infantile, runabout age, during which children do not often complain of minor pains and malaise. Pain may be due to local invasion, hemorrhage and necrosis, or due to ureteral occlusion.[3] Spontaneous intraperitoneal rupture of a Wilms' tumor with massive hemorrhage and wide dissemination of tumor cells within the abdomen has been described.[4-7] Such a case can be mistaken for acute appendicitis. Cachexia, asthenia and anemia are later symptoms. A few cases have been observed in which pulmonary metastases gave the earliest clinical signs of illness, consisting of cough and pleural pain.[8]

Fever may be due to protein liberated by the tumor.[9] "Fever of unknown origin" is one of the commonest non-urologic findings when there is advanced disease, along with weakness and weight loss.[3] Many children have disturbances of urination with frequency, dysuria and albuminuria which may be due to secondary infection from obstruction of the urinary tract. Hematuria is uncommon in Wilms' tumor. The classical triad of symptoms of renal tumors in adults—hematuria, pain, mass—is reversed in order of frequency in Wilms' tumor in children: mass, pain, hematuria. With marked growth of the tumor, effects of compression or displacement of intra-abdominal organs or the diaphragm become manifest.[3]

Hypertension has been found in 50 percent of children with Wilms' tumor.[6] The true incidence may be even higher since blood pressures are not routinely measured in small children. In some cases the hypertension has been relieved by nephrectomy but in other cases it has not.[3] The exact cause of hypertension associated with Wilms' tumor is not known. Renal ischemia due to partial occlusion of the blood supply, the Goldblatt kidney or the independent formation and absorption of pressor substances are possible causes.[10] It is difficult to accept this explanation in view of the fact that severe hypertension sometimes occurs following the development of hepatic and pulmonary metastases, without any involvement of the remaining kidney.[10] Yet, even if the hypertension were due to a pressor substance elaborated by the tumor, it may not be present in every case. All Wilms' tumors are not biochemically the same. In one instance of a child with Wilms' tumor with severe hypertension, marked increase of plasma renin was found.[11] With rare exceptions there have been no long-term survivors among children with Wilms' tumor who had severe hypertension preoperatively.[3,6]

The finding of a mass in the flank or the protrusion of one flank in a well-developed and well-nourished child invites suspicion of the presence of a Wilms' tumor. Because this tumor is characteristically "silent," it may become very large before it is clinically recognized. The tumor commonly presents as a relatively smooth, oval, firm mass extending from one of the upper quadrants. The larger tumors readily extend across the midline so that distinction from a neuroblastoma is not possible on that basis alone. Sometimes a little tenderness can be found on pressure. A Wilms' tumor will remain movable as long as the tumor is contained within the capsule of the kidney. After the tumor has invaded the liver, diaphragm and posterior abdominal wall, the mass becomes fixed. Palpation should be done with great caution in order to prevent dissemination of tumor cells. If the tumor develops at the upper pole of the kidney, early detection is difficult. But as such a tumor grows, pressure on neighboring structures may cause obstruction of the inferior vena cava with development of the collateral circulation, ascites and edema of the legs. Pressure upon the intestines may displace them to one side of the abdomen, resulting in constipation or complete intestinal obstruction.[12]

Plain x-ray of the abdomen will show the mass in most cases and about 10 to 15 percent will show calcification.[10] If the tumor is small, neither abdominal x-rays nor pyelograms may reveal any abnormality. Pyelograms vary greatly, depending on the size of the tumor and its location in the kidney. The renal pelvis may be elongated and distorted in shape or displaced medially and inferiorly (Fig. 5-1). The calyces may show abnormal contours.[3,8,12]

Anemia may be present if the tumor has invaded the bone marrow or if hemorrhage has occurred. There may be leukocytosis. *Metastatic* tumor cells may be found in the bone marrow, but tumor cells are rarely found unless there is antecedent or concomitant bone metastasis visible by x-ray. Hematuria develops in 15 to 20 percent of the cases and is due to invasion of the pelvis or ureter. It is a bad prognostic sign. Cytologic study of the urine may reveal malignant cells in cases where the tumor has ruptured into the renal pelvis.[13]

Biochemical Manifestations

The presence of any disseminated cancer often causes biochemical manifestations that may be useful in diagnosis and management, as well as giving insight into biology of the tumor (Table 5-1). When there is hepatic involvement, the liver func-

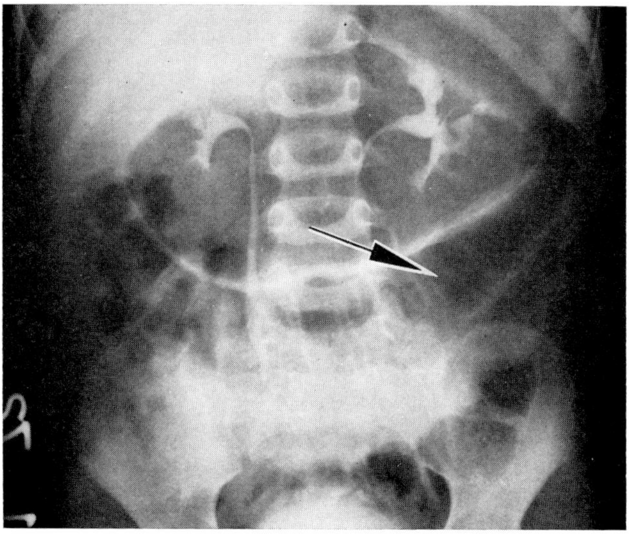

Figure 5-1. IVP of child with Wilms' tumor. The left kidney shows marked distortion of its internal structure, with deviation and splaying of the calyces. There are areas of calcification in the lower portion of the tumor (arrow). (Courtesy of Dr. Richard Rieger.)

TABLE 5-1
CLINICAL AND BIOCHEMICAL ABNORMALITIES THAT MAY BE FOUND IN WILMS' TUMOR

I. *Clinical*
   A. Mass
   B. Pain
   C. Hematuria
   D. Hypertension
   E. Abnormal IVP
   F. Fever
   G. Lung lesions
   H. Hemihypertrophy
   I. Aniridia
   J. Polycythemia

II. *Biochemical*
   A. Elevated SGOT, LDH, alkaline phosphatase
   B. Elevated serum haptoglobin
   C. Elevated plasma renin
   D. Elevated urinary and serum mucopolysaccharides
   E. Elevated urinary of plasma erythropoietin
   F. Elevated blood coagulation factors

tion tests and liver enzymes (SGOT, LDH, alkaline phosphatase) may be abnormal. The lactic acid dehydrogenase (LDH) level is increased with any malignant neoplasm. Liver function tests may be abnormal in patients with extensive replacement of the liver parenchyma by tumor. The average child with Wilms' tumor does not have such extensive dissemination within this organ so that liver function tests may be normal in most patients.[14] With bony metastases the alkaline phosphatase will be increased. Serum proteins show a variety of nonspecific abnormalities including hypoalbuminemia, elevation of alpha- and beta-globulins and either an increase or decrease in the gamma-globulins. The erythrocyte sedimentation rate is increased; the sedimentation rate probably reflects changes in the serum proteins and seems to be more sensitive than the electrophoretic pattern. Hyperuricemia may be present in any disseminated neoplasm.

The serum haptoglobin level is elevated in about half of children with disseminated malignancies. Serum haptoglobin elevation is nonspecific. It is dependent not only on the activity of the malignant disease but also on the type of therapy given.[15,16] Polycythemia which occasionally occurs in Wilms' tumor is accompanied by increased erythropoietin.[17] Further cases of increased erythropoietin have been recorded.[18-20] Persistence of increased levels of erythropoietin in the urine or plasma may be an indication of metastatic disease.[20] Elevated serum and urinary levels of mucopolysaccharide have been demonstrated in children with disseminated Wilms' tumor.[21] Sedimentation velocity studies have revealed an abnormal component in the sera of Wilms' tumor patients. This substance can also be detected by Alcian blue staining after electrophoresis of the sera on cellulose acetate strips and can be precipitated from serum. All of these tests are positive with sera from Wilms' tumor patients. A close similarity between the abnormal serum component and material extracted from the tumor with ethylenediaminetetraacetate is apparent from further studies. Both extracts contain mucopolysaccharide, as revealed by analyses for hexosamines and uronic acids. These findings may be useful for laboratory diagnosis of Wilms' tumor with serum samples.[22]

Many children with disseminated Wilms' tumor show a "hypercoagulable" state, with elevated fibrinogen and a shortened partial thromboplastin time. There may be supernormal levels of factors VIII, IX and XI[23] and increased fibrinolytic activity.[24] It is conceivable that the hypercoagulable state may be a mechanism to counteract the seeding of metastases. Experimental studies in mice showed that administration of an anticoagulant (heparin) increased the incidence of metastases, while giving factors that enhance coagulation (such as epsiloaminocaproic acid) decreased the occurrence of metastases.[25]

Anomalies Associated with Wilms' Tumor

The possibility that Wilms' tumor has prenatal origins is based on the histologic appearance suggesting embryonic maldevelopment, a peak incidence in early childhood, its detection among newborn infants and in the fetus, and its association with congenital malformations. Among the anomalies found to occur excessively in surveys of children with Wilms' tumor are hemihypertrophy[26-30] (Fig. 5-2), aniridia (congenital absence of the iris)[27,31-36] (Fig. 4-3) and genitourinary anomalies. In view of these observations, one might suspect that Wilms' tumor is induced by an agent which is both oncogenic and teratogenic.[37,38]

Patterns of Tumor Growth and Metastasis

Wilms' tumors have the capacity for tremendously rapid growth. They may progress from being undetectable by IVP to a readily palpable abdominal mass in three months.[39] In addition, untreated Wilms' tumors, such as were described one hunderd years ago, often achieved enormous size before the child died.[40] Van der Byl in 1857 described a renal tumor weighing thirty-one pounds in a boy eight years of age.[41]

A Wilms' tumor usually grows to a large size before it is diagnosed. The effect of the tumor on the kidney depends on the site of the tumor. If it arises near the surface it will expand extrarenally and the organ will be displaced rather than distorted, but if it arises near the pelvis it tends to grow down the ureter.[42] Tumors indistinguishable from Wilms' tumor histologically (re-

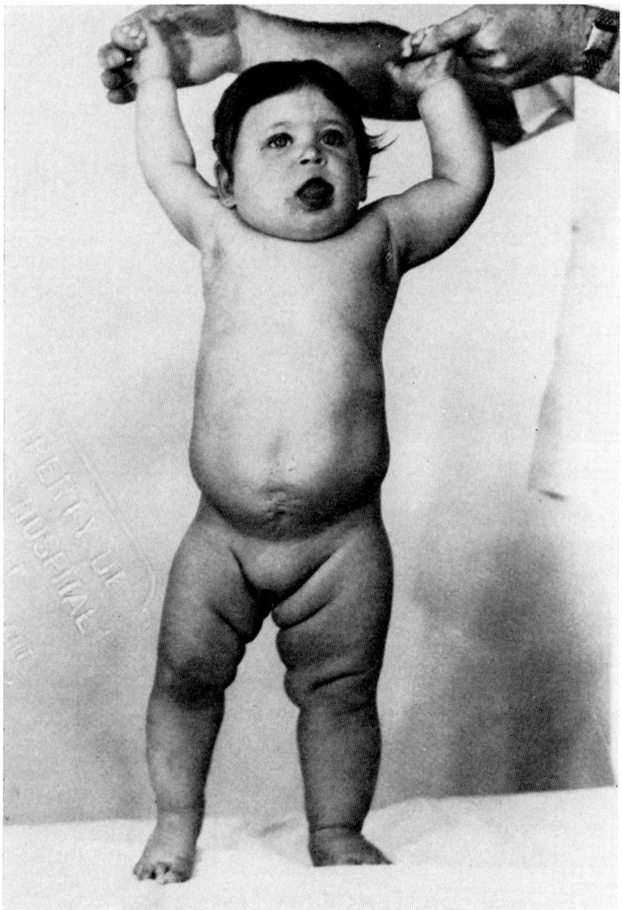

Figure 5-2. A child from whom a Wilms' tumor was removed showing crossed hemihypertrophy. The left extremities and the right side of the face are involved. (Courtesy of Dr. Frank Wilson and the *Journal of Bone and Joint* Surgery.)[26]

troperitoneal embryomas) can rarely arise in retroperitoneal structures quite separate from the kidney. In one case it originated as a separate tumor unattached to the kidney.[43] Usually, however, a Wilms' tumor expands the renal parenchyma and the kidney becomes stretched over the surface of the tumor. The covering of the neoplasm may be very thin and easily torn. When growth

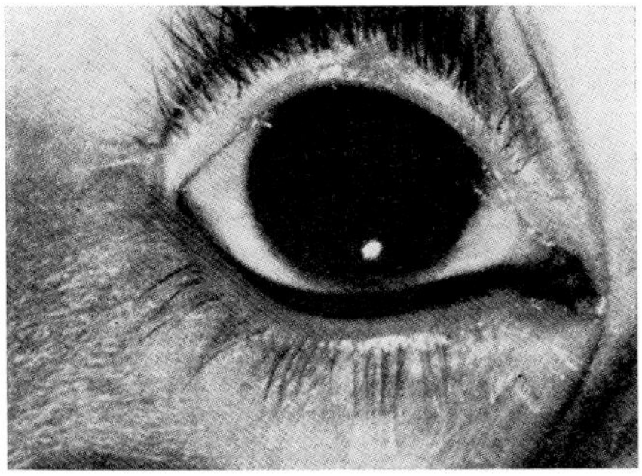

Figure 5-3. Aniridia, absence of the iris, in a child with Wilms' tumor. (Courtesy of Dr. T. Mackintosh and the *British Journal of Ophthalmology, 52*:847, 1968.)[31]

has been very rapid, the tumor is exceedingly vascular and soft, mushy, gelatinous and brain-like in character. Great caution should be taken by the surgeon in removing these soft tumors because of the danger of rupture and tumor dissemination in the peritoneal cavity.

The varied histological picture seen in a Wilms' tumor is in keeping with the concept that it arises from embryonic tissue not definitely committed to one mode of differentiation. The rounded or polygonal hyperchromatic cells with stellate myxomatous tissue are reminiscent of the embryonal rhabdomyosarcoma. Striated muscle fibers may be seen in varying stages of development. This tumor presents varied histologic elements and patterns from case to case and also varies in different parts of the same specimen. However prognosis cannot be correlated with histologic appearance.[3] Unlike neuorblastoma, spontaneous regression of a Wilms' tumor has never been reported.

Wilms' tumors metastasize early, either by direct extension or by way of the bloodstream. The tumors may invade the renal vein and vena cava or spread by way of the lymphatics to the retroperitoneal lymph nodes. Metastases occur most commonly in the lung and next in order of frequency in the liver (Fig. 5-4). Metastases may also occur in the *contralateral kidney* and, rarely, in bone.[3] More common than distant metastases is direct extension from the kidney area which occurs in over 80 percent of cases.

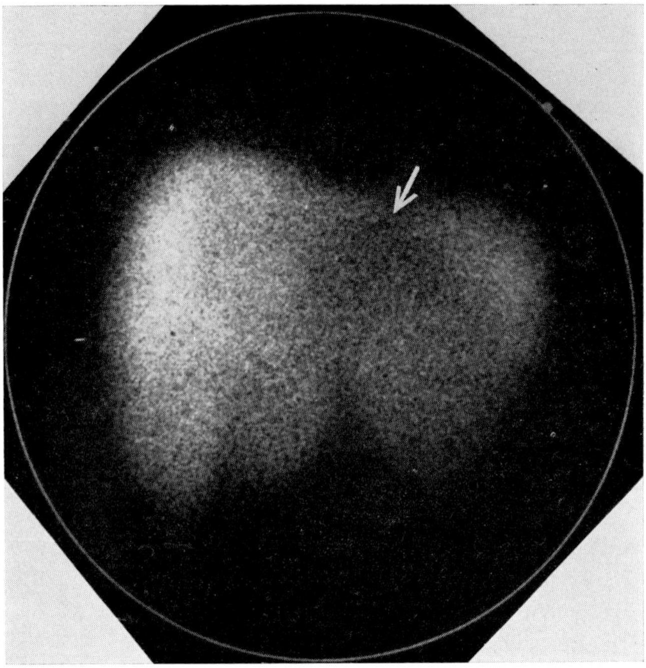

Figure 5-4. Liver and spleen scan using technetium 99m sulfur colloid and and an Anger camera. There is decreased uptake of isotope in the left lobe of the liver (arrow) suggestive of a metastatic lesion. (Courtesy of Dr. S. Goldsmith.)

Local invasion of the perirenal tissues, lymph nodes, liver, diaphragm and posterior abdominal muscles is observed. Local invasion may occur after surgical removal if the tumor escapes from the capsule and seeding of the operative field occurs. Direct invasion of the liver, spleen, intestine and lungs has been reported, and brain metastases may occur. Bone lesions, although rare, have been demonstrated in virtually all bones, including the skull, ilium, scapula, femur (Fig. 5-5) and tibia. Extensions to and involvement of the adrenal gland may cause signs of Addison's disease with pigmentation of the skin.[3] Local invasion of the spine may cause radicular pain, numbness and paraplegia. The epithelial lining of the renal pelvis may rupture and extension may

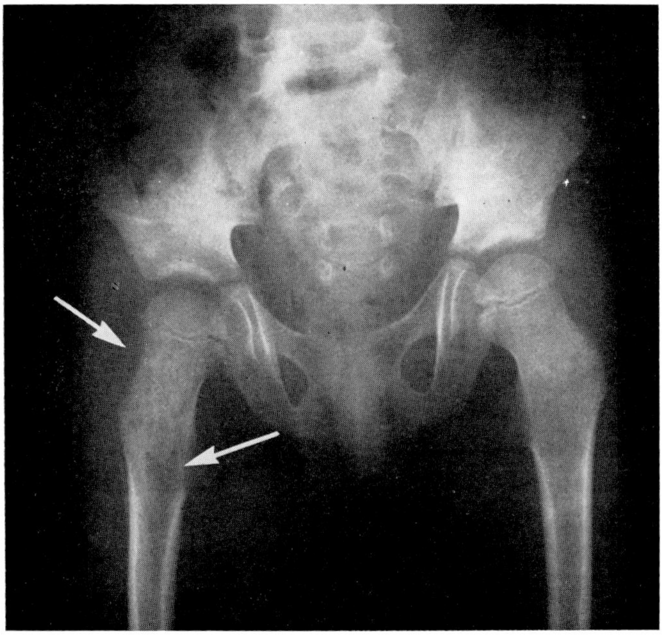

Figure 5-5. Osteolytic bone lesions in the proximal right femur (arrows) of a child with Wilms' tumor.

then occur down the ureter, with "seedling" tumors on the ureteric wall, or even into the bladder.[42,44]

The marked tendency of Wilms' tumors for venous invasion explains the frequency of metastasis to the lung. Because of the extreme tendency of this tumor to invasion of the venous drainage system, a strong rule against excessive palpation of the tumor becomes an important precaution in the preoperative period. Massage of the tumor often causes release of small tumor emboli (microemboli), but occasionally very large tumor emboli are released and give rise to pulmonary embolization. In one case a tumor thrombus filled the entire vena cava; in another case a tumor embolus was dislodged from the renal vein and blocked the atrioventricular orifice.[3] Also, rapid fungating growth may cause the intrarenal tumor to invade the vena cava and extend up as far as the atrium.

Bilateral Wilms' Tumor

Most cases of bilateral Wilms' tumor have been diagnosed at autopsy.[45-50] Since bilateral tumors have been found in a newborn in only one case,[51] their appearance in older children cannot be accepted as positive proof of bilateral independent origin. Involvement of the second kidney may sometimes represent contralateral metastasis. In the past when Wilms' tumors were usually discovered late and often no surgical therapy was given, bilateral involvement was frequently found at autopsy. Since nephrectomy, either alone or in conjunction with radiotherapy, has become the accepted treatment, the proportion of bilateral cases has decreased markedly.[13] The tumor eventually will appear bilaterally in up to 10 percent of cases. Some rare instances suggesting bilateral independent origin are recorded.[52] Still, in any given case of bilateral Wilms' tumor it is difficult to decide whether bilateral tumors are the result of multifocal tumor origin or the result of a single tumor and secondary spread to the other side.

Congenital Wilms' Tumor

From among 309 reported cases of Wilms' tumors occurring in the first year of life, sixty-two were observed in the fetus, premature and full-term infants, and were diagnosed before the third week of life.[53] Of these sixty-two cases with neonatal manifestations of Wilms' tumor, thirty-three were treated surgically and twenty-seven showed apparent cure. None of the stillbirths and none of the older infants who died showed evidence of metastases. On the other hand, in 199 older children (three to twelve months of age) a significant number showed metastases and spread of the tumor. Of the children dying after treatment, as many as 48 percent showed spread.[53] Regional extension or metastasis has not been reported in Wilms' tumors occurring in newborn infants.[2,54-58] For example, one Wilms' tumor occurring in a newborn was so large that it caused dystocia, yet no distant metastases were seen at autopsy.[59] The cause of the lessened degree of malignancy in congenital Wilms' tumor is unknown.

Why do congenital renal tumors, including very large tumors histologically identical with Wilms' tumor, remain localized and curable by simple excision? Similar appearing tumors in older children are metastatic, recur and kill the child in the majority of cases in spite of surgery, x-ray therapy and chemotherapy. It is tempting to postulate some biochemical peculiarity of the internal milieu of the fetus, perhaps endocrine or immunological, which is capable of influencing differentiation of incipient renal tumors toward a benign pattern. Occasionally Wilms' tumors in older children contain areas identical to mesoblastic nephroma. Possibly these are the result of malignant activation of tumors that were formerly mesoblastic nephromas.[60]

Renal tumors present during the first few weeks of life seem to be a distinct entity. They differ from Wilms' tumors occurring in older children in their benign histologic picture and in their inability to metastasize.[61,62] Strictly speaking, the term "congenital Wilms' tumor" may be inaccurate. One can argue that these tumors do not belong to the same group as Wilms' tumor of older children.[62] These benign renal tumors have been called by several names including renal hamartoma, leiomyoma, fibroma, differentiated nephroblastoma, and congenital mesoblastic nephroma.[63] A total of thirty-four such cases have now been reported, some in stillborns.[64-66] All these children have followed a benign course, but some died as a result of surgery or following chemotherapy-induced toxicity. Postoperative x-ray therapy should not be given.[14] Recurrent or metastatic tumors have not been recorded in any of the cases observed so far. The only recommended treatment is surgical removal of the tumor.[67]

Wilms' Tumor in Animals

Wilms' tumor occurs in many domestic animals, including sheep, pigs, dogs, cats, rats, cows, rabbits, parakeets and chickens.[3, 68-73] As is the case in human infants, Wilms' tumors in animals may attain great size but seldom metastasize. Tumors histologically identical with Wilms' tumor may be induced in ovariectomized rats by administration of dimethylbenzanthracene.[74]

Conclusion

Wilms' tumors usually present as a mass, often with pain. Hematuria and hypertension are sometimes seen. Wilms' tumors are occasionally associated with aniridia and hemihypertrophy. This observation suggests that the tumor may be induced by an agent that is not only oncogenic but also teratogenic. The biochemical manifestations of disseminated Wilms' tumor include abnormal liver function tests, elevation of liver enzymes and serum protein abnormalities. In addition, elevation of the serum haptoglobin, increased urinary excretion of mucopolysaccharides, increased plasma renin, increased erythropoietin and the "hypercoagulable" state may be seen in many of these children. Wilms' tumors occurring during the newborn period often show rapid and voluminous local growth but do not metastasize. In addition to their benign behavior, many renal tumors occurring during the newborn period have a benign histological picture. These new findings give broader scope and a more distinctive character to the biological behavior of Wilms' tumor.

DIAGNOSIS AND TREATMENT

The first objectives in managing a child suspected to have a Wilms' tumor is rapid diagnosis and preventing dissemination of the tumor. This tumor must be differentiated from other masses in the flank including neuroblastoma, lymphoma, teratomas, mesenteric cysts, hepatoma, splenomegaly, bezoars, hydronephrosis and polycystic kidneys.

When such a child has been admitted to the hospital, the investigation should proceed with all deliberate speed. The entire work-up from admission to surgery usually can be completed in twenty-four to forty-eight hours. Undue delay in work-up should be avoided, but at the same time, all necessary procedures including blood counts, careful preliminary physical and roentgen examinations, and so forth, should be carried out prior to surgery. The child's bed is signposted to reduce indiscriminate palpation and milking of cancer cells into the circulation. Transillumination of the abdomen may help differentiate a cystic mass.[75] Complete blood count and urinalysis is done. Blood chemical determinations of diagnostic importance include SGOT, BUN, LDH, uric acid and alkaline phosphatase. Bone marrow smears are examined for tumor cells (Fig. 5-6).[76] It is preferable to also

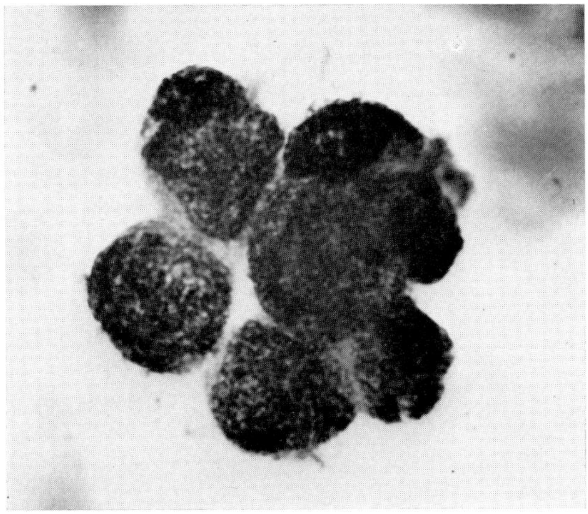

Figure 5-6. Bone marrow smear showing a clump of cells originating from a Wilms' tumor. (Courtesy of Dr. Donald Pinkel and the *Journal of Pediatrics.)* [74]

do a marrow biopsy using the Crosby or Turkell needle.[77] Abdominal x-ray and intravenous pyelogram are done to demarcate the tumor and to assess the status of the opposite kidney. X-ray of the chest and of the skull and long bones are done in search of metastases. Appropriate steps are undertaken to correct any related or unrelated abnormalities, such as electrolyte imbalance, infection or anemia, in anticipation of surgical exploration. Additional studies that may be done include inferior vena cavagram,[78] isotopic scanning of the kidneys and liver,[79] and selective renal angiogram.[80,81] However, abdominal angiography is difficult in small children.[82] Isotopic scan of liver in search of metastases may be done postoperatively. Isotopic scans of the liver are useful preoperatively or immediately postoperatively and before radiation therapy to establish normal baselines. They are very useful in differentiating between postradiation liver damage and metastatic involvement.[14] Even with biopsy, errors in diagnosis may rarely occur, which can prove to be disastrous to the patient. Every diagnostic aid, including selective renal angiogram, in selected cases, should therefore be employed.

Grouping (Staging) the Tumor

Staging is very important as a basis for planning treatment, for estimating prognosis and subsequently, for analysis of survival data. Accurate staging depends on careful observations by the clinician, the radiologist, surgeon and pathologist.[83-87] There are five clinical and anatomical groupings of Wilms' tumors (Table 5-2). In this system the patients are grouped according to clinical findings, x-ray findings and findings at pathology.

TABLE 5-2
GROUPING OF A WILMS' TUMOR*

Group I

Tumor is limited to the kidney and is completely resected. Surface of the renal capsule is intact. Tumor is not ruptured before or during removal and no residual tumor is apparent beyond the margins of resection.

Group II

Tumor extends beyond the kidney but is completely resected. There is local extension of the tumor, with penetration through the renal capsule to the capsular surface (perirenal fat) or beyond, or periaortic lymph nodes are involved. Renal vessels outside the kidney substance, such as the renal vein, contain tumor thrombi, but no residual tumor is apparent beyond margins of resection.

Group III

Residual nonhematogenous tumor is confined to the abdomen. Tumor has been biopsied or ruptured before or during surgery. Implants are on peritoneal surfaces and involved lymph nodes beyond the abdominal periaortic chains. Tumor is not completely resectable because of local infiltration into vital structures.

Group IV

Hematogenous metastases are present in the liver, lung, bone or brain.

Group V

Bilateral renal involvement either initially or subsequently.

*Criteria of National Wilms' Tumor Study Group.[14]

Accurate anatomic grouping of Wilms' tumor is not as easy as it may seem. The surgeon may be unable to dissect out the tumor neatly and intact. It is very difficult to find the anatomical orientation from a mutilated specimen. It may be difficult to decide whether tumor is present in the perirenal fat; whether tumor is invading the normal renal tissue; whether tumor is present in the renal vein or in the regional lymph nodes. Thus, for accurate anatomic grouping, we are dependent upon the success of the surgeon to provide an adequate and anatomically intact specimen, and we are dependent on the pathologist to carefully dissect this specimen and to determine precisely the extent of the tumor and the degree of spread. If we cannot obtain such precise anatomical information, grouping may be inaccurate.

Treatment

One of the important fruits of intensive research of the past twenty years is a more optimistic attitude toward the treatment of children with cancer. Success with new therapy of Wilms' tumor has been an important factor in generating this new optimism. The early studies of Farber and of Gross[88] have special significance in the management of Wilms' tumor and form one of the cornerstones on which the philosophy and principles of caring for childhood cancers in general have been erected.[89] Treatment of Wilms' tumor consists of surgery, chemotherapy and radiotherapy carried out in a combined program and tailored to the specific needs of each child. But early diagnosis of this tumor is still the key to successful treatment.

Surgery, radiotherapy and chemotherapy all have a place in the treatment of Wilms' tumor. Since it has not been possible to cure a large number of cases by one method alone, it is generally agreed that combined treatment is necessary. The therapeutic history of this disease has been one of gradual evolution rather than of controlled clinical trials. Although various authors[5,87,88,90,91] have reported improvement in survival rates over the years, it is often difficult to be certain which alternations in technique have been responsible. It is possible that the better results may be due partly to improved general pediatric and surgical care and not due solely to radical alterations in therapy.[10]

Surgery

The surgeon must take certain precautions to avoid producing hematogenous spread of the tumor and to provide anatomically intact structures for study by the pathologist. The tumor should be handled gently and not squeezed before ligating the renal pedicle to avoid dislodging tumor emboli. Ligation of the pedicle vessels should be done before any manipulation or mobilization of the tumor is attempted. A generous trans abdominal incision is made (Fig. 5-7) so the tumor does not have to be squeezed out through a small opening.[3,92] Regional lymph nodes should be removed at time of surgery both for staging and to prevent recurrence of tumor form local metastases.[1,85,93] If the tumor cannot be completely resected, silver clips should be put in at the outer limits of the tumor to aid the radiation therapist. When the tumor can be completely excised, silver clips are inserted at the periphery, outlining the tumor bed. In some cases radical excision of large infiltrating tumors, with prosthetic replacement of the inferior vena cava, may be curative.[94]

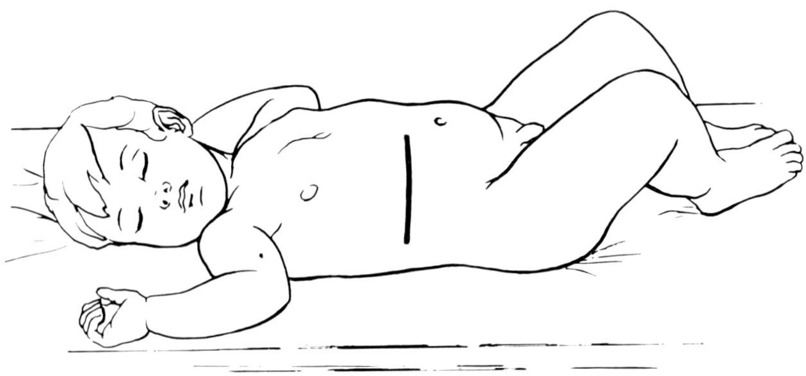

Figure 5-7. Incision for a right-sided Wilms' tumor.[1]

X-ray Therapy

Heimann in 1915 was the first to employ postoperative x-ray therapy in the treatment of Wilms' tumor.[95] X-ray therapy is part of the treatment of all children with Wilms' tumor, except those cases occurring in children less than twelve months of age and which are well encapsulated, stage I.[96] X-ray therapy is initiated shortly after surgery, often on the same day. There is no need to await wound healing since children tolerate radiation therapy very well in the postoperative period.[96]

X-ray therapy is given to the tumor bed and is intended to render nonviable all cells that may have escaped locally from the excised tumor. The size of the field on the body which is radiated depends upon how widely disseminated the tumor appeared to be at the time of surgery and at dissection by the pathologist. If no distant spread is noted or suspected, the child is usually irradiated over a port which encompasses the tumor bed as delineated by the surgeon or encompassing the entire volume in contact with the periphery of the tumor as demonstrated on the preoperative excretory urogram. A quadralateral field similar to that shown in Figure 5-8 is usually employed, depending on the size of the tumor initially. When the portal goes to the dome of the diaphragm, the corner is often "cut" to follow the contour of the diaphragm laterally.[14] The port includes the entire upper and lower quadrants of the abdomen (avoiding the liver or spleen) on the side from which the tumor had been removed and extends across the midline far enough to give effective radiation to the entire para-aortic lymph node chain. Opposing anterior and posterior fields are employed. The field extends across the midline to include the entire width of vertebral epiphyseal plates, but scrupulously avoiding the opposite kidney (Fig. 5-8). Unilateral radiation of the spine of a child may result in growth retardation of the side irradiated, resulting in scoliosis if the child survives long enough.[97] After prolonged follow-up of one series of thirty-four children given x-ray therapy following removal of abdominal tumors, more than one-third showed radiographic changes in the vertebra.[98] These changes included transverse lines in the vertebral bodies and retardation of the axial growth producing scoliosis. Similar changes were observed by others.[99,100] Exostoses of the ribs and ilia have been noted when 2000 rads were given.[12]

The recommended dose of x-ray therapy in a child from two to five years of age with Wilms' tumor is 3,000 rads delivered to the midplane of the tumor bed at the rate of 1,000 rads/week. This dose may be varied according to age. Infants may receive 1,800 rads, while children over five years of age receive 4,000 rads or more.[96] There is a synergistic effect between dactinomycin and x-ray therapy, so that acute skin reactions occasionally occur when

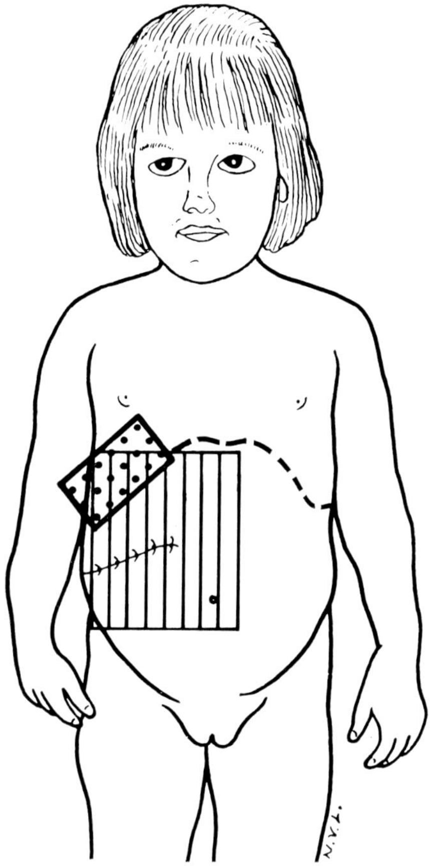

Figure 5-8. Outline of portal for x-ray therapy after removal of a right-sided Wilms' tumor.[14] The portal includes the entire width of the vertebrae and avoids the liver and opposite kidney, as deliniated by previous abdominal x-rays and intravenous pyelogram. A similar portal is drawn on the back. (Drawing by Nicholas Levycky.)

dactinomycin is given concomitantly with or follows the administration of radiation therapy.

Although postoperative x-ray therapy has been used in Wilms' tumor for more than fifty years, it has never been subjected to the test of rigid statistical analysis. However, despite the fact that no randomized prospective study has clearly established the value of postoperative irradiation, few clinicians would deny its use. The only exception is infants under twelve months of age from whom an encapsulated Wilms' tumor was completely excised or from whom a mesoblastic nephroma was removed. The National Wilms' Tumor Study Group has initiated a study in which x-ray therapy is withheld in half of the patients—that is, only dactinomycin is given to this group, to see whether the tumor recurs more frequently in the non-irradiated group. In such a trial, recurrence of tumor in the flank is the index of success or failure. But, obviously, irradiating or not irradiating will have very little influence on the appearance of pulmonary metastases.[14] The results of the National Wilms' tumor study will soon be available. In the meantime we continue to give x-ray therapy to the tumor-free tumor bed, even though theoretically only chemotherapy would need to be given to destroy the micrometastases.

Preoperative x-ray therapy has been advocated and is frequently used, though its value is highly debatable. It is agreed that irradiation of a Wilms' tumor often will result in prompt and considerable reduction in size by causing cytolysis in the tumor. But routine preoperative radiotherapy is not advocated, mainly because an accurate preoperative diagnosis of Wilms' tumor cannot always be made on the basis of physical examination and x-ray examination alone. Preoperative radiotherapy may lead to inordinate delay of surgical intervention in those cases that prove "radioresistant." Also, the tumor may metastasize during the period of x-ray therapy as a result of additional handling of the child and from x-ray–induced hyperemia. There is no proof for the assertion that radiation damages the cells that do escape to the extent that they cannot propagate.[3] However, when the surgeon is confronted with a truly huge tumor in a small baby and the experienced team necessary to bring off the surgical *tour de force* required is not available, he may attempt to reduce the tumor size by preoperative radiotherapy. However prior biopsy through a small incision is advisable.

An alternative that may prove to be better than preoperative x-ray therapy is the preoperative administration of vincristine. Preoperative vincristine has been successful in producing shrinkage and is a method to be preferred to radiation therapy. The reasons are that a dose or two of vincristine is relatively inocuous compared to the postradiation effects of a thousand rads should the preoperative diagnosis be in error and the lesion encountered be benign. Parenthetically, it might be said that the two conditions most commonly mistaken for Wilms' tumor preoperatively are multicystic kidney and neuroblastoma. Vincristine is advantageous in the latter instance because it is an effective agent in the treatment of neuroblastoma as well as for Wilms' tumor; the same cannot be said for actinomycin D. It is for these several reasons then that one would prefer to pretreat these children, thought to be inoperable, with vincristine.[14]

Chemotherapy

In the early 1950's nitrogen mustard was tried in treatment of metastic Wilms' tumor, with little apparent benefit. Since 1955, Farber has pioneered in the use of dactinomycin (also called actinomycin D and Cosmegen®) in the chemotherapy of Wilms' tumor, with or without metastases.[101] This drug has been shown, after extensive trial, to be of considerable benefit to children with Wilms' tumor.[87,91,102,103]

As with all antineoplastic agents, dactinomycin (Fig. 5-9) is a toxic drug, and very careful and frequent observations of the patient for adverse reactions are necessary. A variety of abnormalities of renal, hepatic and bone marrow function have been reported in patients receiving dactinomycin. However, except in instances of bone marrow depression, a causal relationship has not been established. It is advisable to make frequent checks of renal, hepatic and bone marrow function. Toxic effects, excepting nausea and vomiting, usually do not become apparent until two to four days after a course of therapy is stopped and may not be maximal before one to two weeks have elapsed. Usually they are reversible on discontinuance of the drug. Malaise, fever, myalgia, ulcerative stomatitis and pharyngitis may occur. Nausea and vomiting, which occur early during the first few hours after administration, may be alleviated by giving anti-emetics (Tigan® or Thorazine®) . Anemia, leukopenia or pancytopenia may occur.

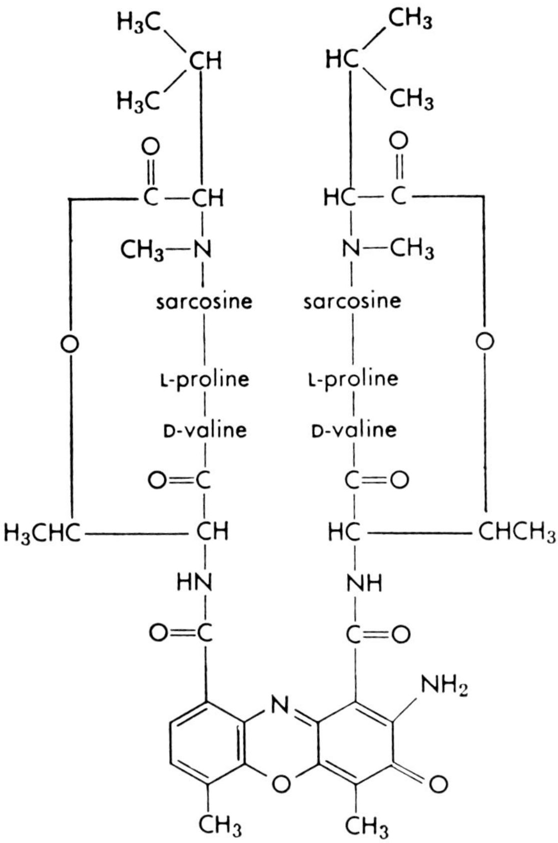

Actinomycin D

Figure 5-9. Molecule of dactinomycin.

While the drug is being given, white blood cell counts should be done daily and platelet counts every three days to detect severe hematopoietic depression. If the white blood cell count falls below $2000/mm^3$ or if the platelet count falls below $100{,}000/mm^3$ the drug should be withheld until recovery occurs. Alopecia, skin eruptions, acne, flare-up of erythema or increased pigmentation of previously irradiated skin is seen. But when properly administered, dactinomycin is usually well tolerated and seldom causes serious complications.

Dactinomycin is a cytotoxic agent. It acts by binding the guanine moiety of deoxyribonucleic acid and thereby prevents the formation of the enzyme, ribonucleic acid polymerase. As a result, synthesis of ribonucleic acid and protein are suppressed and cellular damage occurs.[103] Dactinomycin is the principal component of the mixture of actinomycins produced by *Streptomyces parvullus.* The antibiotic streptomycin is also produced by this group of microorganisms. However, dactinomycin is too toxic to be used in treatment of infectious disease. Because the actinomycins are selectively cytotoxic, they have an antineoplastic effect. This has been demonstrated in experimental animals with various types of tumor implant as well as in human cancers.

The aim of chemotherapy is to achieve maximal kill of tumor cells in children with Wilms' tumor, in order to increase the duration of survival time and to prevent the occurrence of metastasis. Chemotherapy theoretically is more effective than x-ray therapy in preventing or eradicating disseminated metastases. Radiation therapy of the flank cannot be expected to decrease the incidence of remote metastases. Metastases originate as dislodged clusters of tumor cells and are transported in the bloodstream. With the antineoplastic agent present in the blood, the dislodged tumor cells are destroyed before solid implantation and further growth can take place.

What precautions should be observed in administering dactinomycin? This is a very caustic cytotoxic drug and when deposited outside the blood vessels causes acute and necrotizing tissue reactions (Fig. 5-10) . With a uncooperative child, the drug should be carefully administered through a rapidly running, intravenous infusion. Following injection, at least 20 ml of clear solution should be allowed to run into the patient in order to flush the dactinomycin from the infusion tube and needle prior to withdrawing the needle. If this flushing is not done, the amount of dactinomycin remaining in the needle may escape into the subcutaneous tissues when the needle is being withdrawn and result in severe local pain for several days and possibly a slough. In cooperative children with good veins, a plastic infusion set alone may be used for the injection by a skilled operator. The

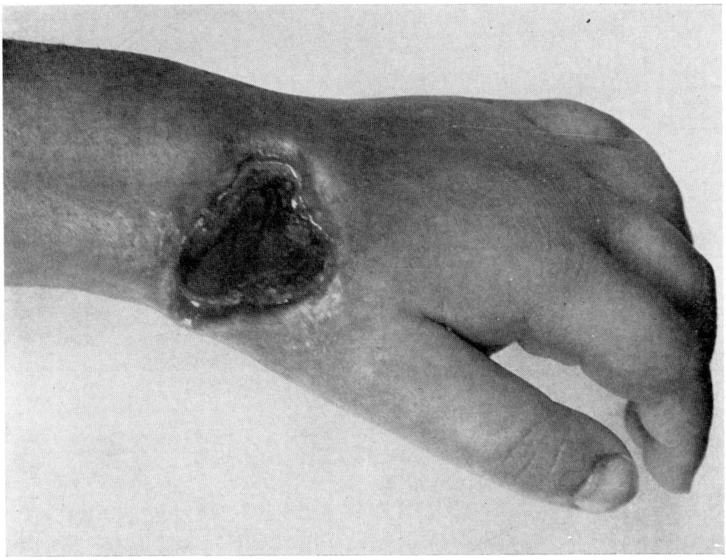

Figure 5-10. Wrist of a child two weeks following extravasation of a minute amount of dactinomycin during injection.

dose of this drug usually given is 0.075 mg/kg, total dose divided into five daily doses. Thus, 15 mg/kg/day is given for five days. These courses should be given intermittently for one to two years. According to the chemotherapy protocol of the National Wilms' Tumor Study Group, the courses of dactinomycin are initiated (a) within twenty-four hours of surgery, (b) at six weeks after surgery, (c) at three months after surgery, (d) at six months, (e) at nine months, (f) at twelve months and (g) at fifteen months after surgery.[14] Other workers give dactinomycin at a larger dose, 0.025 mg/kg (0.6 mg/m^2) and administer the doses every other day for four doses, with courses repeated every six weeks for twelve to eighteen months.[103]

How does the stage of the tumor in a child affect the treatment that should be given? If the tumor is group I and if the child is less than eighteen months old, the patient should be treated with dactinomycin starting immediately postoperatively, then at six weeks, at three months, six months, nine months, twelve months and fifteen months. In group II and III, regardless of age, the patient should be treated immediately with dactinomycin and then intermittently thereafter for the ensuing fifteen months.[104,105] Vincristine may also be added to the chemotherapy regimen in children with group II or group III tumors.[14] In addition, x-ray therapy to the renal bed should be given at a dose appropriate to the size and age of the child. If x-ray therapy is given, the orthopedist as well as the pediatrician or family doctor should follow the child at the same time to prevent or to correct any possible deformity of the spine due to unilateral growth retardation.[95] In group IV, whether or not to use surgery depends on the clinical status. Nevertheless, x-ray therapy combined with chemotherapy should be given as indicated.

FOLLOW-UP

After surgery and after full courses of x-ray therapy and chemotherapy have been given, what follow-up care should the child with Wilms' tumor have? A week after a course of chemotherapy a blood count should be done to detect any delayed depression of the bone marrow. Chest x-ray is done in search of pulmonary metastasis and urinalysis is done to detect any abnormality in the remaining kidney. These examinations should be done monthly for three months after the completion of radiation therapy; then they can be spaced so that they are done with each course of chemotherapy. After that, once every six months for an additional year or year and a half, then once yearly for life together with films of any area that received radiation therapy would seem to be prudent and not excessive.[14] The child's rate of growth and general vitality should be followed to detect any early signs that might suggest that the tumor was recurring. Portal hypertension is a rare late complication of aggressive therapy of Wilms' tumor.[106]

Treatment of Unresectable Tumor

A child with clinically unresectable Wilms' tumor with or without obvious metastases should be started on chemotherapy or radiotherapy, or both, as soon as possible. Preoperative use of vincristine has permitted surgical removal of the tumor within twelve to twenty-one days and without the need for preoperative radiotherapy.[107] Surgery should be performed as soon as the tumor is considered resectable. Careful attention should be taken to prevent serious complications such as postoperative ileus, hemorrhage and infection. Once the tumor has been excised and the child has recovered from the surgical trauma, further chemotherapy or radiotherapy, or both, may be given.

Children with inoperable Wilms' tumors and metastases or with bilateral Wilms' tumors pose the most difficult and serious therapeutic problems. However, there is now hope for some of these cases if aggressive therapy is carried out with radiotherapy and particularly with vincristine or dactinomycin.[2,108]

Treatment of Recurring Tumor

If during or following treatment the child develops a mass in the abdomen or otherwise fails to do well, shows weight loss, unexplained pain or anemia, a thorough work-up should be done. This would be similar to the initial work-up. It would include an intravenous pyelogram, chest x-ray, skeletal survey, blood chemistries (BUN, SGOT, alkaline phosphatase, uric acid and LDH) and bone marrow examination. A liver scan is done to look for evidence of metastases. Cytologic examination of sputum, urine, pleural fluid or peritoneal fluid may reveal metastatic tumor cells. Aggressive, unrelenting attempts to eradicate Wilms' tumor by cooperative efforts by the pediatrician or family doctor, surgeon, chemotherapist and radiotherapist are often rewarded by prolonged survival. Metastases to the lung, liver, bone, omentum, peritoneum and lymph nodes have been controlled permanently in many children.

Twenty to 50 percent of children with Wilms' tumor, depending on the age and stage at time of diagnosis, do poorly following the present-day conventional therapy, consisting of surgery, x-ray therapy and dactinomycin. There is obviously much room for improvement. There is also a continuing search for drugs that might be more effective than dactinomycin. Cyclophosphamide has been studied extensively with and without concommitant administration of vincristine.[107,110] Combination therapy with dactinomycin and vincristine may be tried.[14,111]

What therapy may be tried when the tumor regrows after surgery, x-ray therapy and dactinomycin are given? When the tumor recurs in spite of our best initial efforts, the secondary attack should be aggressive. The solitary metastasis may be excised. However, except in certain large centers, surgeons are not wont to spend long hours dissecting out metastases from children with cancer. Repeat x-ray therapy may be given but the chances of success are greatly reduced. Secondary attack with chemotherapy may include vincristine,[108] cyclophosphamide and vincristine in combination,[107] daunamycin, dactinomycin and vincristine in increasing dosage, BCNU (bis-chlorethyl nitrosourea) or adriamycin.

Pulmonary metastases may be treated by x-ray therapy alone or by a combination of x-ray therapy and dactinomycin. Occasionally pulmonary metastases from Wilms' tumors may be so situated that they can be excised. There are several reports of cures following surgical removal of pulmonary metastases.[5,102,112] Surgical removal of pulmonary metastases may be considered only in the following situations: only one or two isolated deposits are found, their neoplastic nature is confirmed by tomography, and the tumors are not adjacent to the mediastinum or do not involve the pleura. Such pulmonary metastases may be removed by simple wedge resections. Bilateral pulmonary irradiation is indicated in these children prior to any attempts at surgical excision; surgical removal should be reserved for those patients who recur after combined x-ray therapy and chemotherapy.[14] Where deposits are multiple, adjacent to the mediastinum, or involve the pleura, radiotherapy alone is the treatment of choice.[112]

Treatment of Bilateral Wilms' Tumor

The presence of bilateral Wilms' tumors, rarely cured in the past,[47] may yield to bilateral nephrectomy and renal transplantation, coupled with adequate chemotherapy and radiotherapy. Chemotherapy and x-ray therapy serve a dual purpose of destroying residual tumor and early metastases as well as suppressing the immunological reaction of the host to the transplanted kidney.[2] DeLorimier reported the cases of three children who had bilateral nephrectomies and cadaver allotransplantation because of bilateral Wilms' tumors. One of these children was well six months later.[50] Other cases of bilateral Wilms' tumor have been successfully treated by renal transplantation[113]; but nephrectomy followed by x-ray therapy to the remaining kidney and chemotherapy may also produce prolonged survival.[114]

Treatment of Congenital Wilms' Tumor

In a newborn infant with Wilms' tumor, nephrectomy should be postponed until the infant's physical condition has improved sufficiently to withstand the trauma of deep anesthesia and a major operation. In a full-term and healthy baby, this usually takes about forty-eight hours. However, in a premature baby it may take several weeks.[2] Because of poor surgical risk, particularly in premature babies, and also because of the benign behavior of Wilms' tumors presenting during the newborn period,[115] surgery should be postponed and chemotherapy or radiotherapy withheld.[2] However, nephrectomy should be performed as soon as the baby can withstand the anesthetic and surgical stress.[57]

The serious toxic effects of dactinomycin peculiar to infants suggests that this drug should be given only to children over the age of six to twelve months.[2,10] At least four cases of sudden death of infants with renal tumors given a postoperative course of dactinomycin have been reported.[13,63,64,67] The relatively benign behavior of renal tumors in infants is not entirely explainable on the basis that many of the tumors may be hamartomas. In renal tumors of infants, including histologically typical Wilms' tumors, no cases with metastases have been reported.[60,67] However, these facts do not give one the right to undertreat or neglect the infant with Wilms' tumor.[14]

PROGNOSIS

Prognosis is best in children who are less than eighteen months old and whose tumor is anatomically classified as group I. All deviations from this carry a progressively more unfavorable outlook for prolonged survival.[116] But there is need for more objective criteria to gauge the prognosis of each individual patient.[116] The concept of "doubling times" as a measure of growth rate of tumors and its use in estimating prognosis in childhood cancers offers an important new insight. Collins[117] hypothesized that the origin of a cancer is from a single cell which divides to become two cells and these divide to become four, eight, etcetera. If the growth rate of the tumor is assumed to be constant, it could be described in terms of its "doubling time," just as radioisotopic decay is defined by its "half-life."

If one accepts the prenatal origin of childhood tumors, then the time of initial clinical recognition would depend on their growth rate. From this hypothesis, it follows that the time of subsequent clinical recognition of their recurrence would also depend on growth rate, assuming that it is characteristic and constant for each individual tumor. Thus, the "period of risk" would be equal to the age of the patient at the time of the original diagnosis plus nine months. Cure is achieved when the child reaches the "safe period"—that is, twice the age of the child at the time of diagnosis plus nine months. For example, consider a child who is one year of age when an abdominal mass is discovered. If a recurrence is to develop from a single cell which has spread or spilled at or prior to the time of treatment, it should appear within the next year and nine months. If the child reaches the age of two years and nine months and remains free of disease, the "safe period" has been attained (Fig. 5-11). However, more than half of children with Wilms' tumors are over three years old so that the period of risk calculated by Collins' method is often four years or more. In practice the two-year survival rate is almost identical with Collins' variable period survival rate.[118,119]

The prognosis in Wilms' tumor is always guarded. Irrespective of the size of the tumors and the histology, predictions regarding the outcome may be erroneous. Thus, extension of tumor beyond the intrarenal site, either by local infiltration or metastasis, is a very unfavorable sign. But nevertheless some cases showing such spread may recover.

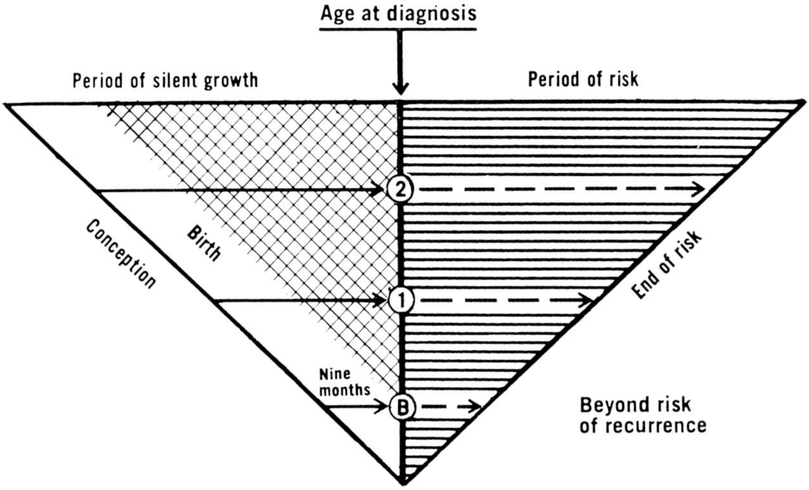

Figure 5-11. Growth of a Wilms' tumor proceeds from left to right. Diagnosis is preceded by a period of silent gorwth that as a minimum is equal to nine month's gestation plus the age of the child at diagnosis. Diagnosis is followed by a period of risk equal to the maximum period of silent growth. If the patient lives beyond the period of risk without recurrence, he should be beyond risk of recurrence. (Adapated from Collins.)[117]

SUMMARY

Current methods used in the diagnosis and treatment of Wilms' tumor are described. The criteria for staging this tumor and clinical significance of these stages are outlined. It is recommended that x-ray therapy be begun within twenty-four to forty-eight hours after surgery and given concomitantly with the first course of dactinomycin. Courses of dactinomycin are then repeated intermittently for the ensuing fifteen months, during which time careful and repeated follow-up examinations are done in search for signs of recurrence of the tumor. Special problems involved when the child has unresectable tumor, recurrent tumor or bilateral tumor are discussed. It is recommended that congenital Wilms' tumor be treated only by simple excision. In evaluating response to therapy and in estimated prognosis, Collins' rule is applicable to very young children; but in older children two-year survival without evidence of recurrence is an adequate criterion for cure.

REFERENCES

1. Pochedly, C.: Current management of the child with Wilms' tumor. *Mod Med, 38:*116-123, January 1970.
2. Uson, A., Wolff, J., and Tretter, P.: Current treatment of Wilms' tumor. *J Urol, 103:*217-221, 1970.
3. Snyder, W., Hastings, T., and Pollock, W.: Wilms' tumor. In Mustard, W. *et al.* (Eds.): *Pediatric Surgery,* (2nd ed.). Chicago, Year Book Medical Publishers, 1969, vol. II, pp. 1024-1937.
4. Tanner, C.: Intraperitoneal rupture of a Wilms' tumor. *Br Med J, 2:* 714, 943.
5. Williams, D.: Nephroblastoma; clinical picture and diagnosis. In Riches, E. (Ed.): *Tumors of the Kidney and Ureter.* Baltimore, Williams & Wilkins Company, 1964, p. 238.
6. Silva-Rosa, M., and Gonzales-Cerna, J.: Wilms' tumor in children; review of 150 cases. *Progr Clin Cancer, 2:*323-337, 1966.
7. Pochedly, C., Waldman, A., and Kenigsberg, K.: Intraperitoneal rupture of a Wilms' tumor with prolonged survival. *JAMA, 216:*334, 1971.
8. Dargeon, H.: *Tumors of Childhood.* New York, Paul B. Hoeber, 1960, pp. 237-246.
9. Brody, S.: Fever associated with neoplastic disease. *Int. Surg, 46:*515-519, 1966.
10. Marsen, H., and Steward, J. (Eds.): Wilms' tumor. In *Tumors in Children.* New York, Springer-Verlag, 1968, pp. 225-249.
11. Mitchell, J., Baxter, T., Blair-West, J., and McCredie, D.: Renin levels in Wilms' tumor; report of a renin secreting tumor. *Arch Dis Child, 45:*376-384, 1970.
12. Deming, C., and Harvard, B.: Nephroblastoma. In Campbell, M., and Harrison, J. (Eds.): *Urology,* (3rd ed.): Philadelphia, W. B. Saunders Company, 1970, vol. II, pp. 913-925.
13. Young, D., and Williams, D.: Malignant renal tumors in infancy and childhood. *Br J Hosp Med, 2:*741-752, 1969.
14. D'Angio, G.: Personal communication, 1972.
15. Owens, J., Smith, R., Podanyi, R., and Martin, J.: Serum haptoglobin in disease. *Clin Sci, 26:*1-6, 1964.
16. Moe, P.: Serum haptoglobin level in disseminated malignant diseases in children. *Acta Pediatr Scand, 59:*381-384, 1970.
17. Thurman, W., Grabstald, H., and Lieberman, P.: Elevation of erythropoietin levels in association with Wilms' tumors. *Arch Intern Med, 117:*280-283, 1966.
18. Murphy, G., Mirand, E., Johnston, G. *et al.*: Erhythropoietin release associated with Wilms' tumor. *Johns Hopkins Med J, 120:*26-32, 1967.
19. Shalet, M., Holder, T., and Walters, T.: Erythropoietin-producing Wilms' tumor. *J Pediatr, 70:*615-617, 1967.

20. Murphy, G., Allen, J., Staubitz, W. *et al.*: Erythropoietin levels in patients with Wilms' tumor. *NY State J Med, 72:*487-489, 1972.
21. Morse, B., and Nussbaum, M.: The detection of hyaluronic acid in the serum and urine of a patient with hephroblastoma. *Am J Med, 42:* 996-1002, 1967.
22. Allerton, S., Beierle, J., Powars, D., and Bavetta, L.: Abnormal extracellular components in Wilms' tumor. *Cancer Res, 30:*679-683, 1970.
23. Miller, S., Sanchez-Avelos, J., Stefanski, T., and Zuckerman, L.: Coagulation disorders in cancer. *Cancer, 20:*1452-1465, 1967.
24. Soong, B., and Miller, S.: Coagulation disorders in cancer. III. Fibrinolysis and inhibitors. *Cancer, 25:*867-874, 1970.
25. Hagmar, B.: Effect of heparin, epsilon-aminocaproic acid and cumarin on tumor growth and spontaneous metastasis formation. *Pathol Eur, 3:*622-630, 1968.
26. Bjorklund, S.: Hemihypertrophy and Wilms' tumor. *Acta Paediatr Scand, 44:*287-292, 1955.
27. Miller, R., F raumeni, J., and Manning, M.: Association of Wilms' tumor with aniridia, hemihypertrophy, and other malformations. *N Engl J Med, 270:*922-927, 1964.
28. Wilson, F., and Orlin, H.: Crossed congenital hemihypertrophy associated with Wilms' tumor. *J Bone Joint Surg [Am], 47-A:*1609-1614, 1965.
29. Fraumeni, J., Geiser, C., and Manning, M.: Wilms' tumor and congenital hemihypertrophy; report of five new cases and review of the literature. *Pediatrics, 40:*886-899, 1967.
30. Boxer, L., and Smith, D.: Wilms' tumor prior to onset of hemihypertrophy. *Am J Dis Child, 120:*564-565, 1970.
31. Fontana, V., Ferrara, A., and Perciaccante, R.: Wilms' tumor and associated anomalies. *Am J Dis Child, 109:*459-461, 1965.
32. DiGeorge, A., and Harley, R.: The association of aniridia, Wilms' tumor, and genital abnormalities. *Arch Opthalmol, 75:*796-798, 1966.
33. Mackintosh, T., Girdwood, T., Parker, D., and Strachan, I.: Aniridia and Wilms' tumor. *Br J Ophthalmol, 52:*846-848, 1968.
34. Flanagan, J., and DiGeorge, A.: Sporadic aniridia and Wilms' tumor. *Am J Ophthalmol, 67:*558-561, 1969.
35. Ghandi, R., Deskmukh, M., and Waingankar, V.: Wilms' tumor with aniridia. *J Pediatr Surg, 5:*571, 1970.
36. Haicken, B., and Miller, D.: Simultaneous occurrence of congenital aniridia, hamartoma, and Wilms' tumor. *J Pediatr, 78:*497-502, 1971.
37. DiPaolo, J., and Kotin, P.: Teratogenesis-oncogenesis; a study of possible relationships. *Arch Pathol, 81:*3-23, 1966.
38. Miller, R.: Relation between cancer and congenital defects in man. *N Engl J Med, 275:*87-90, 1966.
39. Rabinowitz, J., and Bagnasco, F.: Wilms' tumor demonstrating onset and rapid growth. *J Urol, 103:*86-88, 1970.

40. Thomasson, B., and Ravich, M.: Wilms' tumor. *Urol Survey, 11*:83-100, 1961.
41. Reiser, M., and Creevy, C.: Wilms' tumor. *Urol Survey, 2*:413-431, 1952.
42. Watkins, J.: Wilms' tumor with ureteral metastases extending into the bladder. *J Urol, 77*:593-596, 1957.
43. Bhajekar, M., Joseph, M., and Bhat, H.: Unattached Wilms' tumor. *Br J Urol, 36*:187-190, 1964.
44. Ferris, D., and Beare, J.: Wilms' tumor; report of a case with unusual postoperative metastasis. *Proc Staff Meet Mayo Clin, 22*:94-98, 1947.
45. Rickham, P.: Bilateral Wilms' tumor. *Br J Surg, 44*:492-499, 1957.
46. Jagasia, K., Thurman, W., Pickett, E., and Grabstaldt, H.: Bilateral Wilms' tumors in children. *J Pediatr, 65*:371-375, 1964.
47. Bishop, H., and Hope, J.: Bilateral Wilms' tumors. *J Pediatr Surg, 1*: 476-478, 1966.
48. Cochran, W., and Froggatt, P.: Bilateral nephroblastoma in two sisters. *J Urol, 97*:216-220, 1967.
49. Anderson, E., Harper, J., Small, M., and Atwill, W.: Bilateral diffuse Wilms' tumor: A 5-year survival. *J Urol, 99*:707-710, 1968.
50. DeLorimier, A., Belzer, F., Kountz, S., and Kushner, J.: Simultaneous bilateral nephrectomy and renal allotransplantation for bilateral Wilms' tumor. *Surgery, 64*:850-855, 1968.
51. Hou, L., and Holman, R.: Bilateral nephroblastomatosis in a premature infant. *J Pathol Bact, 82*:249-255, 1961.
52. Scott, L.: Bilateral Wilms' tumor. *Br J Surg, 42*:513-516, 1954.
53. Bachmann, K., and Kroll, W.: Wilms' tumor in the first year of life. *D Med Wochenschr, 94*:2598-2602, 1969.
54. Hartenstein, H.: Wilms' tumor in a newborn infant. *J Pediatr, 35*:381-383, 1949.
55. Hoffman, C., Werthammer, S., and Carabia, A.: Congenital Wilms' tumor. *W V Med J, 53*:146-148, 1957.
56. Klapproth, H.: Wilms' tumor; a report of 45 cases and an analysis of 1351 cases reported in the world literature from 1940 to 1958. *J Urol, 81*:633-648, 1959.
57. Sober, I., and Hirsch, M.: Embryoma of the kidney in a newborn infant; case report. *J Urol, 93*:499-551, 1965.
58. Wright, E.: Congenital Wilms' tumor. *Br J Urol, 42*:270-272, 1970.
59. Colepand, L., Welburn, J., and West, O.: Dystocia caused by Wilms' tumor. *Am J Obstet Gynecol, 76*:1329-1333, 1958.
60. Beckwith, J.: Mesenchymal renal neoplasms of infancy. *J Pediatr Surg, 5*:405-406, 1970.
61. Favara, B., Johnson, W., and Ito, J.: Renal tumors in the neonatal period. *Cancer, 22*:845-855, 1968.
62. Richmond, H., and Dougall, A.: Neonatal renal tumors. *J Pediatr Surg, 5*:413-418, 1970.

63. Bolande, R., Brough, A., and Izant, R.: Congenital mesoblastic nephroma of infancy. *Pediatrics, 40*:272-278, 1967.
64. Kay, S., Pratt, C., and Salzberg, A.: Hamartoma (leimyomatous type) of the kidney. *Cancer, 19*:1825, 1826, 1966.
65. Wigger, H.: Fetal hamartoma of kidney. *Am J Clin, Pathol, 51*:323-324, 1969.
66. Waisman, J., and Cooper, P.: Renal neoplasms of the newborn. *J Pediatr Surg, 5*:407-412, 1970.
67. Pochedly, C., Colucci, J., Keingsberg, K., and Loesevita, A.: Hazard of chemotherapy in congenital Wilms' tumor. *J Pediatr, 79*:708-709, 1971.
68. Sullivan, D., and Anderson, W.: Embryonal nephroma in swine. *Am J Vet Res, 20*:324-332, 1959.
69. Moulton, J.: *Tumors in Domestic Animals.* Los Angeles, University of California Press, 1961, pp. 148-151.
70. Feldman, W., and Olson, C.: Neoplastic diseases of the chicken. In Biester, H., and Schwarte, L. (Eds.): *Diseases of Poultry.* Ames, Iowa State University Press, 1965, pp. 913-917.
71. Sandison, A., and Anderson, L.: Tumors of the kidney in cattle, sheep and pigs. *Cancer, 21*:737-742, 1968.
72. Herman, L.: Embryonal nephroma in a parakeet. *Vet Med, 64*:812-813, 1969.
73. Potkay, S., and Garman, R.: Nephroblastoma in a cat; the effects of nephroectomy and occlusion of the caudal vena cava. *J Small Anim Pract, 10*:345-349, 1969.
74. Jasmin, G., and Riopelle, J.: Nephroblastomas induced in ovariectomized rats by 7, 12-dimethylbenzanthracene. *Cancer Res, 30*:321-326, 1970.
75. Mofenson, H., and Greensher, J.: Transillumination of the abdomen in infants. *Am J Dis Child, 115*:428-431, 1968.
76. O'Neill, P., and Pinkel, D.: Wilms' tumor in bone marrow aspirate. *J Pediatr, 72*:396-398, 1968.
77. Pochedly, C.: How to perform bone marrow biopsy in small children. *Clin Pediatr, 9*:226-228, 1970.
78. McCoy, R., Klatte, E., and Rhamy, R.: Use of inferior venacavagraphy in the evaluation of renal neoplasms. *J Urol, 102*:556-559, 1969.
79. Samuels, L.: Combined liver-kidney isotope scans; diagnosis of abdominal masses in children. *JAMA, 204*:630-631, 1968.
80. McDonald, P., and Hiller, H.: Angiography in abdominal tumors in childhood; with particular references to neuroblastoma and Wilms' tumor. *Clin Radiol, 19*:1-18, 1968.
81. Meng, C-H., and Elkin, M.: Angiographic manifestation of Wilms' tumor. *Am J Roentgenol, 105*:95-104, 1969.
82. Nebesar, R., Fleischli, D., Pollard, J., and Griscom, N.: Arteriography in infants and children. *Am J Roentgenol, 106*:81-91, 1969.

83. Garcia, M., Douglass, C., and Schlosser, J.: Classification and prognosis in Wilms' tumor. *Radiology, 80*:574-580, 1963.
84. Beckwith, B., Bishop, H., D'Angio, G., Pickett, L., Sinks, L., Sutow, W., and Wolff, J.: *Minutes of the Wilms' Tumor Integrated Study Group meeting.* May 6, 1968.
85. Fleming, I., and Pinkel, D.: Clinical staging of Wilms' tumor. *J Pediatr, 74*:324-325, 1969.
86. Hilton, C., and Keeling, J.: Staging in relation to treatment of nephroblastoma with actinomycin D. *Br J Urol, 42*:265-269, 1970.
87. Ledlie, E., Mynors, L., Draper, G., and Gorbach, P.: Natural history and treatment of Wilms' tumor; an analysis of 335 cases occurring in England and Wales 1962–1966. *Br Med J, 4*:195-200, 1970.
88. Gross, R., and Neuhauser, E.: Treatment of mixed tumors of the kidney in childhood. *Pediatrics, 6*:843-852, 1950.
89. Rubin, P., Prevention of metastases in Wilms' tumor. *JAMA, 204*:989-990, 1968.
90. Lattimer, J., Melicow, M., and Uson, A.: Wilms' tumor; prognosis more favorable in infants under one year of age. *JAMA, 171*:2163-2168, 1959.
91. Howard, R.: Antinomycin D in Wilms' tumor; treatment of lung metastases. *Arch Dis Child, 40*:200-202, 1965.
92. Martin, L.: Surgical management of solid tumors in childhood. *Am J Roentgenol, 105*:105-109, 1969.
93. Martin, L., and Reyes, P.: An evaluation of 10 years' experience with retroperitoneal lymph node dissection for Wilms' tumor. *J Pediatr Surg, 4*:683-687, 1969.
94. Sarti, L.: Total prosthetic transplantation of the inferior vena cava, with venous restoration of the one remaining kidney on the graft, successfully performed on a child with Wilms' tumor. *Surgery, 67*:851-855, 1970.
95. Whitmore, W.: Nephroblastoma. In Pack, G., and Ariel, I. (Eds.): *Treatment of Cancer and Allied Diseases.* Vol. VII: *Tumors of the Male Genitalia and the Urinary System.* New York, Hoeber Medical Books, 1962, pp. 281-294.
96. D'Angio, G.: Radiation therapy in Wilms' tumor. *JAMA, 204*:987-988, 1968.
97. Rubin, P., Duthie, R., and Young, L.: Significance of scoliosis in post-irradiated Wilms' tumor and neuroblastoma. *Radiology, 79*:539-559, 1962.
98. Neuhauser, E., Wittenborg, M., Berman, C., and Cohen, J.: Irradiation effects of roentgen therapy on the growing spine. *Radiology, 59*:637-650, 1952.
99. Vaeth, J., Levitt, S., Jones, M., and Holtfreter, C.: Effects of radiation therapy in survivors of Wilms' tumor. *Radiology, 79*:560-567, 1962.

100. Schneider, B., Sagerman, R., Wolff, J., and Santulli, T.: Wilms' tumor; the evolution of a treatment program. *Am J Roentgenol, 108*:92-97, 1970.
101. Farber, S.: Chemotherapy in the treatment of leukemia and Wilms' tumor. *JAMA, 198*:826-836, 1966.
102. Fernbach, D., and Martyn, D.: Role of dactinomycin in the improved survival of children with Wilms' tumor. *JAMA, 195*:1005-1009, 1966.
103. Burgert, E., and Glidewell, O.: Dactinomycin in Wilms' tumor. *JAMA, 199*:464-468, 1967.
104. James, D., Hustu, O., Wrenn, E., and Johnson, W.: Childhood malignant tumors; concurrent chemotherapy with dactinomycin and vincristine sulfate. *JAMA, 197*:1043-1045, 1966.
105. Wolff, J., Krivit, W., Newton, W., and D'Angio, G.: Single versus multiple dose dactinomycin therapy of Wilms' tumor. *N Engl J Med, 279*:290-294, 1968.
106. Roback, S., Nesbit, M., Sharp, H. *et al.*: Portal hypertension following surgery, x-radiation, and actinomycin D therapy in nephroblastoma. *J Pediatr, 78*:1031-1033, 1971.
107. Sullivan, M., Sutow, W., Cangir, A., and Taylor, G.: Vincristine sulfate in management of Wilms' tumor. *JAMA, 202*:381-382, 1967.
108. Vietti, T., Sullivan, M., Haggard, M. *et al.*: Vincristine sulfate and radiation therapy in metastatic Wilms' tumor. *Cancer, 25*:12-20, 1970.
109. Hajdu, S.: Exfoliative cytology of primary and metastatic Wilms' tumors. *Acta Cytol (Baltimore), 15*:339-342, 1971.
110. Sutow, W.: Effective chemotherapy in children with Wilms' tumor. *Southern Med J, 60*:254-256, 1967.
111. Sukarachana, K., and Kriesewetter, W.: Wilms' tumor, factors influencing long term survival. *J Pediatr, 69*:747-752, 1966.
112. Martin, J., and Rickham, P.: Pulmonary metastases in Wilms' tumor; treatment and prognosis. *Arch Dis Child, 45*:805-807, 1970.
113. Potter, D., Belzer, F., Rames, L. *et al.*: The treatment of chronic uremia in childhood. I. Transplantation. *Pediatrics, 45*:432-443, 1970.
114. Leen, R., and Williams, I.: Bilateral Wilms' tumor; seven personal cases with observations. *Cancer, 28*:802-806, 1971.
115. Bolande, R.: Benignity of neonatal tumors and concept of cancer repression in early life. *Am J Dis Child, 122*:12-14, 1971.
116. Rubin, P.: Cure and growth rate in childhood tumors. *JAMA, 205*:163-166, 1968.
117. Collins, V.: The treatment of Wilms' tumor. *Cancer, 11*:89-94, 1958.
118. Platt, B., and Linden, G.: Wilms' tumor; a comparison of two criteria for survival. *Cancer, 17*:1573-1578, 1964.
119. Pochedly, C.: Wilms' tumor. *NY State J Med, 71*:1089-1094; 1205-1210; 1526-1528; 1971.

Chapter 6

NEUROBLASTOMA

JERRY Z. FINKLESTEIN AND GERALD S. GILCHRIST

NEUROBLASTOMA is a malignant neoplasm arising from embryonic sympathetic neuroblasts and may originate from the adrenal gland or sympathetic ganglia. With few exceptions it is a tumor of childhood and accounts for 8 percent of deaths from cancer in children. In children it ranks third in frequency to leukemia and central nervous system tumors.[1] Nevertheless, it is a rare condition and the yearly incidence ranges between five and ten new cases per million children under fifteen years of age.[2] Of 1,191 cases located in the United States and Canada between the years 1961 and 1965, 30 percent occurred in the first year of life; proportionate frequency by age group then declined exponentially. In nineteen cases the diagnosis was made at birth and nine more on the second or third day of life.[2]

An increase in diagnosis of neuroblastoma has been reported during the summer months.[3] A seasonal pattern was also documented by Lee,[4] who found an excess of summer deaths from neuroblastoma among children in England and Wales but this could not be confirmed in a mortality study three times larger in the United States.[5] Miller[5] found a slight male preponderance of neuroblastoma deaths, particularly in the younger age groups. Studies on a kindred with multiple congenital disorders including neuroblastomas in four siblings suggested that there may be a hereditary influence.[6] Review of twenty-six cases of neuroblastoma revealed a variety of developmental defects[7]; however, there is no

Note: The authors wish to thank Drs. R. Hittle and R. Lachman of the Departments of Radiology of Childrens Hospital of Los Angeles and Harbor General Hospital respectively for providing and reviewing the x-rays used in the chapter. This study was supported in part by U.S.P.H.S. Grant CA-02649 from the National Cancer Institute.

evidence of familial aggregation of neuroblastoma or of a specific pattern of associated developmental defects. Thus, it is proposed that neuroblastoma is a sporadic postzygotic disorder. Cytogenic studies of neuroblastoma have revealed various abnormal karyotypes but no uniform pattern has been found.[8-10]

PATHOPHYSIOLOGICAL CONSIDERATIONS

There is great variation in the histopathological picture from tumor to tumor and within the same tumor. At one end of the spectrum are undifferentiated cells which are very difficult to distinguish from small cell sarcoma and at the other end are tumors which consist solely of mature cell types. Between these two extremes the tumors may exhibit varying degrees of differentiation.

Neuroblastoma and Ganglioneuroblastoma

Beckwith[11] has devised the following histopathologic grading of neuroblastomas which includes the so-called ganglioneuroblastomas:

Grade I. Predominantly differentiated, over 50 percent differentiating elements.

Grade II. Predominantly undifferentiated, 5 to 50 percent differentiating elements.

Grade III. Slightly differentiated, under 5 percent differentiating elements.

Grade IV. Undifferentiated, no recognizable neurogenesis.

Histologic grade can be related to prognosis. Beckwith found that 5 out of 5 patients with grade I tumors survived beyond two years whereas 3 out or 4 with grade II tumors, 4 out of 13 with grade III and only 1 out of 28 with grade IV tumors survived. Similarly, in another study it was found that approximately 30 percent of patients with well-differentiated or moderately differentiated tumor survived beyond two years without evidence of disease compared with only 9 percent of those with poorly differentiated neuroblastoma.[12]

Ganglioneuroma and Maturation of Neuroblastoma

Ganglioneuromas represent the benign end of the neuroblastoma spectrum. The tumors are usually circumscribed and encapsulated. Their extensions often project from the main tumor and tenaciously entwine adjacent structures. They are often calcified on x-ray examination and can produce elevation in urinary catacholamine excretion.[13]

For many years controversy has existed regarding reports of maturation of neuroblastoma toward the more benign ganglioneuroma.[14-19] The maturation to the more benign form appears to parallel the natural embryogenesis of the sympathetic nervous system.[14] Greenfield and Shelley reviewed sixty-six cases of neuroblastoma and found eleven cases with complete maturation to benign ganglioneuroma.[19] Virtually all reported transformed tumors have been found in a paravertebral position or some other extra-adrenal location.[18,19] The rationale behind Bodian's use of vitamin B_{12} as therapy for neuroblastoma was that since the vitamin is essential for the normal maturation of hematopoietic cells, it might enhance the maturation of neuroblastic cells to ganglioneuroma.[20] This approach did not prove to be successful. Further support for the concept of maturation of neuroblastomas was added when it was found that immature neuroblastoma cells can differentiate into mature ganglion cells in tissue cultures.[21]

Neuroblastoma and Von Recklinghausen's Disease

Chatten and Voorhees[6] in their study of familial neuroblastoma suggested the possibility that a developmental relationship exists between neuroblastoma and neurofibromatosis. This concept is supported by the later finding of ganglion cells and/or ganglioneuromatous tissue within the neurofibromas of several cases of Von Recklinghausen's disease.[22] Ultrastructural similarities were also observed between neurofibroma and neuroblastoma maturing into ganglioneurofibroma. It was then suggested that neurofibromatosis may in some instances be derived from disseminated neuroblastoma or apparently migrating neural crest cells, particularly in the syndrome of congenital neuroblastomas with multiple skin and visceral metastases.[22]

Immunologic Aspects and Neuroblastomas *in situ*

A recent advance in our understanding of neuroblastoma has been the demonstration of cell-bound immune reactions against host neuroblastoma cells when evaluated *in vitro*.[23] Using a colony inhibition assay in which one is able to demonstrate immune reactions against human transplantation antigens, the Hellstroms found that lymphocytes from patients with neuroblastoma inhibited colony formation by neuroblastoma cells. Lymphocytes from mothers of patients with neonatal neuroblastoma were also inhibitory in this system.[23] This work suggests that tumor-specific antigens are present on neuroblastoma cells and that immune mechanisms could play a role in determining the natural history of the disease.

These observations could also partly explain why infants with neuroblastoma have the highest rate of spontaneous regression of any human cancer.[24] It may also provide an explanation for the demonstration of small deposits of neuroblastoma tissue in approximately one in two hunderd autopsies performed on infants up to the age of three months (Fig. 6-1).[25-28] This is forty times

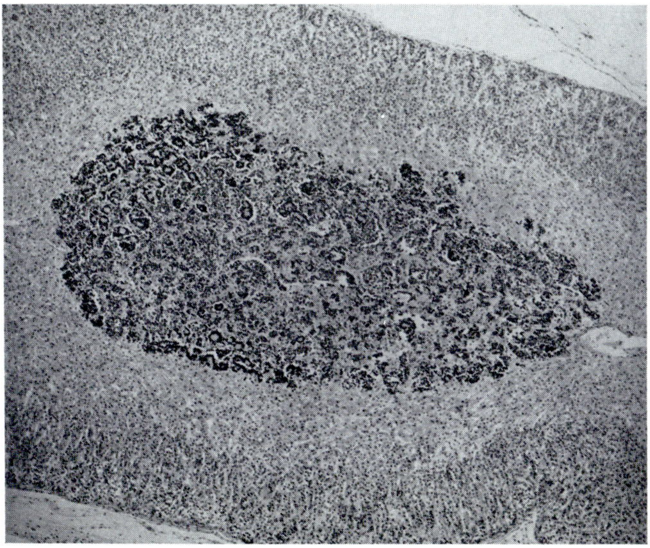

Figure 6-1. Neuroblastoma *in situ* in the adrenal of an infant. (Courtesy of Dr. J. Beckwith.)[25]

the expected rate based on the incidence of the tumor in the childhood population as a whole.[25] Additional evidence related to an immune reaction is provided by the finding that lymphocytic infiltration within the tumor is associated with an improved prognosis.[29]

One can therefore speculate that spontaneous regression of overt tumor or neuroblastoma *in situ* is the result of a cell-mediated immune response. However, this does not provide an explanation of the high incidence of spontaneous regression and "cure" in infants, as opposed to older children. One hypothesis relates to the reduced levels of humoral antibody in young infants and the possibility that their presence in older children could impair the accessibility of tumor cells to the lethal action of lymphocytes.

CLINICAL FEATURES

Presenting Symptoms and Signs

The clinical presentation of children with neuroblastoma is highly variable and is dependent on the site of the primary tumor as well as its pattern of local and metastatic spread. The primary site is often extremely difficult to identify. The presenting symptoms are protean and can include listlessness, diarrhea, bone pain, abdominal pain, shortness of breath, swelling of the orbit, paralysis, vomiting and weight loss. Limp is a fairly common form of presentation. Occasionally, an abdominal mass is palpated by the mother during routine child care. The association of chronic diarrhea and neuroblastoma is well recognized and must be considered in children with otherwise unexplained persistent diarrhea. Although hypertension is not common in children with neuroblastoma, the tumor should be included in the differential diagnosis of a child with unexplained high blood pressure.

The clinical features of the disease can conveniently be categorized according to the anatomical areas involved by tumor.

Head and Neck

Signs and symptoms related to this area are not uncommon as initial presenting features of neuroblastoma. On clinical grounds their differentiation from other malignant and infectious processes can be difficult. One very distinctive sign in neuroblastoma is the fairly rapid onset of periorbital ecchymoses usually associated with varying degrees of proptosis. The involvement can be unilateral or bilateral. When confined to one side it tends to be preferentially on the same side as the adrenal tumor.[30] Other ophthalmologic manifestations include hemorrhage and edema of the eyelids and conjunctivae, blepharitis, ptosis, displacement of the globe and strabismus. Whereas intraocular metastic spread has been documented in several hundred adults, this type of metastasis has never been described in neuroblastoma nor, for that matter, is it a feature of any of the solid tumors of childhood.[31,32] When a retro-orbital mass is present, a bruit may be auscultated. A swelling in the temporal region with proptosis and deviation of the globe is associated with metastatic involvement of the frontal process of the zygomatic bone.

Signs and symptoms of increased intracranial pressure can occur from intracranial disease and thus can result in hydrocephalus, papilledema, retinal hemorrhages and alterations in pupillary reactions. Metastatic spread with subcutaneous nodules is not a usual finding at some time during the course of the disease. Neuroblastoma may also occur as an intranasal neuroepithelial tumor with subsequent intracranial involvement.[33]

Differential diagnosis of masses in the neck include lymphomas, cysts, teratomas, lipomas and intramuscular hemorrhage from trauma. Progressive growth which is painless, demands a biopsy and any mass in an infant under one year of age must be considered as tumor until proven otherwise. Neuroblastomas may originate under the mandible and from the submaxillary ganglion. Others may occur beneath the sternocleidomastoid muscle (Fig. 6-2) or in the retropharyngeal space (Fig. 6-3). Many neuroblastomas in this region will invade the spinal canal and cause cord symptoms unless they are discovered early. Involvement of the cervical nodes is occasionally seen in metastatic neuroblastoma.

Radiographic examination is of great assistance in diagnosis but it may be difficult to distinguish neuroblastoma from other neoplastic disorders such as Ewing's sarcoma, lymphoma and his-

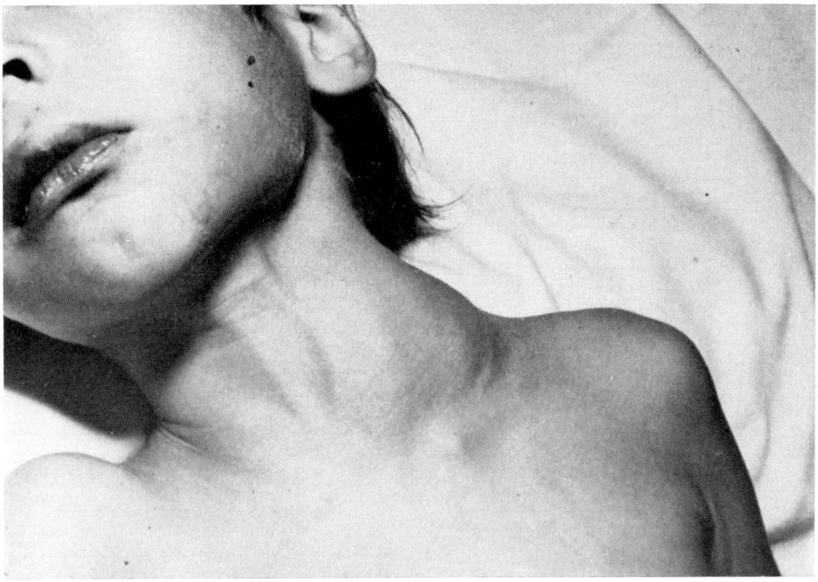

Figure 6-2. A child with neuroblastoma of the neck which was metastatic from a left perirenal primary.

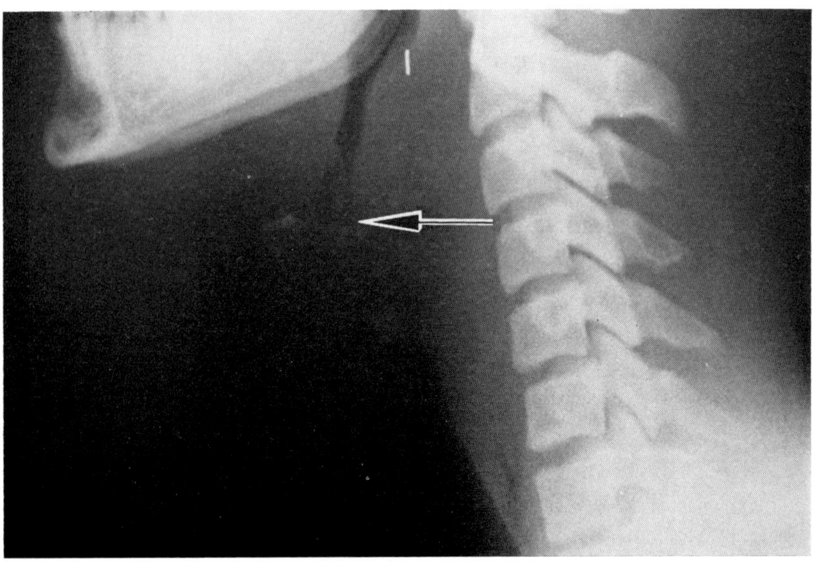

Figure 6-3. Lateral x-ray of the neck showing a precervical neuroblastoma displacing the pharynx and trachea anteriorly (arrow).

tiocytosis X. Roentgenograms of the bony orbit may reveal a destructive lesion and even in the absence of clinical disease in the area, extensive areas of metastatic involvement can be seen in any of the bones of the skull. In patients with intracranial hypertension widening of the sutures may be observed but this has to be distinguished from neoplastic invasion of the suture lines (Fig. 6-4).

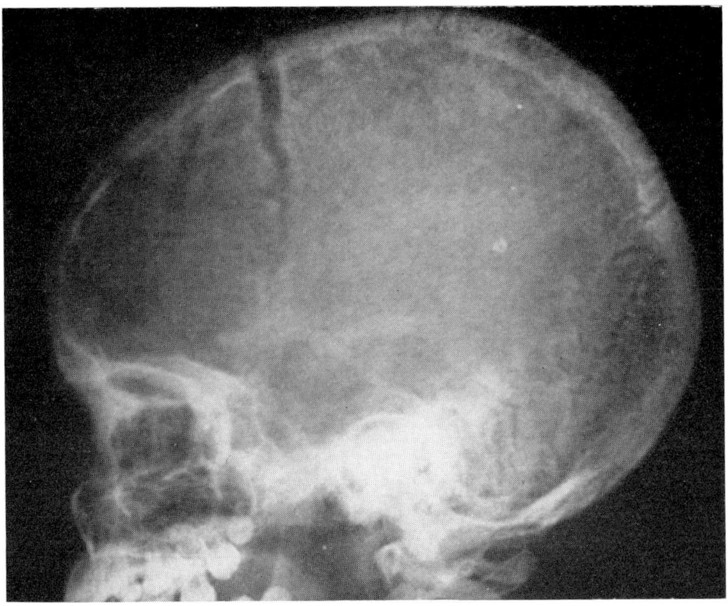

Figure 6-4. Lateral x-ray of the skull of a eleven-year-old boy with metastatic neuroblastoma showing bony destruction involving the entire calvarium. The margins of the sutures also appear to be involved.

Chest

The mediastinum is a common site for primary neuroblastoma and considerable tumor growth can be present before it becomes clinically evident. The primary tumor usually occurs in the superior or posterior mediastinum and the child presents with cough or symptoms of tracheal compression (Fig. 6-5). The tumor may be of the "dumbbell" type and spinal cord compression with re-

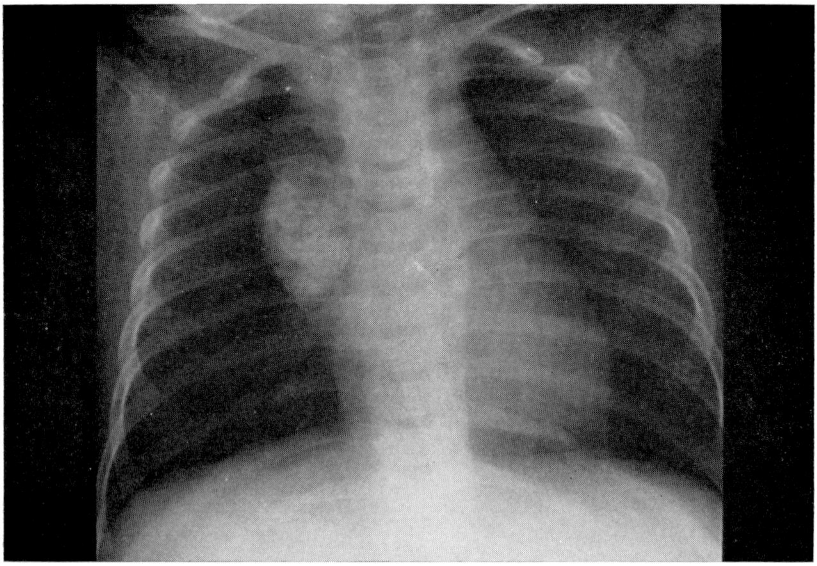

Figure 6-5. Chest x-ray showing a right mediastinal mass containing mottled calcifications. A lateral chest x-ray indicated that the mass was located in the posterior mediastinum.

sultant partial or complete paralysis below the lesion may provide the only clue to the existence of intrathoracic neuroblastoma. Metastatic spread can involve the skeletal structures of the thorax and loss of vertebral height, blurring of the pedicles and widening of neural foramina may be visualized roentgenographically. The ribs may be affected with clinical and/or radiographic evidence of pathological fracture. Pulmonary metastases are not common but do occur and could be mistaken for evidence of other neoplastic diseases, particularly Wilms' tumor (Fig. 6-6).

Abdomen and Pelvis

The presence of an abdominal mass in any child must raise the possibility of neuroblastoma. In a review of 135 cases by Dargeon, thirty-seven were considered to have arisen in the abdominal cavity.[1] The retroperitoneal region is the most common site of origin of abdominal neuroblastomas, and as in the thorax, the

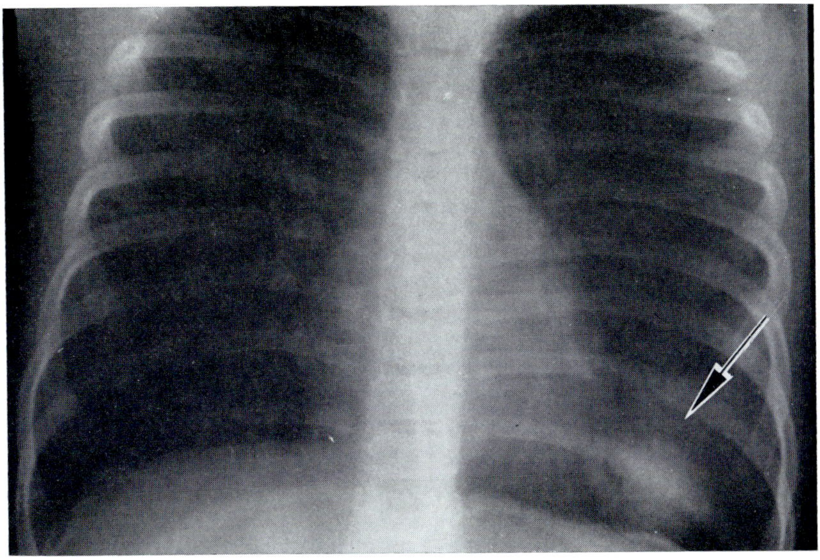

Figure 6-6. Chest x-ray showing two neuroblastoma metastases in the left base. One of the metastases appears to be intrapulmonary and the other extrapleural.

tumor may become inordinately large before any symptoms or signs are noted. It is interesting that in a study of 130 children with a variety of benign and malignant tumors, ten were detected incidental to evaluation of the effects of blunt abdominal trauma.[34] Although hydronephrosis was recognized as the commonest cause of an abdominal mass, neuroblastoma constituted 14 percent of the series.[34] It should be appreciated, however, that hydronephrosis can result from obstruction to the urinary tract by tumor, thus making preoperative evaluation more difficult.

Many of the nonspecific symptoms of neuroblastoma relate to the abdomen and these include anorexia, disturbances of bowel function and abdominal pain. Palpable tumor is undoubtedly the commonest presenting feature of abdominal neuroblastoma and the mass is generally in the flank or subcostal regions. It is usually firm to palpation with poorly defined margins, but there are no unique features which would allow for precise differentiation from other intra-abdominal neoplasms. Abdominal distention is the presenting feature in over 50 percent of children under one year of age.[35] Extension of intra-abdominal tumor into the spinal canal can result in spinal cord compression and varying degrees of paralysis without overt evidence of abdominal disease. Depending on the level of involvement there may be associated bladder or bowel dysfunction.

X-ray examination is invaluable in the diagnosis of intra-abdominal neuroblastoma. In Rice's series[35] calcification within tumors was present in 32 percent of children with an abdominal primary (Fig. 6-7). Intravenous pyelography is essential. In patients with an adrenal primary, the kidney is usually displaced in a downward lateral direction. The kidney is often rotated so that the pelvic calyceal outlines are intact and not distorted thus differ-

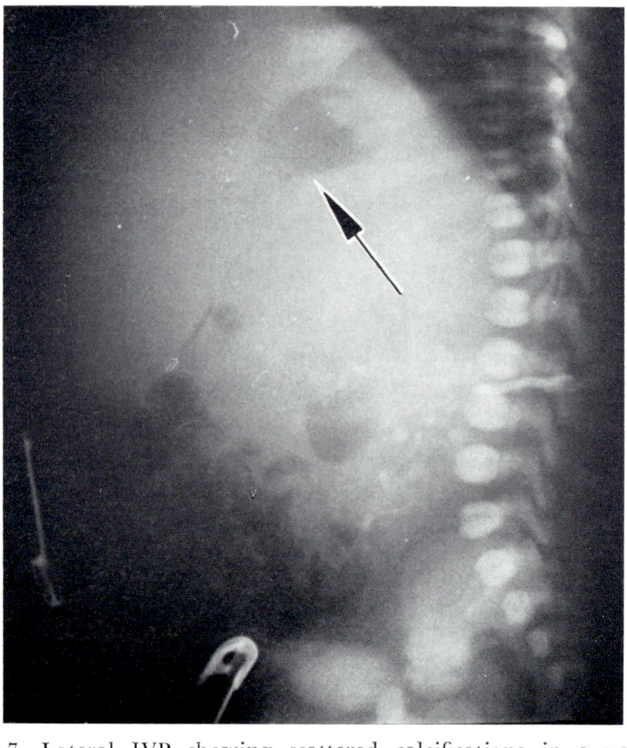

Figure 6-7. Lateral IVP showing scattered calcifications in a very large neuroblastoma which depresses the kidney and displaces the stomach anteriorly (arrow).

entiating it from Wilms' tumor (Fig. 6-8). Occasionally renal circulation is compromised by tumor and kidneys failing to visualize adequately. Paravertebral masses identifiable on routine abdominal x-ray are highly suggestive of neuroblastoma particularly where calcification is present. Their presence makes for easier diagnosis in the occasional case where intravenous pyelography may fail to differentiate between neuroblastoma and Wilms' tumor.

Neuroblastoma arising in the pelvis can result in compression

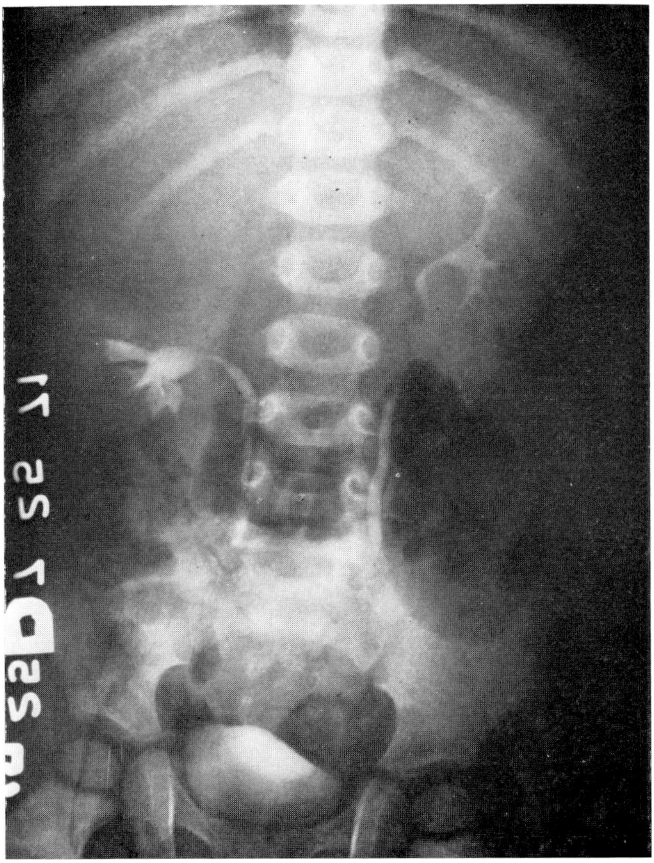

Figure 6-8. IVP showing a large neuroblastoma displacing the right kidney downward and laterally. The right renal calyx shows the typical "drooping lily" deformity.

of the bladder or rectum and may cause symptoms and signs of partial obstruction (Fig. 6-9). Metastases to the scrotum are rare. An occasional infant may present with a primary lesion in the scrotal sac.[36] Intraspinal involvement also occurs and a mass is usually palpable in the buttock, perineum or by rectal examination.

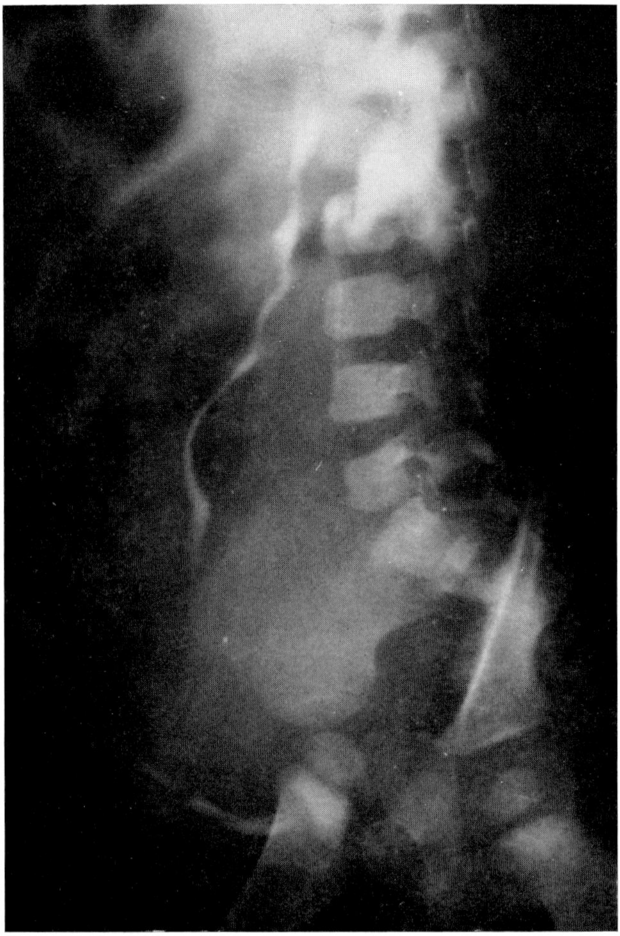

Figure 6-9. An IVP demonstrating a presacral neuroblastoma which displaces the bladder and one ureter anteriorly.

Extremities

Primary lesions arising in the extremities are extremely rare. The authors are personally aware of one patient whose presumed primary arose in a phalanx. Reference is made to a presumed skeletal origin but these are difficult to substantiate because of the known propensity of this tumor to metastasize to bone. Thus the overwhelming majority of symptoms and signs relative to the extremities can be assumed to be the result of metastatic disease usually involving the skeletal structures. Symptoms include complaints of bone pain and limp. Pathological fractures can occur. Radiologic evidence of widespread bony involvement is highly suggestive of neuroblastoma although it is sometimes difficult to distinguish it from other malignant disorders particularly leukemia (Fig. 6-10) .

Skin and Subcutaneous Tissues

Cutaneous and subcutaneous metastases can occur in any area of the body and when widespread have led to speculation regarding multicentric origin for the tumor.[37] This pattern of metastatic disease occurs most frequently in the neonatal period and the term "blueberry muffin" has been used to describe the appearance and characteristic feel of these lesions (Fig. 6-11) .[38] As with all such clinical situations biopsy confirmation is necessary for definitive diagnosis. If sought there is invariably evidence of an intra-abdominal primary.

Central Nervous System

As mentioned previously, neuroblastoma can produce many signs and symptoms referable to the central nervous system. These include the effects of direct tumor invasion of cranial or peripheral nerves and the consequences of spread from the paravertebral area into the extradural space. Extradural primary tumors have been reported to occur, but in our experience there is always evidence of spread from the paravertebral space.

Opsoclonus, or acute cerebellar ataxia, has been described in association with neuroblastoma.[39,40] The pathophysiologic basis

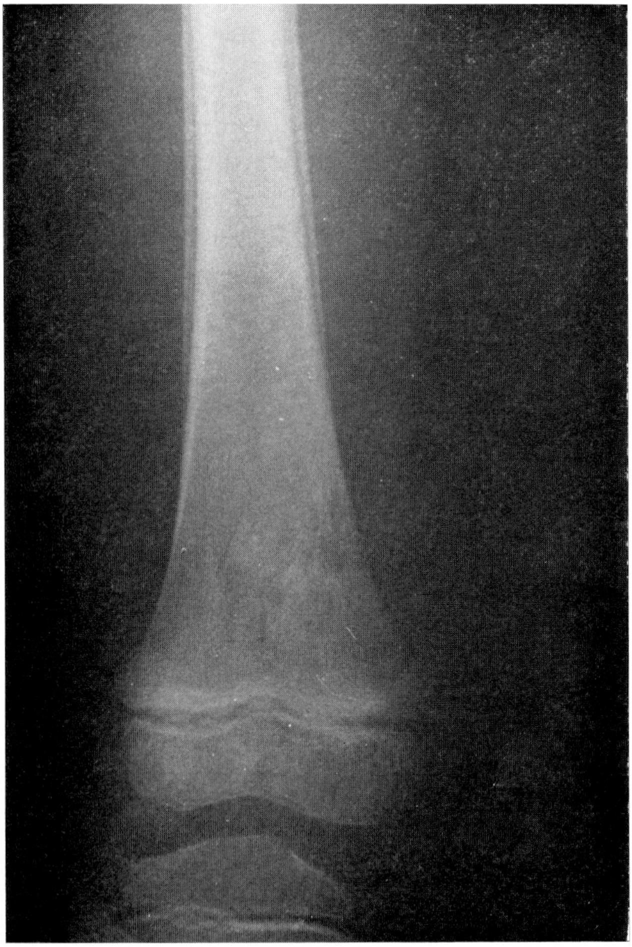

Fgure 6-10. The distal femur of a child with disseminated neuroblastoma. Multiple osteolytic lesions are seen in the metaphysis. Periosteal new bone formation is present along the shaft.

for the cerebellar dysfunction has not been elucidated, but the presence of such cerebellar ataxia usually indicates a bad prognosis for the patient with neuroblastoma. It is recommended that all children with acute cerebellar encehalopathy have a chest x-ray, intravenous pyelogram, skeletal survey, bone marrow examination and measurement of urinary excretion of catecholamines.[40]

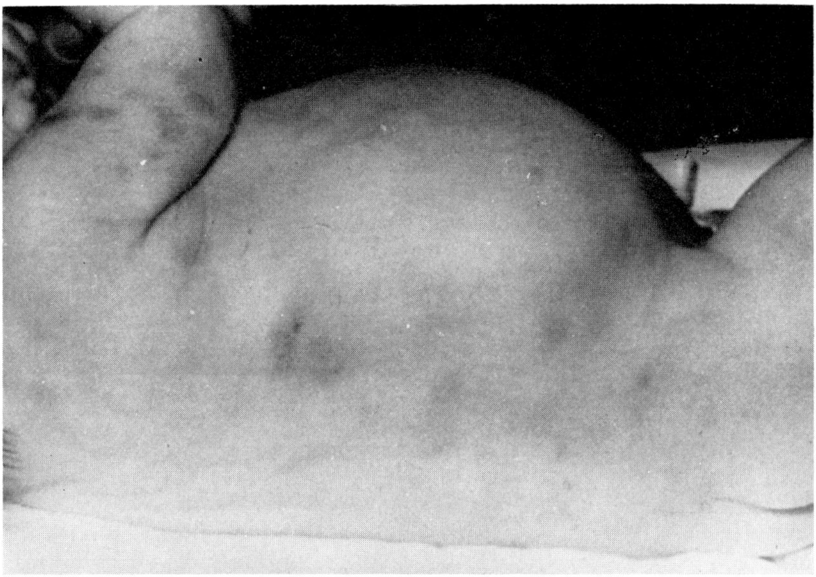

Figure 6-11. A two-day-old infant showing bluish firm subcutaneous nodules scattered over the body. At surgery a very large neuroblastoma was found originating from the left adrenal gland. (Courtesy of Dr. T. E. Shown.)[38]

LABORATORY EVALUATION

Hematologic Findings

The hemoglobin concentration is commonly reduced at the time of diagnosis and this invariably occurs later as a complication of chemotherapy and/or radiotherapy. Anemia at the time of diagnosis was noted in 61 percent of Rice's patients.[36] One or more factors may contribute to the anemia, which is usually normochromic, normocytic but could also reflect varying degrees of iron depletion. Hemorrhage into the tumor may be of sufficient magnitude to account for the drop in hemoglobin and could be further complicated by disseminated intravascular coagulation with attendant hemolysis, depletion of coagulation factors and thrombocytopenia.[41,42] Bone marrow infiltration, infection and nutritional deficiency can all play a role in impairing normal red blood cell production. Occasionally a myelophthisic blood picture with nucleated red cells in the peripheral blood results from metastatic bone marrow invasion.

There is no characteristic leukocyte response in patients with neuroblastoma. Leukopenia or leukocytosis have been observed and reflect the effects of secondary infection or bone marrow invasion. A marked shift-to-the-left with myelocytes in the peripheral blood suggests bone marrow involvement.

Thrombocytopenia is usually a complication of therapy rather than due to the tumor per se. As mentioned previously disseminated intravascular coagulation does occur in these patients particularly in the presence of metastatic disease and the resulting thrombocytopenia may be severe. Occasionally symptomatically significant thrombocytopenia results from bone marrow invasion.

Bone marrow examination should be part of the routine investigation of children with suspected neuroblastoma. Tumor cells can be distinguished from hematopoietic elements without difficulty since they have "an immature appearance" with large nuclei, some of which contain nucleoi. Cytoplasmic vacuoles are often seen. Neuroblastoma cells are usually about the size of small lymphocytes (10μ) and characteristically form syncytia in the marrow (Fig. 6-12). It is not possible to distinguish the type of tumor cell in the marrow with precision by Wright's stain. Forty-nine of 90 patients in one series demonstrated tumor metastases in their marrow aspirates.[43] Of these, 40 patients had a marrow examination within two weeks of diagnosis and 28 demonstrated marrow metastases at that time. Twelve other patients were found to have marrow with metastases from one to twenty-one months after diagnosis. Marrow metastases were found to be in 3 of 17 (18 percent) patients under the age of one year and in 46 of 67 (64 percent) children who presented between the ages of one to six years.[43] Skeletal involvement was usually seen by x-ray examination in patients with positive aspirates.

Biochemical Aspects

Since the cells of the sympathetic nervous system and chromaffin tissue of the adrenal medulla are capable of synthesizing and secreting various catecholamines, it is not surprising that tumors

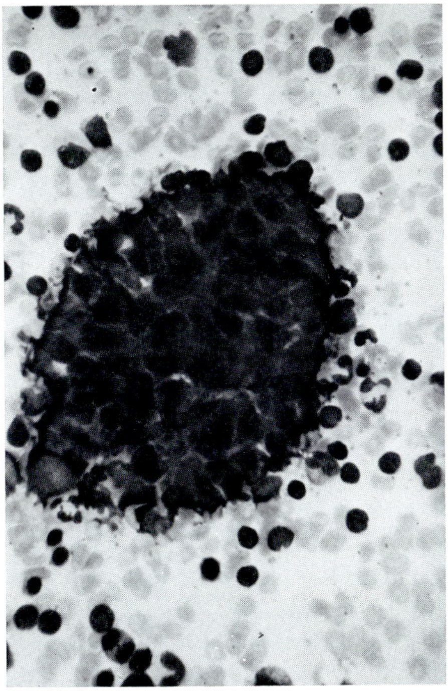

Figure 6-12. A clump of neuroblastoma cells in a bone marrow smear (Wright's stain ×960).

arising from these sites secrete excessive amounts of these compounds. Increased formation of dopa, dopamine, l-norepinephrine and their metabolites are claimed to occur in the majority of patients with neuroblastoma. Table 6-1 outlines the relevant metabolic pathways and demonstrates the wide variety of compounds which might be excreted in excess. These metabolites are identifiable in urine, and although there is great variability in the relative excretion of each compound, one can expect that approximately 90 percent of patients with neuroblastoma will have elevation in the urinary levels of vanillylmandelic acid (VMA) or homovanillic acid (HVA), or both.[44] Thus, determination of these two catecholamines would allow for identification of the majority of neuroblastomas without resorting to more elaborate biochemical procedures. In doubtful cases it may be advantageous

TABLE 6-I

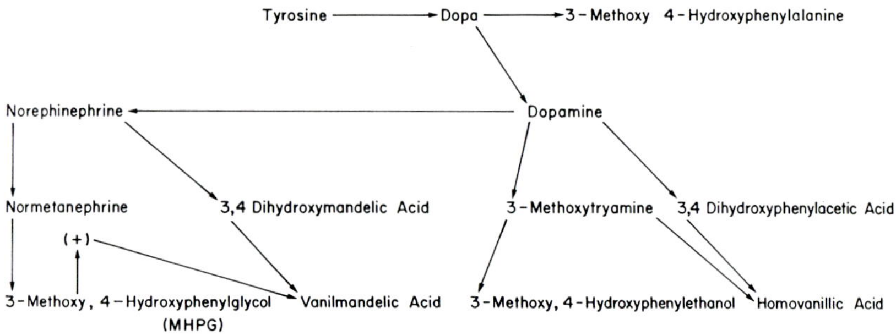

(+) = 3 - Methoxy - 4 - Hydroxy - Mandelaldehyde

to measure the excretion of the other products of dopa metabolism. Measurement of VMA and HVA excretion is not only helpful in diagnosis but can and should be utilized as an index of therapeutic effect since levels of excretion tend to parallel clinical evolution of disease.[45] However, it must be emphasized that one cannot distinguish between ganglioneuroma and neuroblastoma on the basis of catecholamine excretion pattern alone. Neuroblastoma and pheochromocytoma are both neural crest tumors and may excrete similar products of metabolism. One biochemical distinction relates to the fact that pheochromocytomas excrete only VMA and its precursors.

The identification of congenital neuroblastoma in fetuses before birth has been reported.[46] Six mothers presented with symptoms in the eighth or ninth month of pregnancy similar to those of adults with a pheochromocytoma. These symptoms appeared to be caused by fetal catecholamines entering the maternal circulation and included attacks of sweating, paleness, tingling of hands and feet, headaches, decreased sensibility in fingers and toes, heart palpitations and in one case paroxysmal hypertension. The six offspring were diagnosed as having neuroblastoma between day 1 and 9 months of age. All infants had increased levels of urinary excretion of catecholamine metabolites. The symptoms exhibited by the mothers during pregnancy suggests that neurogenic tumors were functioning within the fetus. Analysis of the urine and blood from mothers such as these should provide further information and urinary catecholamines should be assessed whenever pregnant women exhibit the appropriate symptoms during the last months of pregnancy.

A method for rapid determination for catecholamines has been developed and could be adapted as an office procedure.[47] The test is performed as follows:

1. To 4 drops (0.2 ml) of urine in a graduated centrifuge tube add 10% potassium bicarbonate to the 3 ml mark.
2. Add 4 drops of an equivolume mixture of 0.1% paranitroaniline and 0.2% sodium nitrate and shake the mixture.
3. Add isoamyl alcohol to the 4.5 ml mark.
4. Shake tube for one minute.
5. Compare visually against the standard similarly prepared from normal urine to which 5μg of VMA has been added.

A negative urine gives rise to a colorless pale yellow or orange upper layer (isoamyl alcohol), whereas a positive test is one in which this layer has a pink or violet hue equal to or greater than the VMA standard. All the reagents must be refrigerated until immediately prior to use. Paranitroanaline solution is made by dissolving 1 gm of paranitroanaline in 20 ml of concentrated hydrochloric acid diluted to 1 liter with distilled water. Sodium nitrate should be prepared freshly each month. For the VMA standard 10 mg of VMA is diluted in 500 ml of water and 5 drops or 0.25 ml is added to 4 drops of urine. This test gave negative results in 62 children with miscellaneous tumors and positive results in 32 out of 35 patients with neuroblastoma.[47]

Cystathionine, an intermediate metabolite of methionine, is usually found in human brain, liver, kidney and muscle but not normally present in urine. It has been detected in 50 percent of patients with neuroblastoma but its excretion appears to be independent of VMA which could make it a useful diagnostic test in the occasional patient in whom there is no elevation of urinary VMA or HVA. As with the catecholamines, its disappearance from the urine correlates well with clinical improvement.[48] D'Angio has reported preliminary attempts to convert the capacity of neuroblastoma to synthesize cystathionine from methionine through homocysteine by administering Se^{75} labeled methionine to four children with metastatic neuroblastoma.[49] Localization of isotope using the scanning technique was seen within tumor three to six hours after the injection of the radionuclide in three of the patients. In two patients who underwent surgery, incorporation of the radioisotope was seen in excised tumor specimens. This procedure requires further investigation and may become an important diagnostic aid.

Diagnostic Procedures

In situations where neuroblastoma is suspected or even where proven by biopsy it is necessary to document the extent of disease since this allows for a more rational approach to therapy and also provides information of prognostic value.

The following studies are necessary for adequate evaluation:

1. X-rays of the chest, the skull and long bones.
2. Intravenous pyelogram preferably including inferior vena cavagram.
3. Bone marrow examination.
4. Urinary catecholamine determination.
5. Histological confirmation.

Additional studies including radioisotopic scan of liver and spleen; special radiographic views of neural foramina and myelography may be indicated in patients with hepatomegaly or signs of spinal cord compression.

Staging

Prognosis in neuroblastoma is related to age of the patient, the presence or absence of bone marrow metastases, and the degree of differentiation of the tumor cells. Evans[50] proposed a staging scheme which describes the extent of the disease present without reference to resectability, because the latter includes the additional variables of surgical judgement and expertise. Some authors tend to exclude children under one year of age from analysis because of the favorable prognosis in this age group and other authors include the degree of differentiation of the tumor. Evans acknowledges that the age at diagnosis does have prognostic significance but points out that it remains to be shown whether the extent of disease in infants influences their survival. She includes all neuroblastic tumors except pheochromocytoma and ganglioneuroma:

Stage 0. Neuroblastoma *in situ.*

Stage I. Tumor confined to the organ or structure of origin.

Stage II. Tumors extending in continuity beyond the organ or structure of origin but not crossing the midline. Regional lymph nodes on the homolateral side may be involved.

Stage III. Tumors extending in continuity beyond the midline. Regional lymph nodes may be involved bilaterally.

Stage IV. Remote disease involving skeleton, distant organs, soft tissues or distant lymph node groups.

Stage IV-S. Patients who would otherwise be stage I or II but who have disease confined only to one or more of the following sites: liver, skin or bone marrow but without radiographic evidence of skeletal disease.

The proposed staging was applied to one hundred children with neuroblastoma entered into two studies conducted by Childrens Cancer Study Group A. Short-term survival data of this sample demonstrated the staging to be practical and the staging appeared to be of help in estimating prognosis. A special stage IV category (IV-S) was developed because it is recognized that certain findings in children with neuroblastoma do not necessarily indicate a grave prognosis as when similar circumstances occur in patients with other malignancies. Patients in the stage IV-S category, particularly those under twelve months of age, have a good prognosis in spite of the widespread nature of the disease.[51]

TREATMENT

Therapy directed against neuroblastoma must involve a multidisciplinary team approach. Surgeons, radiation therapists and chemotherapists, all play a role in designing the treatment program even when one or other modality is not utilized in the initial plan of therapy. Ideally, a tumor specialist's board consisting of representatives from the various disciplines should review each case from the point of view of adequacy of diagnostic evaluation and in order to plan a rational and consistent treatment regimen. In this way, each patient derives the benefit of in-depth evaluation and ultimately enough data can be collected to allow meaningful review of the success or failure of a particular program.

For convenience we will review the use of each of the current modes of therapy bearing in mind that only close cooperation between the surgeon, radiation therapist and chemotherapist can result in the provision of optimal patient care. Since the approaches with x-ray therapy and surgery have been reasonably well standardized they will be described first. The various drug regimens will be described and approaches being used by the various cancer chemotherapy groups will be outlined. Brief consideration will be given to an immunotherapeutic approach that might be used for treatment, even though it is still considered to be investigational.

Surgery

Completion of the clinical investigation previously described usually requires one to two days. Roentgenographic studies and catecholamine determinations usually provide confirmation of clinical impressions so that the disease can often be diagnosed preoperatively. Anemia, if present, is corrected by blood transfusion prior to operation. In view of the variability of presentation, the role and extent of surgery must be assessed on an individual basis.

Tumors should be completely excised, although most surgeons do not advocate enbloc dissection of contiguous viscera.[52] Whether surgery alone should be considered as definitive therapy in cases where the tumor is completely resected remains to be determined, particularly in the child under one year of age. The role of postoperative chemotherapy in this patient-group is currently under investigation. A surgically resected localized tumor in the infant does not appear to warrant postoperative radiation therapy, although this is also in dispute.

The high probability of early metastasis should not discourage a surgical approach unless x-ray examination, bone marrow examination or lymph node biopsy confirms the widespread nature of the disease. Histologic confirmation of the diagnosis should be made but a bone marrow aspirate infiltrated with tumor cells in a patient with increased urinary excretion of HVA or VMA is sufficient to diagnose neuroblastoma. Often, the resectability of the tumor can be assessed only after laparotomy or exploratory thoracotomy at which time a biopsy reveals metastatic neuroblastoma. However, most radiotherapists and chemotherapists are in favor of removing bulk tumor, leaving a minimum of residual tumor to treat. Thus, surgical resection of as much of the tumor as possible is an acceptable and desirable procedure in children with neuroblastoma, if it can be accomplished without undue hazard. There is insufficient data to answer the question as to whether the removal of the primary affects the growth of metastases.[52]

In addition to evaluation of the tumor from the viewpoint of resectability and the obtaining of adequate tissue for histological examination, the surgeon is in a position to provide information regarding extent of disease which may not be apparent from other diagnostic studies. Even in the presence of metastases initial exploratory laparotomy, or thoracotomy, is often indicated with removal of bulk tumor and marking of residual disease with silver clips that can be followed postoperatively by x-ray examination. Control of disease as evidenced by improvement in clinical, radiologic and biochemical parameters is often an indication for surgical reexploration twelve to eighteen months after the initial surgery. At reexploration the residual tumor, if any, is evaluated by biopsy and removed *in toto,* if possible.

Although there is little in the literature regarding complications secondary to anesthesia in patients with neuroblastoma, these patients can be a problem and blood pressure may have to be controlled with phentolamine and noradrenalin. The postoperative use of an alpha-adrenegic blocking agent such as phenoxybenzamine may be indicated.[53] Adrenocorticoid function may be depressed and additional hydrocortisone may be needed. Patients with secreting tumors may also need extra sedation in the postoperative period.

Radiation Therapy

D'Angio has emphasized that all tissue at risk must be included in the treatment field, but no more than this. He advocates the use of external heavy metal blocks to shape fields appropriately.[54] Radiation dosage is usually adjusted according to age. Midplain doses delivered in the abdomen using 250 KV techniques range from 1800 rads to an infant of less than twelve months to 3500 to 4000 rads to a child four to five years of age.[54] The dose is delivered in $2\frac{1}{2}$ to $4\frac{1}{2}$ weeks time depending on the child's age.[55] Children with neuroblastoma confined to the primary and adjacent lymph nodes should have all areas of tumor included in their treatment field. In planning localized radiation therapy each extra-adrenal site relates to different organs or tissues whose tolerance must be considered. Growing cartilage and growing bones demand attention in all sites. It is usually not possible to completely resect an extra-adrenal neuroblastoma and the radiation therapy recommended uses curative doses with the daily doses of radiation conditioned by the size of the field and the nature of complications.

Radiotherapy is well tolerated by children in the immediate postoperative period, but it seems reasonable to permit the patient to recover for one to two days prior to instituting therapy. Many radiotherapists now recommend inclusion of the entire width of the vertebral body in the irradiated field in order to minimize the incidence of scoliosis which results from asymmetrical irradiation of the vertebral growth centers.[55,56] However, even with this precaution, scoliosis can result from neurogenic involvement and fibrosis and contracture of soft tissues.[55] The liver can also be adversely affected by radiation as evidenced by reduced radioisotope uptake in areas included in the irradiation field. In evaluating 115 children who received irradiation to the liver,

Tefft found abnormalities in liver function with doses as low as 1200 rads.[57] The abnormalities appeared to be dose-related. Generally, those patients who have abnormalities of liver function tests or on liver scans, in the acute phase will show some abnormalities in the chronic phase following irradiation. The incidence of severe clinical dysfunction in children is approximately 5 percent.[57] Care should be taken to exclude the kidneys from the direct radiation beam particularly if the contralateral kidney is outside the area of known tumor involvement. Should the kidneys both be involved one can consider attempting to shield one or both organs to limit the dose to within that tolerated by renal tissue. Another approach would be to attempt to eradicate the tumor surgically, then using only chemotherapy postoperatively and thus eliminating the hazard of radiation nephritis.

Preoperative irradiation is not recommended since it tends to obscure the histological picture, and such therapy does *not* allow for a more definitive surgical procedure to be undertaken, as some have suggested. However, preoperative irradiation can produce clinical regression of tumors and is advocated by Rissanen.[58] We consider that the patient with metastatic disease in whom surgical exploration is not contemplated is usually not a candidate for definitive radiation therapy until such time as chemotherapy or surgery, or both, has restricted the disease so that it is considered accessible to tumoricidal doses of radiation. In patients who have rapid development of spinal cord compression or who develop superior vena caval symptoms, high daily doses of radiation therapy are warranted. A dose of 400 rads daily to a level of 1200 rads has been advocated to assure rapid tumor shrinkage.[59] Increased edema concurrent with the radiation is not a major problem. The "field within a field" technique has been used to concentrate the dose to the critical area.

In cases of widespread dissemination, radiotherapy is administered with a palliative intent and is directed to either the primary site or control of symptoms as with bowel or bladder obstruction, intrathoracic symptoms or spinal cord compression. Palliative doses vary from 200 rads in one treatment to 600 rads on three consecutive days. However, as much as 2000 rads in fourteen days may be required for relief of bone pain, treatment of localized or diffuse intracranial metastases, unsightly scalp masses, or control of intra-abdominal tumors.[55]

Chemotherapy

The two most widely used agents in the treatment of neuroblastoma are cyclophosphamide (Cytoxan) and vincristine (Oncovin). These agents have been used alone in various dosage regimens or in combination as either sequential or alternating chemotherapy.[60-66]

Following James's report in 1965 of 100 percent complete or partial remission rate in children of varying ages with unresectable neuroblastoma,[61] it appeared that a highly effective combination of drugs was now available for treatment of this heretofore, relatively unresponsive tumor. Unfortunately, using a similar regimen of alternating vincristine and cyclophosphamide in children with metastatic neuroblastomia, in a later study by Children Cancer Study Group A objective response was found in only 9 of 29 patients,[65] and of these, only 4 were classified as attaining complete remission. Similarly disappointing results were reported by the Southwest Cancer Chemotherapy Study Group.[64] Certainly vincristine alone has been disappointing in this tumor as evidenced by remission rates of 22 percent in two independent studies.[62,64] On the other hand, cyclophosphamide has produced a much higher response rate even when used in conventional dosage schedules of 2.5 to 5 mg/kg/day.[60] Unfortunately these remission rates are deceptive since they relate to a temporary response; overall survival has not been significantly influenced by chemotherapy. However, it is still necessary to obtain remission data in order to recognize the most effective drugs and then attempt to develop a treatment program to utilize them in a manner which would improve long-term survival.

One approach is to administer larger amounts of an effective drug in order to obtain an improved therapeutic effect. The program is then limited only by an individual's tolerance to the drug. Whereas cyclophosphamide was usually administered in doses of 2.5 to 5 mg/kg/day, we have been impressed by rapid tumor shrinkage when doses of 10 mg/kg were administered daily either by mouth or intravenously.[66] Therapy is continued until the white blood cell count falls to between 1000 and 1500/mm^3, which usually allows for ten to fourteen days of treatment. Objective tumor regression was documented in 9 of 10 patients and complete remission occurred in 8. The treatment can be repeated every three to five weeks.

At the present time, drug treatment with cyclophosphamide alone or in combination with vincristine should be utilized in children with neuroblastoma. Whether or not infants with localized resectable disease should receive chemotherapy is a question currently being evaluated by Children's Cancer Study Group A. In a situation such as where short-term responses to chemotherapy do not influence survival, a continuous search much be made for improved methods of treatment. A few new agents are under investigation: l-sarcolysin and daunomycin have been given to a small number of patients with no dramatic results. Thus far, they have not been shown to be equal to either cyclophosphamide or vincristine as active agents for children with neuroblastoma.[60-70]

Bodian in the early 1960's suggested that patients with neuroblastoma respond to therapy with vitamin B_{12}.[20] However, a survey published in 1965 revealed that American investigators were not able to show any increase in remission rate with either vitamin B_{12} alone or in conjunction with radiation therapy or other chemotherapeutic agents in children with advanced neuroblastoma.[71] Recently the Medical Research Council in England sponsored an analysis of data from various investigators in the United Kingdom in order to evaluate the effect of vitamin B_{12} in children with neuroblastoma.[72] This retrospective study failed to confirm that vitamin B_{12} therapy is beneficial. Forty-three of forty-seven children whose treatment did not include vitamin B_{12} were known to have died compared with 56 of 61 children who received the vitamin in addition to their other treatment. There appears to be no place for vitamin B_{12} therapy in the modern approach to the treatment of neuroblastoma.

Immunotherapy

Stimulated on the one hand by the poor results with conventional therapy in neuroblastoma and by the evidence for the existence of antigens peculiar to the neuroblastoma cell on the other hand, various investigators have attempted to develop treatment programs based on immunotherapeutic principles. Lymphocytes from mothers and older siblings have been infused into patients on the premise that these lymphocytes may react against the tumor cells, as has been suggested might occur on the basis of *in vitro* studies in other centers. Preliminary studies at the New York Memorial Hospital[73] and other centers will, it is hoped, provide data to support or refute this concept.

Treatment Programs Based on Staging

Stage I

Patients with localized disease should have the benefits of complete surgical resection assuming that the primary site is surgically accessible. Although many centers employ radiation and/or chemotherapy in this group of patients, control data is not available to either support or refute their use. If x-ray therapy is given it should be confined to the tumor bed and postoperative chemotherapy should include cyclophosphamide in either conventional or high-dose regimens for twelve to eighteen months.

Stages II and III

Patients with disease extending in continuity beyond the organ of origin are potentially curable. Surgery should be undertaken with a view to removing as much tumor as possible. It is extremely helpful in subsequent management if the surgeon has placed silver clips around the tumor bed or any area of residual tumor. Postoperative radiation therapy should be instituted but could be delayed in situations where chemotherapy is to be used for tumor shrinkage where surgical removal was not accomplished. Chemotherapy utilizing cyclophosphamide with or without vincristine should be continued for at least twelve months. Response to therapy is measured by clinical, radiological and biochemical parameters. Those patients with primary tumors in the abdomen or pelvis, who have responded to therapy and appear controlled, are candidates for a "second-look" operation twelve to eighteen months following the original surgical procedure.

Stage IV

Because of the widespread nature of disease in this group of patients, chemotherapy offers the only approach. Attempts at surgical resection or definitive radiation therapy cannot be expected to alter the poor outcome and these modes of therapy should be utilized for palpation only.

Stage IV-S

The accumulating evidence that these patients have an improved prognosis is apparently not related in any way to therapy. It appears logical to remove the primary and administer chemotherapy postoperatively. Based on a review of twenty-five patients with stage IV-S disease, it was concluded that radiation therapy was not beneficial.[51] Chemotherapy is recommended only in children with demonstrable bone marrow involvement.[51] Unfortunately, it is unlikely that more definitive evaluation of the role of therapy will be forthcoming in this group of patients; they are few in number and most of them are under one year of age and thus have a higher likelihood of spontaneous regression.

PROGNOSIS

Survival is strongly influenced by the patient's age, extent of disease, degree of cell differentiation, the presence of skeletal and bone marrow metastases. Breslow and McCann have analyzed data on 246 children (Table 6-2), treated in institutions affiliated with Children's Cancer Study Group A.[74] Ninety-two percent of infants with stage I disease survived tumor-free, two years from diagnosis compared with only 3 percent of those over twenty-four months of age with stage IV disease. Over 50 percent of patients in this study had stage IV disease and irrespective of age only 6 percent survived two years without disease. Thus, for the majority

TABLE 6-2
CHILDREN WITH NEUROBLASTOMA SURVIVING TWO YEARS FREE OF DISEASE

Age at Diagnosis (months)	*Clinical Stage* I	II	III	IV	IV-S	*All Stages*
0–11	11/12 (92%)	15/16 (94%)	2/4 (50%)	5/18 (28%)	18/19 (95%)	51/69 (74%)
12–23	3/4 (75%)	3/17 (43%)	5/8 (62.5%)	0/25 (0%)	1/3 (33%)	12/47 (25%)
24+	4/5 (80%)	4/12 (33%)	3/15 (20%)	3/93 (3%)	2/5 (40%)	16/130 (12%)
All Ages	18/21 (86%)	22/35 (63%)	0/27 (37%)	8/136 (6%)	21/27 (78%)	79/246 (32%)

From Breslow and McCann.[74]

of newly diagnosed patients the outlook is extremely poor. An improved prognosis has also been observed in patients with mediastinal primaries, but once again the major influence may be age since most of the survivors tend to be in the younger age groups. Also there is a tendency for mediastinal tumors to be less undifferentiated, and as mentioned previously, a number of investigators have been able to relate prognosis to the degree of histopathological differentiation.

In order to evaluate the impact of various modes of therapy on prognosis, a subcommittee of the Solid Tumor Task Force of the National Cancer Institute undertook a comparison of survival following treatment in children with neuroblastoma in each of two years, 1956 and 1962.[75] By 1962 the clinical use of vincristine and cyclophosphamide in patients with solid tumors was common. The data on patients from three chemotherapy study groups were considered together and there were no statistically significant differences in survival of children with neuroblastoma first seen in 1956 as compared to those diagnosed in 1962. The survival pattern of children with or without metastases had not changed. Since radiation and surgical aspects of neuroblastoma management were considered to have been similar during the two study periods, it was concluded that the addition of new antineoplastic agents and the increased use of chemotherapy in 1962 had not improved the survival of children with neuroblastoma. Further investigation of the biology of this unique tumor as well as the continued evaluation of new and improved methods of treatment must be pursued in order to improve the outlook for infants and children with this potentially curable neoplasm.

REFERENCES

1. Dargeon, H.W.: *Tumors of Childhood: A Clinical Treatise.* New York, Harper Medical Books, 1960.
2. Peterson, D.: The epidemiology of neuroblastoma. *J Pediatr Surg, 3 (Part II)*:135-136, 1968.
3. Peterson, D., Bill, A., and Kirkland, I.: Neuroblastoma trends in time. *J Pediatr Surg, 4*:244-249, 1969.
4. Lee, J.: Summer and death from neuroblastoma. *Br Med J, 2*:404-407, 1967.

5. Miller, R., Fraumeni, J., and Hill, J.: Neuroblastoma: epidemiologic approach to its origin. *Am J Dis Child, 115:*253-261, 1968.
6. Chatten, J., and Voorhees, M.L.: Familial neuroblastoma; report of a kindred with multiple disorders, including neuroblastoma in four siblings. *N Engl J Med, 277:*1230-1236, 1967.
7. Sy, W., and Edmonson, J.H.: The developmental defects associated with neuroblastoma; etiologic implications. *Cancer, 22:*234-238, 1968.
8. Whang-Peng, J., and Bennett, J.: Cytogenetic studies in metastatic neuroblastoma. *Am J Dis Child, 115:*703-708, 1968.
9. Levan, A., Manolov, G., and Clifford, P.: Chromosomes of a human neuroblastoma; a new case with accessory minute chromosomes. *J Natl Cancer Inst, 41:*1377-1386, 1968.
10. Cox, D.: Chromosome studies in 12 solid tumors from children. *Br J Cancer, 22:*402-414, 1968.
11. Beckwith, J.B., and Martin, R.: Observations on the histopathology of neuroblastomas. *J Pediatr Surg, 3:(Part. 11):* 106-110, 1968.
12. Surgical Fellows of the American Academy of Pediatrics: Survey of 10 years experience in the management of neuroblastoma. *J Pediatr Surg: 3(Part II):*191-193, 1968.
13. Hamilton, J., and Koop, C.E.: Ganglioneuromas in children. *Surg Gynec Obstet, 21:*803-812, 1965.
14. Haber, S., and Bennington, J.: Maturation of congenital extra-adrenal neuroblastoma. *Arch Pathol, 76:*121-125, 1963.
15. Eyre-Brook, A., and Hewer, T.F.: Spontaneous disappearance of neuroblastoma with maturation to ganglioneuroma. *J Bone Joint Surg, 44:* 882-890, 1962.
16. Visfeldt, J.: Transformation of sympathicoblastoma into ganglioneuroma. *Acta Pathol Microbiol Scand, 58:*414-428, 1963.
17. Wilkerson, J., Van De Water, J.M., and Goepfert, H.: Role of embryonic induction in benign transformation of neuroblastomas. *Cancer, 20:* 1335-1342, 1967.
18. Fox, F., Davidson, J., and Thomas, L.B.: Maturation of sympathicoblastoma into ganglioneuroma; report of two patients with 20 and 46 year survival respectively. *Cancer, 12:*108-116, 1959.
19. Greenfield, L., and Schelley, W.M.: The spectrum of neurogenic tumors of the sympathetic nervous system; maturation and adrenergic function. *J Natl Cancer Inst, 35:*215-223, 1965.
20. Bodian, M.: Neuroblastoma; an evaluation of its natural history and the effects of therapy with particular reference to treatment by massive doses of vitamin B_{12}. *Arch Dis Child, 38:*606-619, 1963.
21. Burdman, J., Goldstein, M., and Journey, L.: Long term tissue culture of neuroblastomas. *J Natl Cancer Inst, 32:*165-169, 1965.
22. Bolande, R., and Towler, W.F.: A possible relationship of neuroblastoma to Von Recklinghausen's disease. *Cancer, 26:*162-175, 1970.

23. Hellström, I., Hellström, K., and Pierce, G.: Cell-bound immune reactions against tumor-specific transplantation antigens. *Can Cancer Conference, 8*:425-442, 1969.
24. Everson, T., and Cole, W.H.: *Spontaneous Regression of Cancer*. Philadelphia, W.B. Saunders Company, 1966.
25. Beckwith, J., and Perrin, E.: *In situ* neuroblastomas; a contribution to the natural history of neural chest tumors. *Am J Pathol, 43*:1089-1104, 1963.
26. Tubergen, D., and Heyn, R.: *In situ* neuroblastoma associated with an adrenal cyst. *J Pediatr, 76*:451-453, 1970.
27. Shanklin, D., and Sotelo-Avila, C.: *In situ* tumors in fetuses, newborns and young infants. *Biol Neonate, 14*:286-316, 1969.
28. Guin, G.H., Gilbert, E., and Jones, B.: Incidental neuroblastoma in infants. *J Clin Pathol, 51*:126-136, 1969.
29. Martin, R., and Beckwith, J.B.: Lymphoid infiltrates in neuroblastomas; their occurrence and prognostic significance. *J Pediatr Surg, 3;(Part II)*:161-164, 1968.
30. Alfano, J.E.: Ophthalmological aspects of neuroblastomatosis: A study of 53 verified cases. *Trans Am Acad Ophthalmol Otolaryngol, 72*: 830-848, 1968.
31. Mortada, A.: Clinical characteristics of early orbital metastatic neuroblastoma. *Am J Ophthalmol, 63*:1787-1793, 1967.
32. Albert, D., Rubenstein, R.A., and Scheie, H.: Tumor metastasis to the eye; clinical study in infants and children. *Am J Opthalmol, 63*:727-732, 1967.
33. Obert, C., Devine, K., and McDonald, J.: Olfactory neuroblastomas. *Cancer, 13*:205-215, 1960.
34. Miller, R., Sterioff, S., Drucker, W.R. *et al.*: The incidental discovery of occult abdominal tumors in children following blunt abdominal trauma. *J Trauma, 6*:99-106, 1961.
35. Rice, M.S.: Neuroblastoma in childhood; a review of 69 cases. *Aust Pediatr J, 2*:1-15, 1966.
36. Simpson, T., Lynn, H., and Mills, S.: Congenital neuroblastoma in the scrotum. *Clin Pediatr, 8*:174-175, 1969.
37. Dargeon, H.: Neuroblastoma. *J Pediatr, 61*:456-471, 1962.
38. Shown, T., and Durfee, M.: Blueberry muffin baby; neonatal neuroblastoma with subcutaneous metastases. *J Urol, 104*:193-195, 1970.
39. Solomon, G., and Chutorian, A.M.: Opsoclonus and occult neuroblastoma. *N Engl J Med, 279*:475-477, 1968.
40. Bray, P.M., Ziter, F., Lahey, M.E., and Myers, G.: The coincidence of neuroblastoma and acute cerebellar encephalopathy. *J Pediatr, 75*: 983-990, 1969.
41. McMillan, C., Gaudry, C.L., and Holemans, R.: Coagulation defects and metastatic neuroblastoma. *J Pediatr, 72*:347-350, 1968.

42. Girolami, A.: A coagulation study in patients with neuroblastoma. *Tumori, 53*:495-502, 1967.
43. Finklestein, J., Ekert, H., Isaacs, H., and Higgins, G.: Bone marrow metastases in children with solid tumors. *Am J Dis Child, 119*:45-52, 1970.
44. Williams, C., Green, M.: Homovanillic acid and vanillylmandelic acid in diagnosis of neuroblastoma. *JAMA, 183*:134-138, 1963.
45. Schweioguth, O.: Excretion of catecholamine metabolites in urine of neuroblastoma patients. *J Pediatr Surg, 3 (Part II)*:118-120, 1968.
46. Voute, P., Wadman, S., and Van Putten, W.: Congenital neuroblastoma symptoms in the mother during pregnancy. *Clin Pediatr, 9*:206-207, 1970.
47. Gitlow, S., Bertani, L., Rausen, A. *et al.*: Diagnosis of neuroblastoma by qualitative and quantitative determination of catecholamine metabolites in urine. *Cancer, 25*:1377-1389, 1970.
48. Geiser, C., and Efron, M.L.: Cystathioninuria in patients with neuroblastoma or ganglioneuroblastoma; its correlation to vanilmandelic acid excretion and its value in diagnosis and therapy. *Cancer, 22*:856-860, 1968.
49. D'Angio, G., Loken, M., and Nesbit, M.: Radionuclear (^{75}Se) identification of tumor in children with neuroblastoma. *Radiology, 93*:615-617, 1969.
50. Evans, A., D'Angio, G., and Randolph, J.: A proposed staging for children with neuroblastoma. *Cancer, 27*:374-378, 1971.
51. D'Angio, G., Evans, A., and Koop, C.E.: Special pattern of widespread neuroblastoma with a favorable prognosis. *Lancet, 1*:1046-1049, 1971.
52. Koop, C.E.: The role of surgery in resectable, non-resectable and metastatic neuroblastoma. *JAMA, 205*:107-108, 1968.
53. Farman, J.V.: Neuroblastomas and anesthesia. *Br J Anaesth, 37*:866-869, 1965.
54. D'Angio, G.: Radiotherapy of Wilm's tumor and neuroblastoma. *Ohio State Med J, 65*:377-380, 1969.
55. Tefft, M., and Wittenborg, M.H.: Radiotherapeutic management of neuroblastoma in childhood. *JAMA, 205*:109-110, 1968.
56. Neuhauser, E., Wittenborg, M., Berman, C., and Cohen, J.: Irradiation effects of the roentgen therapy on the growing spine. *Radiology, 59*:637-650, 1952.
57. Tefft, M., Mitus, A., Das, L. *et al.*: Irradiation of the liver in children; review of experience in the acute and chronic phases and in the intact normal and partially resected. *Am J Roentgenol, 108*:365-385, 1970.
58. Rissanen, P.M.: Radiation therapy in neuroblastoma. *Radiol Clin North Am, 39*:9-19, 1970.
59. Young, L., Rubin, P., and Hanson, R.E.: The extra-adrenal neuroblastoma; high radiocurability and diagnostic accuracy. *Am J Roentgenol, 108*:75-91, 1970.

60. Thurman, W.G., Fernbach, D., and Sullivan, M.: Cyclophosphamide therapy in childhood neuroblastoma. *N Engl J Med, 270*:1336-1340, 1964.
61. James, D., Hustu, O., Wren, E., and Pinkel, D.: Combination chemotherapy of childhood neuroblastoma. *JAMA, 194*:123-126, 1965.
62. Windmiller, J., Berry, D.H., Haddy, T.B. *et al.*: Vincristine sulfate in the treatment of neuroblastoma in children. *Am J Dis Child, 111*: 75-78, 1966.
63. Thurman, W., and Donaldson, M.H.: Cyclophosphamide therapy for children with neuroblastoma. *Cancer Chemother Rep, 51*:399-401, 1967.
64. Sullivan, M., Nora, A., Kulapongs, P. *et al.*: Evaluation of vincristine sulfate and cyclophosphamide chemotherapy for metastatic neuroblastoma. *Pediatrics, 44*:685-694, 1969.
65. Evans, A., Heyn, R., Newton, W., and Leiken, S.: Vincristine sulfate and cyclophosphamide for children with metastatic neuroblastoma. *JAMA, 207*:1325-1327, 1969.
66. Finklestein, J., Hittle, R., and Hammond, G.: Evaluation of a high dose cyclophosphamide regimen in childhood tumors. *Cancer, 23*: 1239-1342, 1969.
67. Pinkel, D., Pratt, C., Holton, C. *et al.*: Survival of children with neuroblastoma treated with combination chemotherapy. *Pediatrics, 73*:928-931, 1968.
68. Sinks, L., and Woodruff, M.: Chemotherapy of neuroblastoma. *JAMA, 205*:111-116, 1968.
69. James, D.: Treatment of neuroblastoma in children by a cyclic program of vincristine and cyclophosphamide. *Cancer Chemother Rep, 51*:411-412, 1967.
70. Fernbach, D., Haddy, T., Holcomb, T. *et al.*: 1-Sarcolysin (NSC-8806) therapy for children with metastatic neuroblastoma. *Cancer Chemother Rep, 52*:293-296, 1968.
71. Sawitsky, A., and Desposito, F.: A survey of American experience with vitamin B_{12} therapy of neuroblastoma; pediatric pharmacology and therapeutics. *J Pediatr, 67*:99-103, 1965.
72. Langman, M.: Treatment of neuroblastoma with vitamin B_{12}. *Arch Dis Child, 45*:385-387, 1970.
73. Helson, L.: Personal communication, 1971.
74. Breslow, N., and McCann, B.: Estimating prognosis in neuroblastoma. *Cancer Res.* (In press, 1971.)
75. Sutow, W., Gehan, E., Heyn, R. *et al.:* Comparison of survival curves, 1956 versus 1962, in children with Wilm's tumor and neuroblastoma; report of the subcommittee on childhood solid tumors, solid tumor task force. National Cancer Institute. *Pediatrics, 45*:800-811, 1970.

Chapter 7

RHABDOMYOSARCOMA

Carl Pochedly

Rhabdomyosarcoma is a malignant tumor originating from rhabdomyoblasts, the embryonic precursors of striated muscle cells. It is the most common type of sarcoma of the somatic soft tissues of infants and children. It ranks fourth in frequency among childhood solid tumors, behind brain tumors, neuroblastoma and Wilms' tumor.[1] Prior to 1958, it was not appreciated that rhabdomyosarcomas might present with any one of several seemingly unrelated histopathological patterns. For this reason, many of the cases were not recognized and the reported incidence of rhabdomyosarcoma in children was inaccurate.[2]

Rhabdomyosarcomas show very variable gross characteristics, rate of growth and histological appearance; they affect individuals of both sexes and all ages. They have been observed to occur in nearly every part of the body but they are found more frequently in certain systems and regions (Table 7-1). They tend to occur in the genitourinary tract, the head and neck, and in the striated musculature of the trunk and extremities. Sporadic occurrence has been noted in the heart, ovary, kidney, upper respiratory tract, upper gastrointestinal tract, biliary tree, breast[3] and brain. They are found in all parts of the body and not only where striated muscle is found. Thus, the tumors occurring adjacent to the bladder, in the kidneys, prostate, spermatic cord and biliary tree do not originate where striated muscle is normally found.

COMMON CLINICAL AND LABORATORY FEATURES

The most common sign and symptom is a "mass," being the presenting complaint in as many as 90 percent of patients.[4] Other signs and symptoms vary with the site of origin of the tumor.

TABLE 7-1
ANATOMIC DISTRIBUTION OF 290 RHABDOMYOSARCOMAS

Location	*Embryonal*	*Alevolar*	*Pleomorphic*	*Total*	
Orbit	66	13		79	
Soft tissue of head and neck	22	10	2	34	
Maxilla	11	5	1	17	52%
Nasopharynx	16	1		17	
Middle ear	2			2	
Larynx	1			1	
Chest wall	5	3	1	9	
Mediastinum	1		1	2	
Diaphragm			1	1	
Upper extremities	7	10	4	21	33%
Lower extremities	19	11	13	43	
Retroperitoneum	19			19	
Common bile duct	3			3	
Abdominal cavity	3	2		11	
Urinary bladder	11			11	
Testis	3	2		5	10%
Vagina	14			14	
Perineum	5	2		7	
Total	208	59	23	290	

From Albores-Saavedra.[30]

Rhabdomyosarcomas of the orbit almost always present with proptosis and diplopia.[5] In rhabdomyosarcoma of the urinary tract patients present with bleeding and obstructive uropathy[6]; in the biliary tract with obstructive jaundice[7]; in the middle ear with bleeding and otitis media.[8]

The multiplicity of these tumor nodules, each discrete and separate, is often not appreciated. Identical small tumors may be encountered in adjacent muscles, although preoperatively only the major lesion was detected. This has led to the conclusion that rhabdomyosarcoma is occasionally multicentric in origin, it offers the logical reason why radical dissection should include removal of the entire muscle in which the tumor develops and even the group of muscles, if more than one are involved by the multicentric tumor process.[9]

Rhabdomyosarcoma in children, despite its highly malignant character, may appear benign when observed early. It may present as an apparently well-demarcated nodule in soft tissue or as a harmless-looking polypoid structure at a body orifice. The most common primary site is in the head and neck region, where it may arise from middle ear, maxillary sinus, palate, nasopharynx, orbit, parotid area, face, neck or upper esophagus. In the pelvic area it may arise from vagina, bladder, prostate or anus. Extremities, trunk and common bile duct may also bear primary tumors. Often the lesion extends far beyond its apparent borders; cell infiltrates may grow along muscle planes to form grossly imperceptible satellite lesions. Rhabdomyosarcomas may be seen at any time during childhood. They spread rapidly, infiltrating locally and metastasizing to lungs, bone and other organs. Bone marrow aspiration may reveal tumor cells even in the absence of x-ray findings.[10]

In general, rhabdomyosarcomas are rapidly growing tumors. Like most types of soft tissue sarcomas, rhabdomyosarcomas are insidiously invasive, although they may appear to be circumscribed or even encapsulated. Local recurrence is frequent, but distant metastasis is even more common. Rhabdomyosarcomas may metastasize either by way of the bloodstream or by way of the lymphatics.[11]

Anemia may be present at the time of the initial diagnosis in children with disseminated disease. When there is hepatic involvement, the liver enzymes (SGOT, alkaline phosphatase and LDH) may be elevated.[12] With disseminated disease there may be elevation of coagulation factor levels (especially factors I, V, VIII, IX and XI) with an associated shortening of the whole blood clotting time and the partial thromboplastin time.[13,14]

Bone marrow examination may reveal metastatic tumor cells (Fig. 7-1).[15,16] Metastatic rhabdomyosarcoma cells may also be found in pleural fluid (pleural effusion), peritonal fluid (ascites) or spinal fluid by cytologic techniques.[17] Hypoglycemia has been reported to occur with large rhabdomyosarcomas. The cause is not known. Improvement of the hypoglycemia frequently occurs after treatment of the tumor by surgery, radiation therapy or chemotherapy.[18-21]

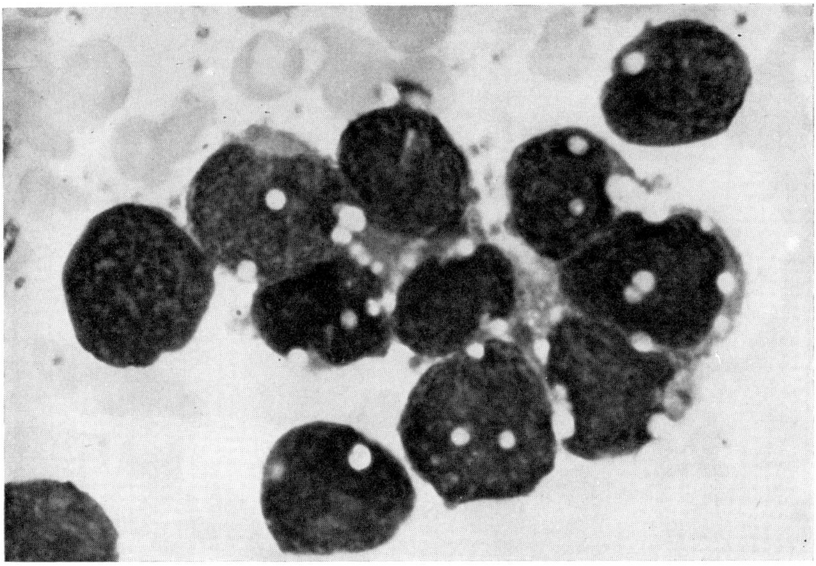

Figure 7-1. Bone marrow smear showing a clump of rhabdomyoblasts in a child with disseminated rhabdomyosarcoma. (Courtesy of Dr. Jerry Finkelstein.)

X-ray examination may reveal metastatic lesions in the lungs or bones.[22] Mediastinal metastases (Fig. 7-2) and bony destruction due to orbital or nasal sinus lesions may be seen on x-ray. Calcific densities may also be present in soft tissue tumors.[23] The skeletal x-ray findings in children with metastatic rhabdomyosarcoma include collapse of vertebrae; destructive lesions in the ileum with compression fracture of the roof of the acetabulum; destructive foci in the skull; calcifications in the kidneys; spinal cord compression (Fig. 7-3); and destruction in the metaphysis of the femurs and tibias.[22] These x-ray changes may also be seen in other common childhood malignancies, neuroblastoma and Wilms' tumor. Isotopic liver scans may reveal discrete liver metastases.

Staging

Determining the antomic extent of the disease, clinical stage, is an important factor in planning treatment, in estimating prognosis and in analysis of survival data in the child with rhabdo-

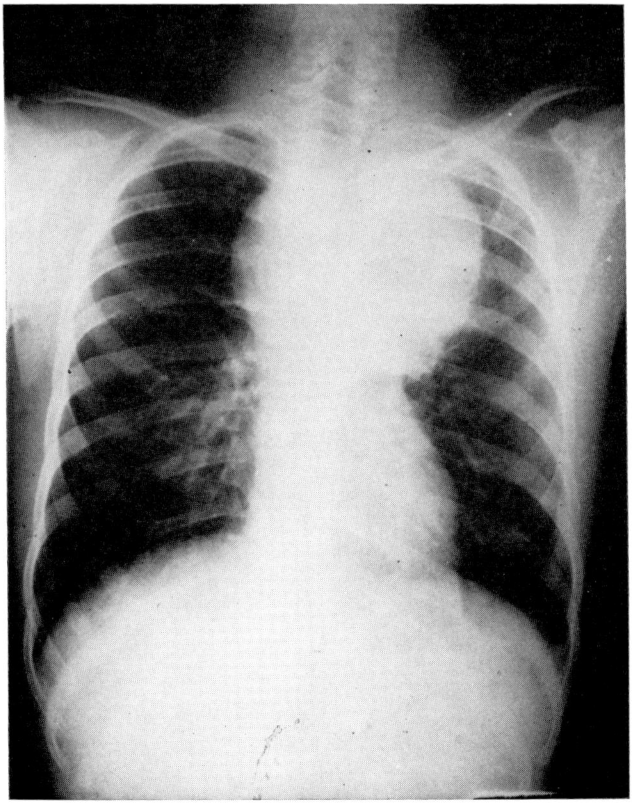

Figure 7-2. Chest x-ray showing a large superior mediastinal metastasis from rhabdomyosarcoma in the right thigh. The child's presenting symptom was cough and chest pain.

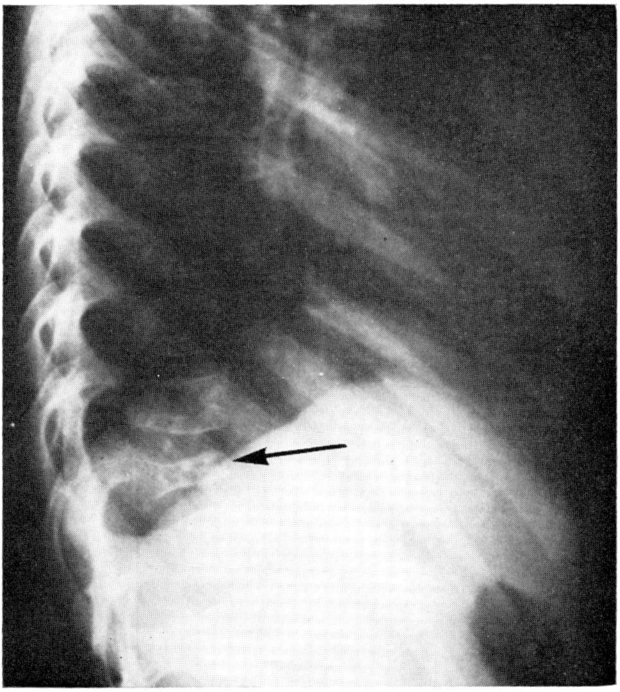

Figure 7-3. Lateral x-ray of spine showing collapse of T-11 (arrow) in a three-year-old child with rhabdomyosarcoma of the hypopharynx. Complete paraplegia ensued. Generalized demineralization is also present.

myosarcoma. The anatomical and clinical criteria for staging of rhabdomyosarcomas[24] are outlined in Table 7-2. Certain studies

TABLE 7-2
CLINICAL STAGING OF CHILDHOOD RHABDOMYOSARCOMA[24]

Stage I — Localized disease, completely resectable

Stage II — Regional disease

A. Completely resectable

B. Nonresectable or partially resectable, for example pelvic lymph node involvement from sarcoma botryoides, infiltration of base of skull from nasopharyngeal primary.

Stage III — Generalized disease

A. Distant metastases with normal bone marrow (pulmonary metastases or disease above and below the diaphragm)

B. Distant metastases with positive bone marrow; pulmonary metastases may or may not be present.

should be completed to accurately stage a tumor in a child in whom a histological diagnosis of rhabdomyosarcoma has been proven:

1. Past history, with careful attention to systemic symptoms, such as fatigue, fever or weight loss.
2. Physical examination, with special attention to palpation of skeletal muscles, genitalia and abdomen.
3. Complete blood count, platelet count, reticulocyte count, red cell sedimentation rate and urinalysis.
4. Liver function tests, especially alkaline phosphatase, SGOT (serum glutamic oxaloacetic transaminase), bilirubin and LDH (lactic dehydrogenase); also determine total serum protein, protein electrophoresis, blood uric acid, and blood glucose.
5. Posteroanterior and lateral x-ray films of chest.
6. X-ray examination of skull and long bones.
7. Intravenous pyelogram.
8. Bone marrow examination, preferably with needle biopsy technic.[25]
9. Isotopic liver scan, if indicated.
10. Liver biopsy, if indicated.

HISTOPATHOLOGY AND TISSUE DIAGNOSIS

In 1946 Stout published his classical paper on the histopathology of skeletal muscle tumors.[4] He studied 121 cases of rhabdomyosarcoma of the soft parts of the head and neck, trunk, and extremities; twenty-five of these cases involved children. But no mention was made of specific tumor subtypes. In 1950, Stobbe and Dargeon reported their concept of an embryonal form of rhabdomyosarcoma that they recognized in the head and neck regions of children.[26] Then Riopelle and Theriault called attention to the alveolar type of rhabdomyosarcoma.[27] Finally, in 1958 Horn and Enterline reported a clinicopathologic study of thirty-nine cases of rhabdomyosarcoma and, on the basis of the gross and microscopic features of the tumors, separated them into four types—namely, embryonal, alveolar, botryoid and pleomorphic.[28] Recognition and accurate diagnosis of some of these tumors, however, is still a matter of considerable concern to pathologists, particularly with those cases that are poorly differentiated and lack clearly discernible rhabdomyoblasts.[29]

Each type of rhabdomyosarcoma has special pathological and clinical features. The pleomorphic variant develops chiefly in the extremities of persons in the older age groups. It is resistant to chemotherapy and radiotherapy.[30,31] The alveolar variant usually arises in the extremities or the head and neck of adolescents and young adults.[32,33] It is almost always intimately associated with striated musculature. The embryonal type, in contrast, rarely occurs in the extremities and tends to involve the region of the orbits, the nasopharynx and the urogenital tract of children below ten years of age.[34,35] Botryoid (grape-like) rhabdomyosarcomas occur in relation to mucous membrane. They occur in the genitourinary tract, common bile duct or the lower rectum and anus, as well as in the ear and nasal cavities. With rare exceptions, these tumors make their appearance before the age of five years and in about half of these cases before the age of two years.[36]

Histologic diagnosis of the rhabdomyosarcoma is often difficult. The presence of cross striations puts the matter beyond doubt, but in those tumors where there are less definite and more primitive rhabdomyoblasts the diagnosis is uncertain. The site of the tumor may support the diagnosis; rhabdomyosarcomas tend to occur in the lower genital tract, orbit, middle ear and pterygoid fossa. In such sites the pathologist may be justified in suspecting a striated muscle origin in a largely undifferentiated sarcoma.[36]

It is presumed that embryonal rhabdomyosarcomas originate from primitive mesenchyme. This presumption is based on the fact that these tumors reproduce certain histological qualities that characterize developmental phases of striated muscle as seen in embryos of three to twelve weeks.[37] Many rhabdomyosarcomas, especially those in young children, contain undifferentiated myxoma-like tissue closely resembling embryonic mesenchyme.[33,38]

The diagnosis of childhood embryonal rhabdomyosarcoma is often difficult or impossible to establish by light microscopy alone. In such cases a tissue diagnosis may be established by use of electron microscopy, immunofluorescent technique to detect myosin and tissue culture of the tumor.[39] The ultrastructure of embryonal rhabdomyosarcoma has been described.[40-43] Only rarely are thick and thin filaments and primitive Z-bands discernible on electron microscopy, but when present they confirm the fact that these are indeed myofilaments and thus establish the diagnosis.[41,44] Thus, electron microscopic examination can support a diagnosis of rhabdomyosarcoma in certain cases of malignant mesenchymal neoplasms which have recognizable diagnostic features except that cytoplasmic striations are not seen.[44] In the immunofluorescent test for myosin, rhabdomyosarcoma cells show a positive reaction.[45] By this technique one can prove that certain filaments seen on electron microscopy are actually myofilaments, thus providing strong evidence for a striated muscle origin of the tumor.[39] Rhabdomyosarcoma cells can readily be grown in tissue culture.[46,47]

CLINICAL MANIFESTATIONS OF RHABDOMYOSARCOMAS IN CHILDREN

The range of clinical manifestations of rhabdomyosarcomas is kaleidoscopic. Rhabdomyosarcomas may occur anywhere in the body since they originate from primitive mesenchymal elements. However they most frequently occur in three locations: head and neck, skeletal muscles of trunk and limbs, and genitourinary tract.

Head and Neck

Rhabdomyosarcoma of the head and neck in children is usually a relentless, progressive tumor which results in the death of a child in a relatively short time. Origin of the primary tumor in the head and neck area is much more common in children than in adults. The histological type of tumor most commonly originating in the head and neck is the embryonal rhabdomyosarcoma. Botryoid rhabdomyosarcomas may occur in the ear, nose and paranasal sinuses. Alveolar rhabdomyosarcomas rarely originate in the head and neck of children.

The first complaint in nearly all patients is a mass, regardless of whether the disease originates in the region of the eye, nasopharynx, ear, side of face, or neck. Bulging of an eye, difficulty in swallowing, obstruction of breathing, nasal obstruction, change in voice quality, cough and discharge from the ear are other symptoms noted. There is pain if the tumor involves a nerve. The rapidity of the expansite and infiltrative growth increases the severity of complaints, and ultimately there may be manifestations of cerebral involvement. When metastases are present, symptoms relating to the organs involved exist.[26] Since these tumors grow rapidly, there is seldom delay of more than a few weeks from the time of discovery of the tumor to the initial examination by a physician.

Rhabdomyosarcoma of the Orbit

Rhabdomyosarcomas may originate in the orbicularis occuli muscles, from any of the extrinsic muscles of the eye, or from the lacrimal glands. Rhabdomyosarcoma of the orbit, once considered a rare tumor, has been recognized with increasing frequency. In fact, recent experience suggests that this is the most common malignant orbital tumor occurring in childhood.[48-52] Rhabdomyosarcoma causes florid and rapidly progressive unilateral exophthalmos in children, usually at the age of seven or eight years. Rhabdomyosarcoma of the orbit appears to be exclusively a disease of infants, children and young adults. In one series 90 percent of the patients were under fifteen years of age.[48] It involves males somewhat more frequently than females.[5,48] A history of trauma to the eye is usually not elicited and there appears to be no definite hereditary or familial influence.[5] Because of its relative frequency and very poor prognosis, rhabdomyosarcoma is one of the most important orbital lesions to be considered in the differential diagnosis of unilateral proptosis in childhood.

Nearly all patients exhibit exophthalmos and usually this is the first sign or symptom to appear (Fig. 7-4). The most striking feature of the exophthalmos is its rapid and even alarming progression. Either at onset or shortly thereafter about one-third of the patients show a drooping of the upper lid. In about one-quarter of the patients a discrete mass can be palpated. But the ability to palpate a discrete mass depends to some extent on the length of time after onset when the palpation is attempted; the

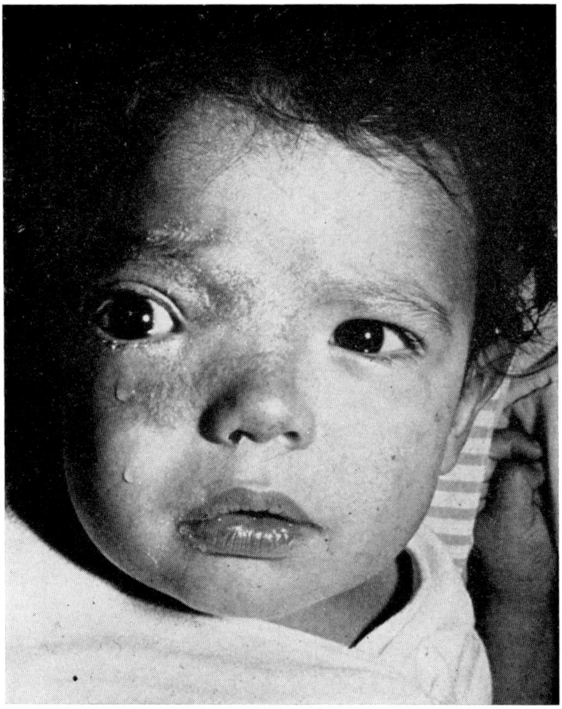

Figure 7-4. Unilateral proptosis erythema, and tearing in a child with rhabdomyosarcoma originating in the right ethmoid sinus. The affected eye is displaced laterally. The tumor is also seen projecting from the right nostril. (Courtesy of Dr. Otto Campos.)

longer the growth has progressed, the less likely it is that a discrete mass will be detected. About 10 percent of the patients complain of pain or headache, usually not well localized, being referred to the forehead over the affected eye. Tearing may also be complained of, often very early in the course of the disease.[5] The clinical evidence in favor of a diagnosis of orbital rhabdomyosarcoma includes the age of the patient and the rapidity of progression of the exophthalmos. Laboratory studies may be of little help. Some cases show slightly increased orbital dimensions by x-ray examination on the affected side as compared to the unaffected side, others show erosion of bone on x-ray examination (Fig. 7-5).

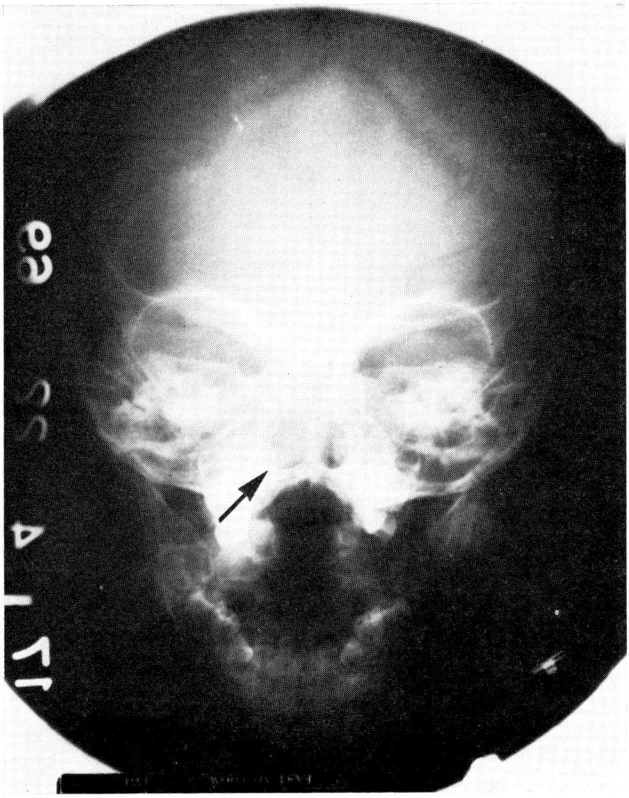

Figure 7-5. Anteroposterior view of the skull (Towne's view) of the child in Figure 7-4. An osteolytic lesion is seen in the right ethmoid area. There appears to be a homogeneous mass filling the right nasal cavity as well as the ethmoid sinus and possibly protruding into the medial wall of the right orbit. There is decalcification of bone in this region.

The differential diagnosis includes infantile hemangioma, leukemia and neuroblastoma. The possibility of infantile hemangioma will usually be considered only in patients in the newborn period or within the first five or six months of life since this is the period during which the florid phase of an orbital hemangioma may occur. The majority of such cases will show skin stigmas which make the diagnosis clear, but an occasional hemangioma will be obscure and might be confused with rhabdomyosarcoma.

Leukemia, of course, often occurs in the same age group as that affected by rhabdomyosarcoma; this diagnosis can usually be confirmed or excluded by examination of the blood and bone marrow. Neuroblastoma most commonly does not involve the orbit until the disease is well advanced in other locations, notably in the abdomen. Consequently, the diagnosis will usually have been made before the orbit becomes involved. The diagnosis in rhabdomyosarcoma of the orbit, however, must always be a tissue diagnosis. A child with unilateral exophthalmos should have a detailed neurological examination, including carotid angiography and brain scan, even in the absence of symptoms and signs of intracranial extension.[53]

Multilating surgery to the eye of a child is entered upon with great reluctance. For this reason, many earlier reports of the results of surgery in orbital rhabdomyosarcoma have been unduly pessimistic.[54,55] There appears to be no doubt that orbital exenteration cures about half the cases of rhabdomyosarcoma of this region. But cure is possible only if the tumor is confined to the orbit and no distant matastases are present. The ophthalmologist may be urged to withhold surgery until a trial of radiation therapy,[56] or chemotherapy, or both, has been carried out. This procrastination may have a disastrous effect on the final outcome.[5,57] A few cases or orbital rhabdomyosarcoma were treated initially by regional perfusion followed by exenteration. The results were not better than exenteration alone.[58]

Rhabdomyosarcoma of the Ear

Rhabdomyosarcoma may occur in the external auditory canal, the middle ear, the mastoid or the paranasal sinuses.[59,60] The tumors may be either the embryonal or botryoid type. Rhabdomyosarcomas account for the vast majority of malignant temporal bone tumors in children.[61]

Embryonal rhabdomyosarcoma frequently presents as a painless tumor in the axis of the eustachian tube or the first branchial pouch and cleft. There is usually a lytic lesion in the adjacent bony structure of the head. This tumor may be associated with a drainage from the ear similar to a chronic otitis media.[62,63] It often presents with a painless, foul-smelling discharge and mass of granulation tissue in the external or middle ear, the appearance of which is not unlike inflammatory polyps of the ear.[61] In case where ear infections do not promptly improve on antibiotic therapy, this unusual tumor should be suspected, especially in young children.[8]

Embryonal rhabdomyosarcoma affects one ear only, the other being normal. The most common presenting symptoms are a triad of otitis media, polypoid mass in the external ear and bloody discharge from the ear. Less commonly the presenting symptom is an external mass posterior to the ear. The mass usually grows very rapidly. Even though it is first noted as a small insignificant soft prominence, it may have grown to an alarming degree before the next observation. The absence of pain may explain why the tumor frequently progresses rapidly to an advanced stage before it is discovered. Occasionally, paralysis of paresis of the facial nerve is a presenting symptom. Even when the facial nerve is not affected when the patient first presents, it is involved almost invariably during the course of the disease due to the progressive destruction of the contents of the middle ear. Vertigo is a relatively late symptom which follows facial paralysis.[62,63] Hearing loss is often present but may not be noted in a child because it is unilateral.

The biological behavior of this tumor is such that it is invasive locally and has a tendency for early spread out of the temporal bone into surrounding structures. The tumor spreads from the middle ear to involve the mastoid and from there breaks through the inner cortex to the posterior fossa.[64-66] The tumor may invade the brain stem and cause unilateral cranial nerve paresis.[67]

Radiological examination should consist of a regular skull examination, including the Towne and Caldwell views and both lateral projections. Axial and semiaxial views of the skull are important because they demonstrate the carotid canal and jugular fossa to the best advantage. These areas are the first involved with direct extention of the tumor from the middle ear. Furthermore, in some cases in which the skull x-rays are normal when the patient is first seen, extensive destruction in the area of the mastoid process and petrous pyramid may take place within a few weeks.[8]

In some cases the routine skull films fail to demonstrate bone destruction but laminagrams of the petrous bones taken at the same time reveal extensive destruction of the bony external auditory canal and the bony wall of the middle ear. This would suggest that in all cases involving a polyp of the external auditory canal, otitis media and bloody discharge, a complete radiological examination including the skull films and laminagraphic studies of the petrous pyramid should be done.[8] Demonstration of bone destruction by x-ray helps confirm the histopathological diagnosis. Also, demonstration of bone destruction preoperatively will enable the surgeon to plan a more rational surgical attack and enable the radiotherapist to plan his treatment portals more accurately.

Rhabdomyosarcoma of the middle ear is an aggressive and lethal tumor of children. The benign early symptoms are followed by local and regional recurrence and distant metastasis. Early and radical surgery combined with x-ray therapy and chemotherapy is indicated.[66] Surgery almost always consists of radical mastoidectomy. The dose of radiation therapy has varied from 2,200 to 9,000 rads to the base of the skull. With this therapy early rapid regression of the visible tumor usually follows. Unfortunately, there is also rapid recurrence of the local tumor. Treatment usually has no effect on tumor which has invaded bone.[8]

Rhabdomyosarcomas of Mouth and Neck Muscles

Rhabdomyosarcomas may originate in any of a large number of foci in the mouth and neck. They may originate in the floor of the mouth,[68,69] tongue,[2,70,71] uvula,[72] soft palate,[26,73] hard palate,[31] nasopharynx,[74] larynx,[2,31,75-77] lip,[79,80] nose,[1] gingiva,[73,82] temple,[74] cheek,[10,31,73,82-84] muscles of the mandible (masseters),[4,26,46,68,73,79] area of the parotid gland[26,73] and muscles of the neck.[26,46,73,86] The tumors are usually embryonal rhabdomyosarcomas, but occasionally the alveolar type occurs. Superficial tumors are discovered as simply painless masses. They may appear deceptively benign when first noted.[11,35] Tumors in the larynx in small children may present with hoarseness and acute respiratory obstruction requiring tracheostomy (Fig. 7-6).[77,78,87] Therapy consists of ablative surgery, x-ray therapy and chemotherapy; but prolonged survival is rare.

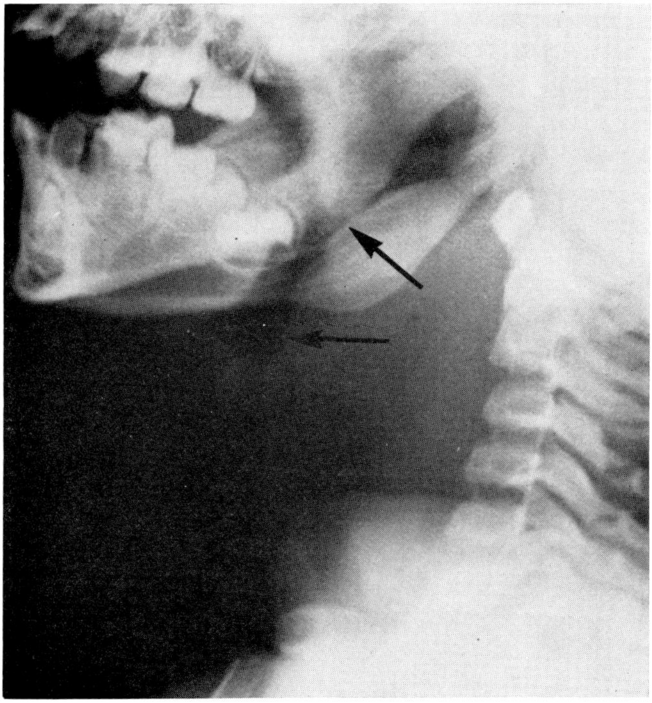

Figure 7-6. Lateral x-ray of the pharynx showing a very large soft tissue mass displacing and compressing the trachea anteriorly. Arrows indicate anterior borders of the mass.

Trunk, Limbs and Limb Girdles

Rhabdomyosarcomas of the trunk and extremities may be any of three types: embryonal, alveolar or pleomorphic. The embryonal type is most common, especially in children; the alveolar type is more malignant; the pleomorphic type occurs at all ages, but is much more common in the older age groups. The lesions are rapid growing and are usually fairly large by the time the patient comes to clinical attention. Trauma plays no role in the causation of rhabdomyosarcomas, but the limb or part containing the tumor is more predisposed to injury. In fact, treatment has often been delayed due to a presumptive diagnosis of "charley-horse." Some patients may be able to recall trauma to the approximate location in the body where a muscle tumor subsequently developed.[88] But when we consider the number of bruised arms and shins which fall to the lot of the average child, it seems safe to disregard trauma as an etiological factor.[9] In addition to those occurring in the limbs and limb girdles, rhabdomyosarcomas not uncommonly occur in skeletal muscles of the chest, abdominal wall and back (retroperitoneum).* Similar tumors of skeletal muscles occur in domestic animals.[91,96]

As in most instances of soft tissue sarcoma, symptoms contribute little of diagnostic significance for this group of tumors. The first symptom is usually a mass; pain may also be present. There may be brawny edema of the distal portion of the involved extremity; there may be ulceration of the skin overlying the tumor mass.[97] Metastasis may be demonstrable at the time of diagnosis.

It is surprising that metastases do not invariably occur, if we consider the fact that the involved muscles contract forcibly on the enclosed rhabdomyosarcoma. Spread of the tumor occurs both by local infiltration and by distant metastases. Locally the tumor spreads readily along the fascial planes and along the intermuscular spaces.[9] Rhabdomyosarcomas have an abundant vascular supply and tend to metastasize early to the lungs. Generalized metastases to bone, skin, brain and viscera are rare. The spinal column is sometimes secondarily involved. Rhabdomyosarcomas also metastaze through lymph vessels to regional lymph nodes.[9] The anatomic sites of metastases in a series of 204 patients with rhabdomyosarcoma of the trunk and extremities in one series[98] were lungs 30 percent; regional lymph nodes, 15 percent; liver, 7 percent; bone, 7 percent; and subcutaneous tissues, 6 percent. The tumor may also metastasize to the pleura, kidney, adrenal glands, mediastinum, pericardium, pancreas, ovary and brain.[72] The clinical course of rhabdomyosarcomas varies greatly. Some tumors run a fulminating course with early distant metastasis and

*See the following references: 1, 4, 9, 10, 28, 30, 89, 90.

death within a year, while others display an indolent potential and metastasize only after several local recurrences.

In one series of one hundred cases of untyped rhabdomyosarcomas, the upper extremity including the shoulder was involved in thirty-four cases and the lower extremity, including the buttocks and groin, was the site of the tumor in fifty-four cases.[9] There was thus a predilection for the lower extremity and particularly for the thigh muscles. Other large series of embryonal rhabdomyosarcomas[34,97] gave similar findings. A striking finding regarding site of origin of embryonal rhabdomyosarcoma is a predilection for lesions of the extremities in female patients and a high frequency of retroperitoneal lesions among male patients.[34] As is the case with many types of malignant neoplasms, some of these tumors have extremely rapid growth while under observation and others are slower in terms of clinical "growth rate." Retroperitoneal and pelvic lesions often demonstrate rapid growth, while tumors in other sites usually have a more indolent growth pattern.[34]

In one series of 109 cases of *alveolar* rhabdomyosarcoma, the median age of all patients at time of diagnosis was fifteen years.[32] The muscles and surrounding soft tissues of the upper extremities, the lower extremities and the trunk were almost equally affected. A slightly smaller number involved the head and neck region. The forearms and the hands, especially the flexor muscles and the muscles of the hypothenar eminance, were commonly affected. In the perianal, perineal and perirectal region there were sixteen cases. The median survival time following diagnosis was only nine months.[32]

Twelve cases of rhabdomyosarcoma arising within the skeletal muscle of the hand were studied.[99] The cell type in nine was alveolar; two, pleomorphic; and one, embryonal. These tumors have been uniformly fatal regardless of treatment. Alveolar rhabdomyosarcomas located in the head and neck region, chest wall and perineum have a higher incidence of local recurrence than those located in the extremities. If the tumor is treated conservatively, it will invariably recur, regardless of the anatomic site, and later will metastasize. The regional lymph nodes, lungs and bones are the most common site of metastasis. Massive bone marrow replacement and compression of the spinal cord, resulting from metastases to the vertebral bodies, are seen fairly often.[31,100]

In one study 204 patients with *pleomorphic* rhabdomyosarcoma were reviewed.[98] This is a tumor of advancing years, only 6.3 percent of these patients were under fifteen years old. In another series, eighty-seven patients with pleomorphic rhabdomyosarcoma in the extremities were studied.[101] Lesions of the upper extremity had a better prognosis than those of the lower extremity, and the more distal lesions had a better prognosis than the more proximal lesions. The survival rate was higher among patients having superficial tumors than among those having deeply-seated tumors. Pleomorphic rhabdomyosarcomas exhibit a wide spectrum of growth and metastatic potential. There does not seem to be any correlation between clinical behavior and the histological pattern.[101]

There is a high rate of local recurrence of rhabdomyosarcomas after local excision. Radical surgical ablation by *en bloc* excision or amputation affords the best chance for survival.[101] Rhabdomyosarcomas are often multicentric; palpable tumor nodules may exist in superior segments of the muscle, which may grow and be discovered later if the muscle is not entirely removed.[9] Although these tumors are encapsulated, microscopic tumor tissue extends far beyond the tumor's apparent boundaries. Thus, surgical excision should include all the tissue proximal to the insertion and origin of the muscle and also the fascial structures that surround them.[90,102] About one-third of treated cases survive for five years.[98]

Genitourinary Tract

Rhabdomyosarcomas may occur in association with nearly all the organs of the genitourinary tract, but they occur most commonly in the urinary bladder and vagina. In boys they also occur in the testes, prostate and spermatic cords. In girls they occur in the cervix, uterus and ovaries. Tumors occurring in the bladder and in the vagina are the botryoid type. In other locations the tumors are embryonal in type. Botyroid rhabdomyosarcoma is usually a tumor of infancy. These grape-like tumors often show a close resemblance to the gross and histologic appearance of allergic polyps of the nasal mucosa. Thus, their malignant nature may not be immediately recognized. Tumors with similar gross and microscopic features have also been found in the common bile duct, anus, nasopharynx, middle ear and maxillary antrum. They also occur in the bladder of dogs.[103-105] In portions of botryoid rhabdomyosarcomas invading viscera or in visceral metastases, the usual histologic features of the embryonal type of tumor are seen.[37]

Botryoid Rhabdomyosarcoma of the Urinary Bladder

While these tumors are rare in terms of overall bladder malignancy, they constitute the most common form of bladder malignancy in children.[6] The great majority of botryoid rhabdomyosarcomas of the bladder appear during the first three to four years of life. There is a male predominance of 2.5:1.[107] The tumors originate in the submucosal and superficial muscular layer at the base of the bladder. The bulk of the tumor is a mass of pearly-grey grape-like lobules (Fig. 7-7). The tumors may also extend down the urethra through the membranous portion of the male or for the whole length of the female urethra. Similar extension upwards into the ureters may occur. A vaginal or labial tumor

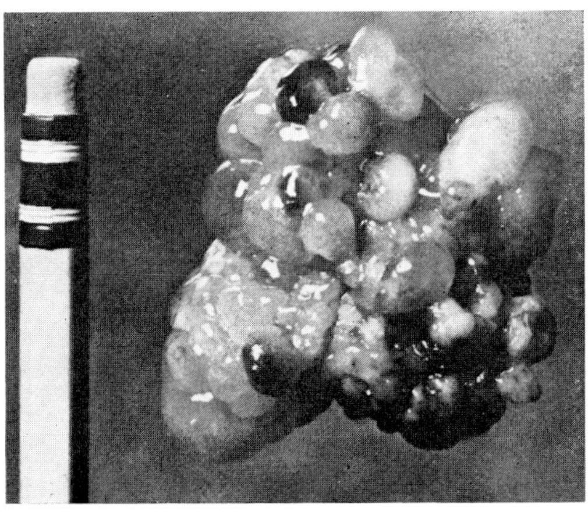

Figure 7-7. Botryoid rhabdomyosarcoma removed from the urinary bladder of a child, showing the typical "bunch of grapes" appearance. (Courtesy of Dr. R. Flocks and the *Journal of Urology, 73*:300, 1955.)[109]

may involve the bladder by upward expansion. The lobules may extend into the posterior urethra, causing obstruction.[108] In girls the tumor, in a high proportion of cases, prolapses down these urethra to present at the vulva.[106] The initial complaint in small children with botryoid rhabdomyosarcoma of the bladder may be recurring abdominal pain, pain on urination, hematuria, retention of urine, straining on urination, or recurring cystitis. The obstructive element is often severe and may be complicated by infection. Some degree of upper tract dilatation is the rule and uremia may be present on admission.

On physical examination the bladder is palpably distended and tense; the suprapubic mass does not disappear on catheterization. On rectal examination the bladder is evidently firmer than would be expected in simple retention. Most infants and children with this tumor manifest early hematuria, dysuria and a palpable, tender suprapubic mass, not reduced by catheterization.

In the intravenous pylogram the upper urinary tract shows dilation from back pressure.[109] Cystogram reveals multiple, smooth filling defects at the bladder base (Fig. 7-8).[110] On cystoscopic examination the typical grey, polypoid, edematous grape-like

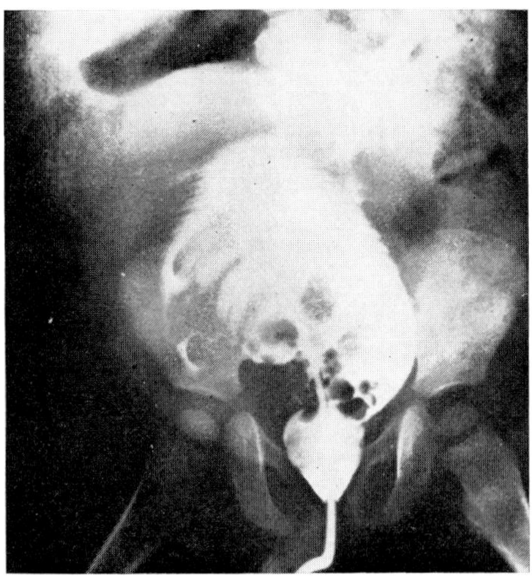

Figure 7-8. Cystogram showing lobulated filling defect in the bladder due to botryoid rhabdomyosarcoma. (Courtesy of Dr. D. Innes Williams and the *British Journal of Urology, 36*:51-55, 1964.)[108]

tumors are seen filling the bladder. But the cystoscope may fail to negotiate the vesical neck if the latter is obstructed by the neoplasm.[111]

Gross examination of the bladder shows multiple, soft, myxomatous, polypoid, grape-like clusters arising from the trigone, the bladder neck, the vesical orifice, or sometimes covering the entire inner surface of the bladder.[6,112] The term "rhabdomyosarcoma" implies, of course, that striated muscle cells are present, but fundamentally, these tumors are embryonic sarcomas; much of the tissue consists of immature mesenchyme which undergoes a variable degree of differentiation to striated muscle, to connective tissue and possibly to smooth muscle.[6,108] Many hypotheses have been suggested regarding the histogenesis of botryoid rhabdomyosarcomas.[107] Some have suggested dysontogenetic origin from embryonal cell rests along the course of the wolffian or mullerian ducts. Others believe the tumors originate from the mesenchyme of the urogenital ridge.[113]

Botryoid rhabdomyosarcomas of the bladder usually do not have metastases at time of initial diagnosis. When spread occurs it may be to the local lymph nodes or by bloodstream to the lungs and liver as well as by direct invasion of adjacent organs.[108]

Radical surgery is indicated. In boys this means cystectomy, prostatectomy, possibly including removal of the bulbous urethra.[114,115] In girls, total cystectomy and anterior exenteration would seem to be the procedure of choice.[111,116] This tumor is comparatively insensitive to irradiation and furthermore, the presence of an obstructed and infected urinary tract renders radiation therapy an unsatisfactory form of preoperative treatment. The possibility that chemotherapy may be useful is still being explored.[117]

Once the diagnosis is established, radical surgery should be carried out as early as possible. Although the tumor spreads into the lumen, the infiltration is minimal. Thus, it will fill up the bladder and urethra; and in girls, it may present at the external urethral meatus. If a suprapubic cystostomy is done, the tumor fungates through it with great rapidity. Lymphatic and hematogenous metastases occur relatively late in the course of the disease, death usually resulting from hydronephrosis, pyelonephritis and uremia. Hence prompt, radical extirpative surgery will give the patient the best chance of cure.[110]

Botryoid Rhabdomyosarcoma of the Vagina

Botryoid rhabdomyosarcomas may arise from the lower part of the female genital tract both in adult women and in little girls. The large majority of cases make their appearance before the age of five years. There is a definite difference in the average age at which the tumor is first seen and in the number of cases reported from each of the three sites: body of the uterus, cervix and vagina. Tumors of the body of the uterus appear in the older age groups (from forty to sixty years) whereas tumors of the vagina appear in infants and in young children.[118,119] The vaginal tumor may originate in the anterior wall, the posterior wall or in the region of the hymen.[33] The tumor appears as flesh-like, pinkish, moist, edematous polyps which are friable and show superficial areas of necrosis and hemmorrhage. In appearance they resemble a hydatidiform mole.[119]

The first symptoms may be a serosanguineous, mucoid or bloody discharge with or without a foul odor. As the tumor progresses in size, it fills the vagina and protrudes through the vulvar orifice. As a result of erosion and infection, hemorrhage and necrosis are common complications. The growth may distend the vagina or infiltrate the rectovaginal or vesical-vaginal septum. The tumor also infiltrates the tissues of the pelvic floor and fills the pelvic cavity, compressing the bladder anteriorly and the uterus laterally or posteriorly.[33] It may penetrate and perforate the uterine wall and cause fatal peritonitis. Spread may occur into the parametrium and the pelvis. Ureteric dilation follows obstruction of the bladder outlet.[120] Dissemination of the tumor to the regional pelvic and para-aortic lymph nodes has been reported, but this too is relatively uncommon. Distant metastases seldom occur. The clinical course shows it to be extremely malignant, quickly recurring and progressing locally. By local extension the tumor may invade the spinal canal, the iliac vein and the inferior vena cava.[33] Death usually results from pressure on the ureters by the tumor with a resultant hydronephrosis. The average duration of life without surgery is less than one year.[119,121,122]

Polypoid or grape-like masses in the vagina give rise to the clinical impression of botryoid rhabdomyosarcomas, particularly when found in infants or children, however, benign vaginal polyps with a similar appearance also occur. They not only may raise the specter of botryoid rhabdomyosarcoma in the clinician's mind but also may have bizarre histogical features suggesting malignancy.[123] On the other hand botryoid rhabdomyosarcomas may at first appear benign on both clinical and histological examination.[124] Thus great care should be exercised to exclude malignancy in all vaginal polyps in little girls.

Radium and x-ray therapy have been given an extensive trial and have nearly always been followed by rapid recurrence of the tumor.[124] Radical surgical extirpation may occasionally produce a cure.[120,124-126] The key to successful surgical treatment is early diagnosis, while the tumor is still localized to the subepithelial tissue of the vagina. In such cases vaginectomy and hysterectomy may produce a cure,[127,128] but if the tumor has spread it may not be possible to obtain a wide margin of excision without excising the urethra, the vulva, the bladder and sometimes, the rectum.[120,121]

Prostate

Prostatic rhabdomyosarcomas occur at all ages, but about half of the cases appear during the first five years of life.[129] These tumors usually produce few early symptoms. Pain is usually absent, and the onset of frequency and nocturia is insidious. The urinary stream becomes weak and narrow. Later dysuria and a urethral discharge may develop, followed by urinary retention, hematuria and straining on urination. After the mass reaches some size, there may be difficulty in defecation and presence of backache, tenesmus and hemorrhoids. The tumor may be readily palpated by rectal examination. Late in the disease the abdomen becomes swollen; there may be edema of the penis and lower extremities, priapism, anemia, cachexia, weight loss and a bulging perineum. Sepis may overshadow this progression of events, and the child's symptoms on admission may be those of acute urinary retention, cystitis or pyelonephritis.[130,131] In prostatic rhabdomyosarcomas the urinary obstruction is more gradual in onset than in bladder tumors. The average age at initial diagnosis is higher than in the bladder tumors and the tumor is further advanced with local spread as well as distant metastases when first seen.[108]

The diagnosis does not present any real difficulty. A smooth, firm or tensely cystic mass fills the pelvis and projects upwards into the abdomen, closely resembling the distended bladder. Rectal examination reveals the tumor to be anterior to the bowel, distinguishing it from a sacral neuroblastoma or teratoma. Cystourethrography confirms the prostatic position of the tumor and shows the distortion of the urethra. Endoscopy is usually impossible, or at least unrewarding, because of the extreme displacement of the bladder. The only other important cause of swelling of the prostate at this age is abscess, which is accompanied by leucocytosis, fever and systemic disturbances. Biopsy of the tumor is best performed by a needle introduced from the perineum.[108]

The frequent presence of undifferentiated mesenchyme-like tissue as well as muscular elements in the tumors and the homology of the upper vaginal and prostatic regions, together suggest that prostatic rhabdomyosarcomas of boys are homologous with the vaginal and cervical rhabdomyosarcomas of girls.[33] Spread of the neoplasm has already occurred in most children before they are brought for treatment.[132] Rhabdomyosarcomas of the prostate usually spread by way of the lymphatics, but hematogenous metastasis to distant organs may also occur to the lung or to the brain.[133]

If this tumor is found at an early stage, prompt radical cystoprostatectomy and urethrectomy may occasionally effect a cure. Pelvic lymphadenectomy, generous excision of the lower ureters, and removal of subsymphysial periosteum may reduce the high local recurrence rate.[129] Although total cystectomy yields a significant salvage rate for rhabdomyosarcomas of the bladder, those of prostatic origin remain incurable because extensive local tumor spread usually precedes the appearance of symptoms.[129] Treatment recommended by some is total pelvic exenteration, urethrectomy, bilateral pelvic lymphadenectomy, and ileal conduit urinary diversion.[129] Pelvic exenteration with lymph node excision and extensive removal of the perineal structures, penis and rectum, is advised by others.[134] Prolonged survival even following radical surgery for rhabdomyosarcoma of the prostate is rare.[134,135] Rhabdomyosarcomas of the prostate are resistant to present modes of chemotherapy and radiation therapy.[117] The average survival after the appearance of the first symptom is only seven months.[129]

Spermatic Cord and Paratesticular Tissues

The testicular appendages—namely the vaginal tunics and spermatic cord—are affected by occurrence of rhabdomyosarcoma. They are rapidly growing, highly malignant neoplasms observed chiefly within the first two decades of life. Since these tumors are often rapidly invasive, the exact tissue of origin may be difficult to determine. If the testis itself is compressed but not involved, the lesion presumably arose in one of the paratesticular tissues.[136] Nearly all rhabdomyosarcomas of the paratesticular tissues are embryonal in type. Some are botryoid or pleomorphic and rare cases are alveolar in type.[137] About thirty cases of rhabdomyosarcoma of the spermatic cord have been reported.[39,137-151]

Unlike other soft tissue sarcomas, rhabdomyosarcomas tend to metastasize to lymph nodes, usually to the nodes of the renal hilum. Thus, it is necessary to perform radical periaortic lymph node dissection as part of the definitive therapy for rhabdomyosarcomas of the testis and paratesticular tissues.[136] The entire mass of nodes surrounding both renal pedicles and lying along the aorta up to the level of the superior mesenteric artery should be excised *en bloc*. Since the normal lymphatic flow may be altered or even reversed once the primary channels have been obstructed by tumor, the lower aortic lymph nodes and iliac nodes must also be excised.[136] Postoperative x-ray therapy should be given.[39,151] Chemotherapy has also been utilized but with little benefit.[147,158] The majority of the patients are dead within one year after surgery. However, some cases have shown prolonged survival.[139,145,152]

Testis, Ovary and Kidney

Thirteen cases of pure testicular rhabdomyosarcoma have been described.[153-155] The fairly frequent finding of striated muscle elements in testicular teratomas may be taken as evidence that testicular rhabdomyosarcomas arise as a unilateral development; care must always be taken to exclude the presence of other tissues in the tumor before a diagnosis of pure testicular rhabdomyosarcoma is made. A review of reported cases of paratesticular rhabdomyosarcoma led Alexander[155] to the conclusion that these tumors, unlike those occurring in other sites, have a better prognosis in early childhood. Teratomas in infants may behave in a benign manner.[33]

Testicular rhabdomyosarcomas metastasize to the retroperitoneal lymph nodes. Therefore, retroperitoneal node dissection is recommended for all intrascrotal rhabdomyosarcomas, even when no metastases are found.[154] Thus, radical orchiectomy is the basic treatment; but because of the site of origin, the extent of the tumor and the frequent existence of metastases, chemotherapy should also be given. Dactinomycin and cyclophosphamide have been used. The patients usually die of pulmonary metastases within a year of the original diagnosis.[153]

Rhabdomyosarcoma of the *ovary* is extremely rare, probably not more than seven authenticated cases have been described.[156,157] Only one case occurred in a child.[156] The diagnosis of ovarian rhabdomyosarcoma has not been accepted by many pathologists unless evidence of high degree of differentiation, such as cross striations, could be demonstrated. Many believe such tumors should be regarded as teratomas.[157]

Rhabdomyosarcoma of the *kidney* is a highly malignant but very rare tumor. Only four cases have been reported, two were in children.[158-160] Constance described a one-year-old infant, who died with rhabdomyosarcomas of both kidneys. Some authors believe that the renal rhabdomyosarcoma is a Wilms' tumor where striated muscle is the dominant cell type, or the element which grew the fastest.[161]

Gastrointestinal Tract

The most common location for rhabdomyosarcoma in the gastrointestinal tract is in the biliary tree. Davis[162] reviewed twenty-three cases of botryoid rhabdomyosarcoma of the biliary tree in the pediatric age group.[7,163,167] Symptoms at the onset of the disease include malaise, fever and jaundice, suggesting the presence of infectious hepatitis. Progression in the intensity and duration of jaundice and the appearance of right upper quadrant abdominal pain and mass of variable size suggest obstruction as the etiology of the jaundice. In several cases, the obstruction was substantiated by x-ray studies of the upper gastrointestinal tract and biliary tree. Nearly all cases showed elevation of both the direct and indirect reacting serum bilirubin and elevation of serum alkaline phosphatase.

At laparotomy the biliary tree is found to be distended either with pale, gelatinous material or grape-like polypoid structures. When these are removed from the biliary tree, there is resumption of the bile flow for a short period of time. Occasionally distant metastases occur, but botryoid rhabdomyosarcomas have a greater tendency for local invasion of contiguous structures within the abdomen. Death is usually due to direct invasion of the liver, pancreas, omentum and nearby structures by the tumor.[162,167] Wide surgical resection of the tumor and the use of chemotherapy and x-ray therapy may result in significant prolongation of life, with diminution in the size of residual tumor and palliation of tumor effects.[162] one apparent cure was reported.[168]

An eighteen-month-old boy underwent abdominal exploration because of an enlarging mass in the right upper abdomen.[169] At surgery, a 19 by 18 cm tumor mass almost completely occupied the right lobe of the liver. Complete right hepatic lobectomy was performed. Microscopically, the neoplasm was identified as a rhabdomyosarcohepatoma, being a combination of rhabdomyosarcoma and hepatocellular carcinoma. Additional cases of such tumors have been reported.[170-172]

Several cases of rhabdomyosarcoma of the upper gastrointestinal tract have been reported.[173-175] One of these was in a child who had a rhabdomyosarcoma of the stomach.[174] Radical excision of the tumor may occasionally lead to prolonged survival. X-ray therapy and chemotherapy may be tried. Rhabdomyosarcoma of the perirectal tissues is treated by abdominoperineal resection.[176, 177] in these cases rhabdomyosarcoma occurs below the peritoneal reflection, in the presacral region, with inseparable involvement of the rectum and anal canal.[178] In the botryoid type, the tumor may present as an anal papilloma.[177,179]

Bronchi, Heart and Brain

Ten cases of primary rhabdomyosarcoma of the bronchi and lungs have been reported, all were in adults.[180-184] In only three cases could definitive therapy be carried out.[187] Primary tumors of the heart are uncommon. Approximately 25 percent of all primary cardiac tumors are malignant neoplasms of the sarcoma group. The most common are the spindle-cell and the primitive fusocellular types, while rhabdomyosarcomas are rare. Primary tumors of the heart may be manifested clinically by a variety of symptoms and signs, depending on the location, size and growth characteristics of the tumor.[185-189] Rhabdomyosarcomas may also originate in the pericardium.[190]

A small number of primary neoplasms of the nervous system that have contained rhabdomyosarcomatous elements in whole or in part have been described. In seven instances the site of origin was the cerebellum and two examples arose from the region of the third ventricle and the lumbar spinal cord, respectively. All examples, except one, occurred in children. On four occasions the lesional tissue comprised pure rhabdomyosarcoma whereas a teratoid origin could be ascribed to the remainder.[191] One case of primary cerebellar rhabdomyosarcoma occurred in a $3\frac{1}{2}$-year-old boy.[192] The tumor arose in the cerebellar vermis, was locally resected, and after temporary remission led to the patient's death within two years. The brain and spinal cord showed massive surface spread. There was no parenchymal penetration or true extracranial metastasis. An additional similar case was described.[193]

CONGENITAL RHABDOMYOSARCOMA

A series of fifteen infants with congenital rhabdomyosarcomas was described.[194] The following was the anatomical distribution of the rhabdomyosarcomas: head and neck, six cases; urogenital system, three cases; upper extremity and perineal region, two each; and lower extremity and trunk, one each. Of the eight cases studied histologically, four tumors were well-differentiated embryonal type and four were poorly differentiated, two of these suggested the botryoid type. Eight of the fifteen infants survived without known recurrence; six died of their tumor and one was lost to follow-up. Examination of the eight infants surviving suggests that radical surgery effected a cure in five. However, in the other three, followed from sixteen months to 13½ years, treatment was limited to local excision. Although recurrence took place in one infant, surgical excision gave prolonged survival. All three had well-differentiated embryonal tumors which may account for the excellent results of local excision only. This finding contrasts sharply with the very high mortality rate in rhabdomyosarcomas occurring in older children and adults. Thus, congenital mesenchymal tumors usually do not show a malignant course. It appears that congenital rhabdomyosarcomas differ biologically from those occurring in older children, even though they are histologically similar.[194]

THERAPY OF RHABDOMYOSARCOMAS

Therapy of rhabdomyosarcomas must be tailored to the individual child, according to the site and size of the primary tumor and the degree of spread. Comments regarding therapy are included under the various sites of primary tumors as discussed above. The combined use of surgery, x-ray therapy[195-199] and chemotherapy is recommended.

Many drugs have been tried in chemotherapy of these tumors.[200] Intermittent high doses of cyclophosphamide produced tumor regression in several cases.[201] Other series have shown effective tumor regression with actinomycin D and vincristine[202] and with combined use of vincristine, actinomycin D and cyclophosphamide (VAC).[203,204]

REFERENCES

1. Baily, W., Holaday, W., Kontras, S., and Clatworthy, W.: Rhabdomyosarcoma in childhood; a review of 14 cases. *Arch Surg, 82*:943-949, 1961.
2. Mahour, G., Soule, E., Mills, S., and Lynn, H.: Rhabdomyosarcoma in infants and children; a clinicopathologic study of 75 cases. *J Pediatr Surg, 2*:402-409, 1967.
3. Mikulowski, P., and Berge, T.: Alveolar rhabdomyosarcoma. *Acta Pathol Microbiol Scand, 75*:282-290, 1969.
4. Stout, A.: Rhabdomyosarcoma of skeletal muscles. *Ann Surg, 123*:447-472, 1946.
5. Jones, I., Reese, A., and Krout, J.: Orbital rhabdomyosarcoma. *Am J Ophthal, 61*:721-736, 1966.
6. Mostofi, F., and Morse, W.: Polypoid rhabdomyosarcoma (sarcoma botryoides) of the bladder in children. *J Urol, 67*:681-687, 1952.
7. Farinocci, C., Fairchild, J., Sulak, M., and Gilpatrick, C.: Sarcoma botryoides of the common bile duct; report of two cases. *Cancer, 9*:408-417, 1956.
8. Potter, G.: Embryonal rhabdomyosarcoma of the middle ear in children. *Cancer, 19*:221-226, 1966.
9. Pack, G., and Eberhart, W.: Rhabdomyosarcoma of skeletal muscle; report of 100 cases. *Surgery, 32*:1023-1064, 1952.
10. Pinkel, D., and Pickren, J.: Rhabdomyosarcoma in children. *JAMA, 175*: 292-298, 1961.
11. Horn, R.: Sarcomas of the soft tissues. *JAMA, 183*:511-514, 1963.
12. Oliver, J., El Hilali, M., Belitcky, P. and MacKinnon, K.: LDH isoenzymes in benign and malignant prostate tissue. *Cancer, 25*:863-866, 1970.
13. Soong, B., and Miller, S.: Coagulation disorders in cancer. III. Fibrinolysis and inhibitors. *Cancer, 25*:867-874, 1970.
14. Miller, S., Sanchez-Avalos, J., Stefanski ,T., and Zuckerman, L.: Coagulation disorders in cancer. *Cancer, 20*:1452-1465, 1967.
15. Delta, B., and Pinkel, D.: Bone marrow aspiration in children with malignant tumors. *J Pediatr, 64*:542-546, 1964.
16. Finkelstein, J., Ekert, H., Isaacs, H., and Higgins, G.: Bone marrow metastasis in children with solid tumors. *Am J Dis Child, 119*:49-52, 1970.
17. Hajdu, S., and Koss, L.: Cytologic diagnosis of metastic myosarcomas. *Acta Cytol, 13*:545-551, 1969.
18. Papaionnau, A., and McPeak, C.: Rhabdomyosarcoma of the buttock producing hypoglycemia. *Ann Surg, 161*:553-561, 1965.

19. McPeak, C., and Papaionnau, A.: Nonpancreatic tumors associated with hypoglycemia. *Arch Surg, 93:*1019-1024, 1966.
20. Rothenberg, A., and Pilz, C.: Unusual manifestations of rhabdomyosarcoma. *Arch Intern Med, 118:*446-452, 1966.
21. Bizer, L.: Rhabdomyosarcoma. *Am J Surg, 118:*453-458, 1969.
22. Caffey, J., and Anderson, D.: Metastatic embryonal rhabdomyosarcoma in the growing skeleton. *Am J Dis Child, 95:*581-600, 1958.
23. Moskowitz, M., Rosenbaum, H., Sweet, R., and McLeod, C.: Calcified embryonal rhabdomyosarcoma with local bone invasion; an unusual case. *Radiology, 91:*121-122, 1968.
24. Pratt, C.: Response of childhood rhabdomyosarcoma to combination chemotherapy. *J Pediatr, 74:*791-794, 1969.
25. Pochedly, C.: How to perform bone marrow biopsy in childern. *Clin Pediatr, 9:*226-228, 1970.
26. Stobbe, G., and Dargeon, H.: Embryonal rhabdomyosarcoma of head and neck in children and adolescents. *Cancer, 3:*826-833, 1950.
27. Riopelle, J., and Theriault, J.: Sur une forme meconnue de sarcome des parties malles; le rhabdomyosarcoma alveolare. *Ann Anat Pathol (Paris), 1:*88-94, 1956.
28. Horn, R., and Enterline, H.: Rhabdomyosarcoma; clinico-pathologic study and classification of 39 cases. *Cancer, 11:*181-199, 1958.
29. Enzinger, F.: Recent trends in soft tissue pathology. In *Tumors of Bone and Soft Tissue.* A collection of papers presented at the Eighth Annual Clinical Conference on Cancer, 1963, at the University of Texas M.D. Anderson Hospital and Tumor Institute, Houston, Texas. Chicago, Year Book Medical Publishers, 1965, pp. 315-332.
30. Albores-Saavedra, J.: Rhabdomyosarcoma. *Progr Clin Cancer, 1:*683-691, 1965.
31. Albores-Saavedra, J., Martin, R., and Smith, J.: Rhabdomyosarcoma; a study of 35 cases. *Ann Surg, 157:*186-197, 1963.
32. Enzinger, F., and Shiraki, M.: Alveolar rhabdomyosarcoma; an analysis of 110 cases. *Cancer, 24:*18-31, 1969.
33. Willis, R.: *Pathology of Tumors* (3rd ed.). London, Butterworths, 1960, pp. 743-761.
34. Lawrence, W., Jegge, G., and Foote, F.: Embryonal rhabdomyosarcoma; a clinicopathological study. *Cancer, 17:*361-376, 1964.
35. Masson, J., and Soule, E.: Embryonal rhabdomyosarcoma of the head and neck; report of eighty-eight cases. *Am J Surg, 110:*585-591, 1965.
36. Marsden, H., and Steward, J.: *Tumors in Children.* New York, Springer-Verlag, 1968, pp. 197-207.
37. Patton, R., and Horn, R.: Rhabdomyosarcoma; clinical and pathological features and comparison with human fetal and emybryonal skeletal muscle. *Surgery, 52:*572-584, 1962.

38. Willis, R.: *The Borderland of Embryology and Pathology*. London, Butterworths, 1962, pp. 437-440.
39. Tanimura, H., and Furuta, M.: Rhabdomyosarcoma of the spermatic cord. *Cancer, 22*:1215-1220, 1968.
40. Kroll, A.: Fine-structural classification of orbital rhabdomyosarcoma. *Invest Ophthal, 6*:531-543, 1967.
41. Freeman, A., and Johnson, W.: A comparative study of childhood rhabdomyosarcoma and virus-induced rhabdomyosarcoma in mice. *Cancer Res, 28*:1490-1500, 1968.
42. Perk, K., Shachat, D., and Maloney, J.: Pathogenesis of a rhabdomyosarcoma (undifferentiated type) in rats induced by a murine sarcoma virus (Moloney). *Cancer Res, 28*:1197-1206, 1968.
43. Toker, C.: Embryonal rhabdomyosarcoma; an ultrastructural study. *Cancer, 21*:1164-1170, 1968.
44. Horvat, B., Caines, M., and Fisher, E.: The ultrastructure of rhabdomyosarcoma. *Am J Clin Pathol, 53*:555-564, 1970.
45. Johnson, W., Jurand, J., and Hiramoto, R.: Immunohistologic studies of tumors containing myosin. *Am J Pathol, 47*:1139-1155, 1965.
46. Chatty, E., and Hawk, W.: Clinicopathologic assessment of 26 cases of rhabdomyosarcoma. *Cleveland Clin Q, 35*:97-113, 1968.
47. McAllister, R. *et al.*: Cultivation *in vitro* of cells derived from a human rhabdomyosarcoma. *Cancer, 24*:520-526, 1969.
48. Porterfield, J., and Zimmerman, L.: Rhabdomyosarcoma of the orbit; a clinicopathological study of 55 cases. *Virchows Arch [Pathol Anat], 335*:329-344, 1962.
49. Frayer, W., and Enterline, H.: Embryonal rhabdomyosarcoma of the orbit in children and young adults. *Arch Ophthal, 62*:203-210, 1959.
50. Calhoun, F., and Reese, A.: Rhabdomyosarcoma of the orbit. *Arch Ophthal, 27*:558-578, 1942.
51. Howard, G., and Casten, V.: Rhabdomyosarcoma of the orbit in brothers. *Arch Ophthal, 70*:319-322, 1963.
52. Ashton, N., and Morgan, G.: Embryonal sarcoma and embryonal rhabdomyosarcoma of the orbit. *J Clin Pathol, 18*:699-714, 1965.
53. Sevel, D.: Intracranial extension of a non-striated embryonal rhabydomyosarcoma of the orbit. *Br J Ophthal, 53*:180-184, 1969.
54. Spaeth, E., and Cleveland, A.: Rhabdomyosarcoma in infancy and childhood. *Am J Ophthal, 53*:463-466, 1962.
55. Kirk, R., and Zimmerman, L.: Rhabdomyosarcoma of the orbit in a survivor of rhabdomyosarcoma of the kidney. *Arch Ophthal, 81*:559-564, 1969.
56. Landers, P.: X-ray treatment of embryonal rhabdomyosarcoma of orbit; case report of 13-year survival without recurrence. *Am J Ophthal, 66*:745-747, 1968.

57. Greer, C.: Rhabdomyosarcoma of the head and neck with special reference to the orbit. *Trans Ophthalmol Soc Aust, 25:*80-83, 1966.
58. Dayton, G., Langdon, E., and Rochlin, D.: Management of orbital rhabdomyosarcoma. *Am J Ophthal, 68:*906-909, 1969.
59. McCuaig, D.: Rhabdomyosarcoma of the maxillary sinus. *Ann Otol Rhinol Laryngol, 61:*146-153, 1952.
60. Pastore, P., Sahyoun, P. and Mandeville, F.: Rhabdomyosarcoma of the maxillary antrum. *Arch Otolaryngol, 52:*942-947, 1950.
61. Gross, C., Bikhazi, H., and Hoffman, P.: Rhabdomyosarcoma of the ear; a cause for suppurative ear diseases in children. *Arch Otolaryngol, 90:*609-616, 1969.
62. Blanchard, C., and House, H.: Two case reports of embryonal rhabdomyosarcoma with primary presentation in the ear. *Arch Otolaryngol, 66:*588-591, 1957.
63. Mehra, Y.: Embryonal rhabdomyosarcoma of the ear. *J Laryngol Otol, 74:*114-116, 1960.
64. Karatay, S.: Rhabdomyosarcoma of the middle ear. *Arch Otolaryngol, 50:*330-334, 1949.
65. Davidson, R. :Rhabdomyosarcoma of the middle ear. *Laryngoscope, 76:* 1889-1920, 1966.
66. Myers, E., Stool, S., and Weltschew, A.: Rhabdomyosarcoma of the middle ear. *Ann Otol Rhinol Laryngol, 77:*949-958, 1968.
67. Solomon, G., *et al.*: An extra-axial brainstem tumor of childhood. *Am J Dis Child, 117:*338-340, 1969.
68. Arean, V., and Marcial-Rojas, R.: Rhabdomyosarcoma in children. *Am J Surg, 93:*143-146, 1957.
69. Kauffman, S., and Stout, A.: Congenital mesenchymal tumors. *Cancer, 18:* 460-476, 1965.
70. Ulin, A., Showmaker, W., and Froio, G.: Rhabdomyosarcoma of the tongue. *N Engl J Med, 250:*98-104, 1954.
71. Wood, G., and Williams, G.: Rare tumor of tongue of newborn child. *Ear, Eye, Nose & Throat Month, 31:*83-85, 1952.
72. Bowman, J.: Rhabdomyosarcoma of striated muscle in preadolescent children. *J Pediatr, 55:*620-634, 1959.
73. Moore, O., and Grossi, C.: Embryonal rhabdomyosarcoma of the head and neck. *Cancer, 12:*69-73, 1959.
74. Dito, W., and Batsakis, J.: Rhabdomyosarcoma of the head and neck; an appraisal of the biologic behavior in 170 cases. *Arch Surg, 84:*582-588, 1962.
75. Glick, H.: Unusual neoplasm in the larynx of a child (rhabdomyosarcoma). *Ann Otolaryngol Chir Cervicofac, 53:*699-704, 1944.
76. Pearson, R., Gammel, E., and Thayer, W.: Rhabdomyosarcoma of the hypopharynx. *Arch Otolaryngol, 64:*238-240, 1956.

77. Harris, H.: Rhabdomyosarcoma of the larynx; report of a case. *Arch Otolaryngol, 74*:205-209, 1961.
78. Batsakis, J., and Fox, J.: Rhabdomyosarcoma of the larynx; report of a case. *Arch Otolaryngol, 91*:136-140, 1970.
79. Koop, E., and Tewarson, I.: Rhabdomyosarcoma of the head and neck in children, *Ann Surg, 160*:95-103, 1964.
80. Tucker, A.: Rhabdomyosarcoma and its rare occurrence in the lower lip. *Plast Reconstr Surg, 24*:369-379, 1959.
81. Kaloyannides, T.: Pleomorphic rhabdomyosarcoma of the gingiva. *J Oral Surg, 27*:150-155, 1969.
82. Henny, F., and Downs, J.: Treatment of embryonal rhabdomyosarcoma of the maxilla with combined therapy. *J Oral Surg, 26*:316-320, 1968.
83. Farra, C.: Rhabdomyosarcoma of the naso-orbital angle. *Arch Otolaryngol, 70*:500-501, 1959.
84. Alli, A., and Oluwasanmi, J.: A case report of rhabdomyosarcoma of the cheek. *West Afr Med J, 18*:62-65, 1969.
85. Sippel, H., and Nyberg, C.: Embryonal rhabdomyosarcoma of the mandible and maxilla; report of a case. *J Oral Surg, 27*:731-734, 1969.
86. Dito, W., and Batsakis, J.: Intraoral, pharyngeal, and nasopharyngel rhabdomyosarcoma. *Arch Otolaryngol 77*:123-128, 1963.
87. Pochedly, C., Suwansirikul, S., and Orodile, A.: Rhabdomyosarcoma as a cause of acute respiratory obstruction. *JAMA, 217*:969, 1971.
88. Cureton, R., and Griffiths, J.: Rhabdomyosarcoma of the hand following severe trauma. *Br J Surg, 44*:509-513, 1957.
89. Specht, R., Walker, J., and Faxon, H.: Rhabdomyosarcoma of the chest wall. *Arch Surg, 68*:687-692, 1954.
90. Phelan, J., and Juardo, J.: Rhabdomyosarcomas. *Surgery, 52*:585-591, 1962.
91. Krough, G.: Two cases of rhabdomyosarcoma in chickens. *Nord Vet Med, 5*:232-236, 1953.
92. Worley, G., and Gorham, J.: The comparative pathology of rabdomyosarcoma with a report of a case in a dog. *Am J Pathol, 30*:836-849, 1954.
93. Moulton, J.E.: *Tumours in Domestic Animals*. Berkeley and Los Angeles, University of California Press, 1961, p. 65.
94. Campbell, J., and Appleby, E.: Tumors in young chickens bred for rapid body growth (broiler chickens); a study of 357 cases. *J Pathol Bact, 92*:77-90, 1966.
95. Finocchio, E., Coffman, J., and Strafuss, A.: Rhabdomyosarcoma in a
96. Sah, R., and Sharma, R.: A case of rhabdomyosarcoma in poultry. *Indian* horse. *Vet Med, 64*:494-496, 1969.
Vet J, 46:377-380, 1969.
97. Soule, E., Geitz, M., and Henderson, E.: Embryonal rhabdomyosarcoma of the limbs and limb-girdles. *Cancer, 23*:1336-1346, 1969.

98. Keyhani, A., and Booher, R.: Pleomorphic rhabdomyosarcoma. *Cancer, 22*:956-967, 1968.
99. Potenza, A., and Winslow, D.: Rhabdomyosarcoma of the hand. *J Bone Joint Surg, 43*:700-708, 1961.
100. Viets, H., and Wittenborg, M.: Rhabdomyosarcoma eroding spinal column and compression of spinal cord. *Arch Pathol, 40*:179-181, 1945.
101. Linscheid, R., Soule, E., and Henderson, E.: Pleomorphic rhabdomyosarcomata of the extremities and limb girdles. *J Bone Joint Surg, 47-A*:715-726, 1965.
102. Catin, J., McNeer, G., Chu, F., and Booher, R.: The problem of local recurrence after treatment of soft tissue sarcoma. *Ann Surg, 168*:47-53, 1968.
103. Stamps, P., and Harris, D.: Botryoid rhabdomyosarcoma of the urinary bladder of a dog. *J Am Vet Med Assoc, 153*:1064-1068, 1968.
104. Osborne, S., Low, D., Perman, V., and Barnes, D.: Neoplasms of the canine and feline urinary bladder; incidence, etiologic factors, occurrence and pathologic factors. *Am J Vet Res, 29*:2041-2055, 1968.
105. Teunissen, G., and Misdorp, W.: Rhabdomyosarcoma of the urinary bladder and fibromatosis of the extremities in a young dog. *Zentralbl Veterinaermed, 1*:81-88, 1968.
106. Whitaker, B.: A case of embryonal sarcoma of the bladder of an infant. *Br J Surg, 46*:289-291, 1959.
107. Leiger, J.: Botryoid sarcoma and rhabdomyosarcoma of the bladder. *J Urol, 86*:583-490, 1961.
108. Williams, D., and Schistad, G.: Lower urinary tract tumors in children. *Br J Surg, 36*:51-65, 1964.
109. Flocks, R., and Culp, D.: Polypoid fibromyxosarcoma of the urinary bladder in a child. *J Urol, 73*:299-306, 1955.
110. Bhansali, S.: Sarcoma botryoides of the bladder in infancy and childhood. *J Urol, 87*:871-875, 1962.
111. Jarman, W., and Kenealy, J.: Polypoid rhabdomyosarcoma of the bladder in children. *J Urol, 103*:227-231, 1970.
112. Maletta, T., and Horton, B.: Botryoid sarcoma of the bladder in children; a case report. *J Urol, 82*:490-493, 1959.
113. Batsakis, J.: Urogenital rhabdomyosarcoma; histogenesis and classification. *J Urol, 90*:180-186, 1963.
114. Parker, P., Smith, P., and Rathmell, T.: Sarcoma botryoides of the bladder; successful therapy by cystectomy. *J Urol, 82*:494-496, 1959.
115. Kafka, V., Krolupper, M., and Palecek, L.: Rhabdomyosarcoma of the bladder in childhood; report of a successfully treated case. *J Urol, 96*:210-213, 1966.
116. Thompson, I., and Coppridge, A.: The management of bladder tumors in children; a study of sarcoma botryoides. *J Urol, 82*:590-595, 1959.

117. Miller, H., Benjamin, J., and McEnvoy, R.: Sarcoma botryoides; a 7-year survival. *J Urol, 101*:567-569, 1969.
118. McFarland, J.: Dysontogenetic and mixed tumors of the urogenital region; with a report of a new case of sarcoma botryoides vaginae in a child, and comments upon the probable nature of the sarcoma. *Surg Gynecol Obstet, 61*:42-57, 1935.
119. Spademan, L., Cohen, E., and Girton, F.: Sarcoma botryoides. *Am J Obstet Gynecol, 65*:203-207, 1953.
120. Shackman, R.: Sarcoma botryoides of the genital tract of female children. *Br J Surg, 38*:26-30, 1950.
121. Daniel, W., Koss, L., and Brunschwig, A.: Sarcoma botryoides of the vagina. *Cancer, 12*:74-84, 1959.
122. Sternberg, W., Clark, W., and Smith, R.: Malignant mixed mullerian tumor (mixed mesodermal tumor of uterus); study of 21 cases. *Cancer, 7*:704-724, 1954.
123. Norris, H., and Taylor, H.: Polyps of the vagina; a benign lesion resembling sarcoma botryoides. *Cancer, 19*:227-232, 1966.
124. Duncan, A., and Fahmy, E.: Sarcoma botryoides of the vagina and cervix in children. *J Obstet Gynaecol Br Commonuy, 60*:87-91, 1953.
125. Ulfelder, H., and Quan, S.: Sarcoma botryoides vaginae; complete excision of tumor in infant by combined abdominal-perineal approach. *Surg Clin North Am, 27*:1240-1244, 1947.
126. Ober, W., and Egcomb, J.: Sarcoma botryoides in the female urogenital tract. *Cancer, 7*:75-91, 1954.
127. Richmond, E.: Sarcoma botryoides of cervix. *Am J Obstet Gynecol, 65*:201-202, 1953.
128. Ober, W., Smith, J., and Rouillard, F.: Congenital sarcoma botryoides of the vagina. *Cancer, 11*:620-623, 1958.
129. Lemmon, W., Holland, J., and Ketcham, A.: Rhabromyosarcoma of the prostate. *Surgery, 59*:736-740, 1966.
130. McPhail, J.: Rhabdomyosarcoma of the prostate. *J Urol, 87*:617-622, 1962.
131. Kohler, F., and Murphy, J.: Rhabdomyosarcoma of male genital tract. *J Urol, 82*:500-503, 1959.
132. Grier, E., and Phillips, F.: Rhabdomyosarcoma of the prostate. *J Urol, 69*:695-702, 1953.
133. Johnson, W.: Rhabdomyosarcoma of prostate with extensive central nervous system metastases; a case report. *J. Urol, 84*:758-760, 1960.
134. Marshall, V.: A 5-year cure of rhabdomyosarcoma of the prostate in childhood, *J Pediatr Surg, 4*:366-369, 1969.
135. Goodwin, W. *et al.*: Rhabodomyosarcoma of the prostate in a child; first five year survival. *Trans Am Assoc Genito urin Surg, 59*:186, 1967.

136. Burrington, J.: Rhabdomyosarcoma of the paratesticular tissues in children; a report of 8 cases. *J Pediatr Surg, 4*:503-510, 1969.
137. Arean, V., and Kraeger, J.: Paratesticular rhabdomyosarcoma. *Am J Clin Pathol, 43*:518-427, 1965.
138. Gray, C., and Biorn, C.: Rhabdomyosarcoma of the spermatic cord. *J Urol, 74*:402-406, 1955.
139. Cannon, E., Altheide, J., and Allen, H.: Malignant tumors of the spermatic cord and testicular tunics. *South Med J, 49*:17-23, 1956.
140. Satter, E., Heidder, F., and Wear, J.: Primary sarcoma of the spermatic cord and epididymis. *J Urol, 82*:148-154, 1959.
141. Hoffman, W., and Baird, S.: A rare tumor of the spermatic cord, rhabdomyosarcoma. *J Urol, 84*:376-381, 1960.
142. Walker, W., and Cameron, H.: Rhabdomyosarcoma of the epididymis. *Br J Surg, 49*:319-322, 1961.
143. Irvine, E., Berg, O., and Nelson, R.: Rhabdomyosarcoma of paratesticular tissues; report of case. *N Engl J Med, 266*:994-995, 1962.
144. Bhansali, S.: Rhabdomyosarcoma of the spermatic cord. *Br J Surg, 50*:883-884, 1963.
145. Gowing, N., and Morgan, A.: Paratesticular tumours of the connective tissue and muscle. *Br J Urol, 36:(Suppl. 2)*:78-84, 1964.
146. Irisawa, S., Shirai, M., Matsushita, S., Kagayama, M., and Ichijo, S.: A case of the paratesticular rhabdomyosarcoma. *Dermatol Urol, 20*:759-762, 1966.
147. Stanton, M.: Rhabdomyosarcoma of the paratesticular tissues; report of a case. *N Zeal Med J, 65*:389-391, 1966.
148. Fox, T., and Collier, R.: Rhabdomyosarcomas of the spermatic cord; a review and case presentation. *Am Surg, 33*:483-489, 1967.
149. Arlen, M., Grabstald, H., and Whitmore, W.: Malignant tumors of the spermatic cord. *Cancer, 23*:525-532, 1969.
150. Assini, M., Otero, G., and Canton, J.: Rhabdomyosarcoma of the vaginal tunic. *J Urol, 101*:732-734, 1969.
151. Ross, L.: Rhabdomyosarcoma of the spermatic cord. *Pediatrics, 43*:890-892, 1969.
152. Holtz, F., and Abell, M.: Testicular neoplasms in infants and children. II. Tumors of non-germ cell origin. *Cancer, 16*:982-992, 1963.
153. Davis, A.: Rhabdomyosarcoma of the testicle. *J Urol, 87*:148-154, 1962.
154. Ravich, L., Lerman, P., Drabkin, J., and Foltin, E.: Pure testicular rhabdomyosarcoma. *J Urol, 94*:596-599, 1965.
155. Alexander, F.: Pure testicular rhabdomyosarcoma. *Br J Cancer, 22*:498-501, 1968.
156. Sandison, A.: Rhabdomyosarcoma of the ovary. *J Pathol Bacteriol, 70*:433-438, 1955.
157. Payan, H.: Rhabdomyosarcoma of the ovary; report of a case. *Obstet Gynecol, 26*:393-395, 1965.

158. Weisel, W., Dockerty, M., and Priestly, J.: Sarcoma of the kidney. *J Urol, 50*:564-570, 1943.
159. Constance, T.: Bilateral rhabdomyosarcoma of the kidney. *J Pathol Bacteriol, 59*:492-495, 1947.
160. D'Antonio, G., and Leonetti, P.: Malignant rhabdomyoma of the kidney. *Rass Inst Clin Ter, 48*:1204-1210, 1968.
161. Seabury, J.: Renal rhabdomyosarcoma. *JAMA, 201*:1043-1044, 1967.
162. Davis, G., Kissane, J., and Ishak, K.: Embryonal rhabdomyosarcoma (sarcoma botryoides) of the biliary tree; report of 5 cases and a review of the literature. *Cancer, 24*:333-342, 1969.
163. Horn, R., Yakovac, W., Kaye, R., and Koop, C.: Rhabdomyosarcoma (sarcoma botryoides) of the common bile duct; report of a case. *Cancer, 8*:478-487, 1955.
164. Hays, D., and Snyder, W.: Botryoid sarcoma (rhabdomyosarcoma) of the bile ducts. *Am J Dis Child, 110*:595-605, 1965.
165. Delany, H., Driscoll, P., and Ainsworth, H.: Sarcoma botryoides of the common bile duct. *J Pediatr Surg, 1*:571-578, 1966.
166. Virenque, J.: A case of botryoid sarcoma of the bile ducts. *Am Chir Infant, 7*:25-38, 1966.
167. Soper, R., and Dunphy, D.: Sarcoma botryoides of the biliary tree. *Surgery, 63*:1005-1011, 1968.
168. Akers, D., and Needham, M.: Sarcoma botryoides of the bile ducts with survival. *J Pediatr Surg, 6*:474-479, 1971.
169. Wuester, W., and Knauer, W.: Complete right hepatic lobectomy for rare teratoid liver cancer in infancy. *Cancer, 14*:361-368, 1961.
170. Williams, A.: Liver tumor of mixed type. *Br J Surg, 41*:13-15, 1953.
171. Goldman, R., and Friedman, N.: Rhabdomyosarcohepatoma in an adult and embryonal hepatoma in a child. *Am J Clin Pathol, 51*:137-143, 1969.
172. Misugi, K., Okajima, H., Misugi, N., and Newton, W.: Classification of primary malignant tumors of liver in infancy and childhood. *Cancer, 20*:1760-1771, 1967.
173. Thorek, P., and Neiman, B.: Rhabdomyosarcoma of esophagus. *J Thorac Cardiovasc Surg, 20*:77-89, 1950.
174. Templeton, A., and Heslin, D.: Primary rhabdomyosarcoma of stomach and esophagus. *Am J Roentgenol, 86*:896-899, 1961.
175. Moses, I., and Goodley, E.: Rhabdomyosarcoma of the duodenum. *Am J Gastroenterol, 51*:48-54, 1969.
176. Pack, G., Miller, T., and Trinidad, S.: Pararectal rhabdomyosarcoma; report of two cases. *Dis Colon Rectum, 6*:1-6, 1963.
177. McGregor, J., and Jewett, T.: Perianal rhabdomyosarcoma in an infant. *Dis Colon Rectum, 8*:52-55, 1965.
178. Fisher, E., and Gruhn, J.: Perianal rhabdomyosarcoma. *Arch Surg, 77*:230-234, 1958.

179. Sharp, W., and Helwig, E.: Sarcoma botryoides (embryonal rhabdomyosarcoma) of the anus. *Am J Dis Child, 97:*845-848, 1959.
180. Forbes, G.: Rhabdomyosarcoma of the bronchus. *J Pathol Bateriol, 70:* 427-431, 1955.
181. Gordon, L., and Bass, H.: Primary rhabdomyosarcoma of the lung; report of a case. *Cancer, 8:*588-592, 1955.
182. Drenna, J., and McCormack, R.: Primary rhabdomyosarcoma of the lung. *J Pathol Bacteriol, 79:*147-149, 1960.
183. Conquest, H., Thornton, J., Massie, J., and Coxe, J.: Primary pulmonary rhabdomyosarcoma; a report of three cases and literature review. *Ann Surg, 161:*688-692, 1965.
184. Bariffi, F., Del Bono, M., and Natali, P.: A case of primary rhabdomyosarcoma of the lung. *Arch Tisiol Mal Appar Resp, 22:*123-145, 1967.
185. Hallermann, F., Kincaid, O., Brown, A., and Dougherty, G.: Rhabdomyosarcoma of the heart. *JAMA, 184:*939-942, 1963.
186. Berge, T.: Rhabdomyoma and rhabdomyosarcoma of the heart. *Acta Pathol Microbial Scand, 56:*113-120, 1962.
187. de Saint-Florent, G., *et al.*: A primary malignant tumor of the mitral valve with surgical removal. *J Thorac Cardiovasc Surg, 58:*71-78, 1968.
188. Kuehl, K., Perry, L., Chandra, R., and Scott, L.: Rhabdomyoma causing subaortic stenosis. *Pediatrics, 46:*464-468, 1970.

189. Engle, M., and Glenn, F.: Primary malignant tumor of the heart in infancy; case report and review of subject. *Pediatrics, 15:*562-574, 1955.
190. Ohta, G., Ohe, K., Nishivo, T., and Oda, K.: Primary rhabdomyosarcoma of the pericardium. *Acta Pathol Jap, 19:*223-228, 1969.
191. Goldman, R.: Gliomyosarcoma of the cerebrum; report of a unique case. *Am J Clin Pathol, 52:*741-744, 1969.
192. Legier, J., and Wells, H.: Primary cerebellar rhabdomyosarcoma; case report. *J Neurosurg, 26:*437-438, 1967.
193. Shuangshoti, S., Pitaratn, P., and Viriyapanich, P.: Primary rhabdomyosarcoma of cerebellum; necropsy report. *Cancer, 22:*367-371, 1968.
194. Kauffman, S., and Sout, A.: Congenital mesenchymal tumors. *Cancer, 18:*460-476, 1965.
195. del Regato, J.: Radiotherapy of soft-tissue sarcomas. *JAMA, 185:*216-218, 1963.
196. Cassady, J.R., Sagerman, R., Tretter, P., and Ellsworth, R.: Radiation therapy for rhabdomyosarcoma. *Radiology, 91:*116-120, 1968.
197. McNeer, G., Cantin, J., Chu, F., and Nickson, J.: Effectiveness of radiation therapy in the management of sarcoma of the somatic soft tissues. *Cancer, 22:*391-397, 1968.
198. Nelson, A.: Embryonal rhabdomyosarcoma; Report of 24 cases and

study of the effectiveness of radiation therapy upon the primary tumor. *Cancer, 22:*64-68, 1968.

199. Hermens, A., and Barendsen, G.: Changes of cell proliferation characteristics in a rat rhabdomyosarcoma before and after x-irradiation. *Eur J Cancer, 5:*173-189, 1969.

200. Haddy, T., Nora, A., Sutow, W., and Vietti, T.: Cyclophosphamide treatment for metastatic soft tissue sarcoma. *Am J Dis Child, 114:* 301-308, 1967.

201. Finklestein, J., Hittle, R., and Hammond, G.D.: Evaluation of a high-dose cyclophosphamide regimen in childhood tumors. *Cancer, 23:* 1239-1242, 1969.

202. Grosfeld, J., Clatworthy, H.W., and Newton, W.: Combined therapy in childhood rhabdomyosarcoma; and analysis of 42 cases. *J Pediatr Surg, 4:*637-645, 1969.

203. Sutow, W.: Chemotherapeutic management of childhood rhabdomyosarcoma. In *Neoplasia in Childhood.* Chicago, Year Book Medical Publishers, 1969, pp. 201-208.

204. Wilbur, J., Sutow, W., Sullivan, M. *et al.*: Successful treatment of rhabdomyosarcoma with combination chemotherapy and radiotherapy. *Proc Am Soc Clin Oncol (VII).* Chicago. April 7, 1971. Abstract #56.

Chapter 8

TREATMENT AND PROGNOSIS OF CENTRAL NERVOUS SYSTEM TUMORS

MARILYN J. SONLEY

THE BRAIN is the commonest site of childhood tumors. The annual incidence of brain tumors in children is fifteen to twenty per million of the total population.[1]

GENERAL PRINCIPLES OF THERAPY

The cornerstone of successful therapy is early diagnosis. Unfortunately, young children are often unable to appreciate minor changes in sensation, power and coordination and to verbalize their complaints. Consequently, they may not be brought to a physician until the tumor has enlarged sufficiently to produce signs gross enough to be noticed by the parents. The physician should consider the diagnosis of brain tumor whenever a child presents with headache, especially if the headache occurs in the morning; vomiting, particularly if unaccompanied by nausea; alteration in personality, intellect, vision, coordination or motor activity; endocrinologic disturbances such as diabetes insipidus; or simply failure to thrive.

Many physicians retain an excessively pessimistic view about the prognosis of brain tumors and in the face of classical symptoms will diligently search for an extracranial cause before reluctantly accepting the possibility of a brain tumor. Actually the prognosis varies considerably with the pathological classification of the tumor. With the possible exception of glioblastoma multiforme, no histopathologic type of brain tumor is always fatal; and in some tumors, such as astrocytoma of the cerebellum, a near-normal life expectancy is possible for the majority of patients. Even if a tumor does eventually cause death, early diagnosis and appropriate treatment may permit a relatively normal life for several years.

Surgical Treatment

The tumor's location should be defined as precisely as possible by neurological examination and by neuroradiological techniques. The surgical approach depends on the site, possible histopathology and the presence or absence of increased intracranial pressure. If the flow of cerebrospinal fluid is obstructed, causing hydrocephalus, the increased pressure may be relieved by shunting the CSF via a catheter from a ventricle to the peritoneal cavity or right atrium. A few days later, when the child has recovered from the dehydration and cerebral anoxia, craniotomy will be associated with a reduced morbidity and mortality rate.[2] Shunts may become blocked by tumor debris, fibrin clots or kinking, so when a patient with a shunt develops headache and vomiting, the cause may be a blocked shunt rather than recurrence of the tumor.

Edema of brain tissue adjacent to the tumor may contribute to the increased intracranial pressure. The intravenous administration of steroids or an osmotic diuretic such as urea or mannitol will usually decrease the edema. With diuretics this effect is temporary and corrective surgery should be performed within hours of their administration.

Brain tumors rarely metastasize outside the craniospinal cavity. However in two tumors, medulloblastoma and ependymoma, malignant cells float freely in the CSF; in such cases a shunt into the atrium or peritoneal cavity provides a route for these cells to reach the rest of the body. Such metastatic spread through a shunt occurs relatively frequently in children with medulloblastoma[3,12] but rarely in ependymomas. Ventriculoperitoneal or ventriculoatrial shunts should not be used in children with medulloblastoma unless some method of filtering the cells or irradiating the tumor cells as they pass through the shunt can be developed.

Surgical excision should be complete if it can be accomplished safely. This is possible more frequently now with improvements in anesthetic techniques, fluid and electrolyte balance, and cortisone replacement therapy and with new surgical aids such as the dissecting microscope. If the tumor is sensitive to radiotherapy, complete resection is not always necessary. However even in radiosensitive tumors removal of the bulk of the tumor relieves the symptoms of increased pressure, reduces the total amount of tissue to be destroyed by radiotherapy, and may eliminate the less radiosensitive anoxic areas of the tumor.[4]

If the tumor involves vital areas such as the brain stem or thalamus, resection is impossible and sometimes even a biopsy may seriously compromise the patient's neurological status, if not his life. With such tumors the surgeon frequently makes the diagnosis on clinical grounds and refers the patient for radiotherapy.

Radiotherapy

The degree of sensitivity of brain tumors to radiation varies with the pathologic type. The value of radiation in the treatment of specific tumors will be discussed later. During the course of radiotherapy, children are usually as active as their neurological status will allow. Nausea and occasionally vomiting may occur briefly after each treatment but may be relieved by antiemetics. Depression of the bone marrow within the radiation field produces changes in the peripheral blood counts only if the whole spine or the whole CNS is irradiated. Interruption of the treatment for two or three days is usually followed by a return of the peripheral blood counts to low normal levels.

Edema of the tumor or adjacent brain tissue may occur during the first week of radiation and the associated deterioration in the neurological signs may be attributed mistakenly to tumor growth or hemorrhage into the tumor. Intravenous steroids may relieve the edema, but if the CSF pathway is blocked a shunt may be necessary. Alopecia develops two to three weeks after starting radiation. Regrowth of hair is often complete but depends on the dosage, type of radiation (supervoltage spares the skin), and the individual's sensitivity.

Future growth of irradiated tissue will be less than normal, but when radiation is confined to the skull, this is usually not clinically significant except in very young infants. If the whole spine is irradiated the adult height will be a few inches shorter than anticipated, the amount depending on the age of the child at the time of treatment. No damage to the brain or to the pituitary has been attributed to irradiation at currently acceptable therapeutic dosages.[5] The disability shown by some young infants in later life is more likely due to damage caused by the tumor because of late diagnosis.

Late sequelae are rare. Demyelination of the neurons in the irradiated tissue may occur two to nine months after radiation. The symptoms are often similar to those of the original tumor, so recurrence of tumor during the first year after radiation should be verified by radiological techniques or, if necessary, by biopsy. Cancer has rarely developed in irradiated tissue many years after radiotherapy.[4,6]

In summary, if a brain tumor is radiosensitive the beneficial effects of discriminately applied radiation outweigh the rare potentially adverse effects.[5]

Chemotherapy

Three barriers protect the brain from toxic substances: (a) the blood-brain barrier, probably situated in the glial cells surrounding the capillaries; (b) the blood-CSF barrier in the choroid plexus; and (c) the CSF-brain barrier in the ependyma. Unfortunately, these "protective" barriers also prevent most of the chemotherapeutic agents from reaching the tumor. Brain cells, unlike tumor cells, do not synthesize desoxyribonucleic acid or undergo mitosis. A drug which interferes with either activity should attack the tumor cells almost exclusively if it could but reach them in sufficient concentration. The following drugs have demonstrated some anti-tumor effect in brain tumors.

Methotrexate by intravenous or intra-arterial infusion has been relatively unsuccessful,[7] but when injected intrathecally it is absorbed through the ependyma into the brain and tumor tissue. It may be given by lumbar puncture, by intraventricular injection through a needle or an indwelling catheter, or even directly into the tumor.[7-9] One dosage schedule is 0.25 mg/kg intrathecally daily for five days,[10] repeated at intervals of from four to twelve weeks depending on the clinical course and response. Other regimens are also used.[8] Methotrexate enters the systemic circulation from the CSF and may cause mouth ulcers, diarrhea and pancytopenia.

Vincristine injected intravenously in a dosage of 0.05 mg/kg weekly has caused temporary regression of some brain tumors.[11-13] The side effects include alopecia, marrow depression, constipation, paresthesia, jaw pain, loss of deep tendon reflexes and occasionally muscle weakness, especially foot and wrist drop. Some of these symptoms may be difficult to differentiate from those due to recurrence of the tumor.

Bis-chlorethyl nitrosourea (BCNU) is a lipid-soluble agent which readily crosses the blood-brain barrier when given intravenously. The usual dosage is 100 mg/sq m of body surface given by push injection daily for two or at the most three days and repeated approximately every six weeks depending on the rate of bone marrow recovery. Immediate side effects include pain on injection, vomiting and flushing of the face and conjunctiva. Depression of the bone marrow results in a fall in the peripheral blood counts commencing three or four weeks after the injection and persisting for two to three weeks.

Bromouridine (BUDR) makes cells which have incorporated it into their nucleus more sensitive to radiotherapy. It is given in conjunction with methotrexate which promotes its uptake by the cells. It has been used clinically for some time[14] but its value is still not clear.

Chemotherapy trials in childhood brain tumors have been few, but many children with medulloblastomas, and a few with astrocytomas, have had partial or complete disappearance of signs and symptoms following the administration of vincristine, BCNU or methotrexate. Few children with ependymomas have had a trial of chemotherapy. Tumor regression following chemotherapy is temporary and is usually measured in weeks or months.

The response rates of the various tumors to chemotherapy will be given in the discussion of the individual tumors, but they are sufficiently low that no newly diagnosed tumor should be treated only with chemotherapy. Chemotherapy has been used primarily when tumors have recurred or progressed after radiotherapy and surgery. It is possible that chemotherapy, given in addition to radiation and surgery at the time of diagnosis might increase the cure rate, but this has not yet been adequately studied. The prime need, however, is the discovery of new, more effective chemotherapeutic agents.

TREATMENT OF SPECIFIC BRAIN TUMORS

Infratentorial Tumors

In children approximately 70 percent of brain tumors are situated in the posterior fossa (Table 8-1).

Cerebellar Astrocytomas

These tumors are usually benign and have the best prognosis of all brain tumors in children. Fortunately, they are the commonest tumors found in the posterior fossa.[15] They are seen throughout childhood, with a peak incidence between five and eight years of age. Usually well differentiated and well demarcated, they are often cystic. The presenting symptoms are usually those of cerebellar malfunction and increased intracranial pressure.

Complete excision is frequently possible, with a low operative mortality.[15] Cystic astrocytomas consist of a mural nodule surrounded by a wall which usually is not composed of tumor tissue. If the mural nodule is removed the lesion rarely recurs even when the cyst wall is left in place, whereas failure to remove the nodule almost always results in recurrence.

Of 130 children treated by Matson, 112 are alive and free of disease from three months to thirty-eight years later.[15] Five-year survival rates of 70 to 75 percent have been reported by several other investigators,[5,16,17] with some patients alive and well thirty-nine years after diagnosis.[18] The majority of the long-term survivors are neurologically normal or have minor residual disabilities and are self-supporting. Even after incomplete resection of solid astrocytomas long-term survival is possible.[17] Seven of nine patients who had incomplete resection are alive twelve to twenty-nine years later.[18] So tumor fragments attached to the brain stem or to the floor of the fourth ventricle and presenting a hazard in removal should be left unexcised.

TABLE 8-1
CLASSIFICATION OF BRAIN TUMORS

		Number in Tumor Registry, Hospital for Sick Children	
I. *Infratentorial*			
A. Cerebellar astrocytoma		135	413
B. Medulloblastoma		116	
C. Ependymoma		60	
D. Brain stem tumors		95	
E. Miscellaneous and unclassified		7	
II. *Supratentorial*			
A. Cerebral hemispheres			
1. Astrocytomas	86		
*glioblastoma multiforme	22	108	285
2. Ependymoma		22	
3. Miscellaneous and unclassified		25	
B. Tumors of chiasma-sella turcica region			
1. Craniopharyngioma		39	
2. Optic nerve glioma		35	
3. Diencephalic syndrome		4	
C. Tumors of pineal area		21	
D. Tumors of thalmus or floor of third ventricle		31	
III. *Miscellaneous*			
A. Choroid plexus tumors		12	22
B. Meningeal			
1. Meningioma		2	
2. Leptomeningeal sarcoma		2	
3. Melanosarcoma		2	
4. Unclassified		4	
IV. *Spinal Cord Tumors*			
A. Extradural (primary)		3	24
B. Intradural			
1. Extramedullary		*	
2. Intramedullary			
Astrocytomas		11	
Ependymomas		8	
Miscellaneous and unclassified		2	
			744

*Not recorded in registry.

Radiotherapy is said to have no role in the treatment of benign cerebellar astrocytomas.[1,15,18] However, if repeated recurrences develop, radiotherapy should be tried.[5,12] Infrequently, astrocytomas of the cerebellum are malignant on histological examination. Since they tend to recur quickly even after apparently complete resection, radiotherapy should be given postoperatively.[19]

Medulloblastomas

These malignant tumors have a peak incidence between the ages of two and seven years.[20] Arising in the cerebellum, they usually extend into the fourth ventricule and often obstruct the CSF pathway, causing hydrocephalus. The presenting symptoms are the same as for cerebellar astrocytomas. Tumor cells float freely in the CSF and tend to seed diffusely throughout the entire CNS. Metastases of medulloblastoma to bone marrow, bone and lung occur occasionally,[3,21] more commonly than in any other brain tumor.

The increase in intracranial pressure usually present at diagnosis may be reduced with steroids or diuretics. Shunting procedures allow the entry of tumor cells into the systemic circulation and should be avoided whenever possible. The tumor can rarely be completely resected, but because it is radiosensitive and often radiocurable, complete resection is not essential for cure. Simple decompression and biopsy, followed by radiotherapy, has produced survival figures comparable to those achieved by radical surgery followed by radiation.[4,22] Where feasible though, the bulk of the tumor should be removed, since eradicating necrotic anoxic areas facilitates the destruction of the residual tumor by radiation.[4] The whole CNS must be irradiated if the tumor cells floating in the CSF are to be destroyed. If only the tumor site is radiated the tumor always recurs.

Medulloblastomas are the most sensitive to chemotherapy of all brain tumors. Vincristine frequently causes partial or complete regression of signs and symptoms for periods of from one to twenty-two months.[11-13] Metastases outside the CNS may also disappear temporarily following intravenous vincristine.[12,21]

Methotrexate given intrathecally or intraventricularly has caused regression of signs for several months,[7,23] and BCNU has also been effective.[12] BCNU should be used cautiously in children with medulloblastomas because it causes depression of the marrow and previous radiation to the whole CNS will have reduced the bone marrow reserve.

Long-term survivals were unknown until the necessity of radiating the whole CNS was recognized.[24] The five-year survival after surgery and whole CNS irradiation has been reported to be 38 percent[3] to 50 percent[20] with one report as high as 77 percent.[25] However, the actual survival for all cases diagnosed is less because these reports include only those patients who completed a course of radiotherapy and exclude those who died prior to or during radiotherapy or who had irreparable damage and were not suitable for radiation therapy. Of the forty-six patients seen at the Hospital for Sick Children from 1955 to 1965, 28 percent have survived at least five years and are apparently free of disease; whereas if only those who completed a course of radiation therapy to the whole CNS are considered, 50 percent are alive five to thirteen years later. The surviving children are at the lower limit of height for their age; but all the surviving children are attending school or working and have minimal or no neurological abnormalities.[26]

Ependymoma

Ependymomas arise wherever ependymal cells occur within the ventricular system, the central canal of the spinal cord or the filum terminale. Seventy percent are infratentorial.[27,28] Usually arising within the fourth ventricle, they may occasionally extend over the upper cervical cord or extend anteriorly to occlude the aqueduct. The initial symptoms may be entirely those of increased intracranial pressure. Limitation of neck motion and tenderness over the cervical spine may occur if the cervical cord is involved. Ependymomas metastasize through the CSF but less frequently than medulloblastomas.[12,29] Metastases outside the CNS are very rare.[30,31] Excision of the tumor should be complete, but frequently a thin layer of tumor must be left on the floor of the fourth ventricle to avoid damaging cranial nerve nuclei.

Radiotherapy should be directed to the posterior fossa at least. Some authors never radiate the whole CNS prophylactically,[27] while others[1] do so only if the cells are undifferentiated. However, the degree of differentiation of the tumor cannot be correlated with the clinical course.[28] Because of the frequency of metastatic spread via the CSF, we irradiate the whole CNS in a manner identical to that for medulloblastoma.[32]

If the tumor recurs, re-irradiation or repeat resection on one or more occasions can produce a significant prolongation of useful life.[1] The response to chemotherapy is not known.

The five-year survival rate is less than that found in medulloblastoma. From 17 to 33 percent are alive five years after diagnosis.[12,27,28] If those who complete their course of radiation are considered separately, the five-year survival rate ranges from 28 to 58 percent.[5,12,27] Late recurrences are frequent. In one series, one-half of those patients surviving ten years later died of local recurrence; one as long as twenty-four years after diagnosis.[27]

Brain Stem Tumors

Arising anywhere between the hypothalamus and the upper cervical spinal cord, these tumors are found most commonly in the region of the pons. Although seen throughout childhood, most are found in children five to eight years of age.[15] Usually present at the time of diagnosis are palsies of several cranial nerves (most frequently the VIth and VIIth), spastic hemiplegia or quadriplegia due to involvement of the corticospinal tracts, and occasionally ataxia from infiltration or compression of the cerebellopontine tract. Brain stem tumors rarely obstruct the CSF pathway, so signs of increased intracranial pressure are uncommon. They are usually astrocytomas of various grades of malignancy. An air encephalogram typically shows a thickened pons with the aqueduct and the fourth ventricle displaced upwards and backwards.

Infiltrative rather than encapsulated, they are always unresectable because of their location near vital structures. Even a small biopsy can cause hemorrhage and severe damage to the cranial pathways and can be obtained safely in less than 25 percent of those children who undergo craniotomy.[12,15] Surgical exploration allows visualization of the tumor if the diagnosis is in doubt and an attempt at aspiration of the lesion if the clinical signs or angiography suggest a cystic lesion. But in the majority of cases the diagnosis is made on clinical grounds.

Irradiation offers the only possibility of permanent control. Temporary responses have been seen, but rarely, with vincristine,[11] BCNU[33] and intrathecal methotrexate.[8,10] The value of giving vincristine and BCNU in conjunction with radiotherapy for newly diagnosed brain stem tumors is being studied.[12]

Without radiation almost all patients are dead within one year of diagnosis,[12,15] and even with radiation the survival of the majority of children is short. Of 42 children treated at the Hospital for Sick Children between 1955 and 1966, 9 are alive five years or more after diagnosis, and all 9 were treated with radiation. Four of the 9 survivors had their diagnosis made on clinical grounds only; 5 children underwent surgical exploration, and in 3 of them in whom a biopsy was possible, all were low-grade astrocytomas. For those who died, the median duration of survival was only six months. Similar results have been reported from other centers.[5,34] These tumors may recur many years after diagnosis.

Supratentorial Tumors

Astrocytomas

Astrocytomas arising in the cerebral hemispheres are quite unlike those in the cerebellum. Usually infiltrative rather than encapsulated, they are infrequently cystic and commonly malignant. They may be subdivided on the basis of their microscopic appearance into four grades,[35] grade I being the most benign and grade IV (also called glioblastoma multiforme) the most malignant, while grades II and III are intermediate. Glioblastoma multiforme is characterized by a tendency to subcortical infiltration and rapid growth. It often spreads beyond the involved lobe and may even invade the opposite hemisphere. The brain tissue adjacent to the tumor is usually very edematous.

Because of the infiltrative nature, large size and deep location of astrocytomas, total removal is rare; but total removal should be attempted whenever possible because astrocytomas are relatively resistant to radiation. If the tumor is detected early and is confined to a lobe, whether frontal, temporal or occipital, then radical lobectomy may be curative. It is impossible, without a randomized study, to determine the precise role of radiotherapy in the treatment of astrocytomas of middle grades of malignancy.[5,17,19] However retrospective analyses of patients with glioblastoma multiforme have shown that the duration of survival is prolonged by radiation,[35] and the quality of survival is better,[37] even though the actual cure rate is not increased. We currently radiate all incompletely resected or inoperable astrocytomas of any grade.

Anticonvulsant medication should be given postoperatively for at least one year to all patients with hemispheral tumors and indefinitely if the electroencephalogram shows seizure activity or if convulsions occur.[15] Chemotherapy has been tried in some patients with recurrent tumors. In adults with astrocytoma or glioblastoma multiforme treated with BCNU, approximately half showed regression of their tumor for periods of one to ten months.[33,38] BCNU has also demonstrated some activity against astrocytomas in children.[38] Vincristine[21,40] and intrathecal methotrexate[8,10] have produced temporary tumor regression less frequently. The value of giving BCNU and vincristine in addition to radiotherapy to children with newly diagnosed astrocytomas of grades III and IV is being assessed.[12]

Approximately 50 percent of children with supratentorial astrocytomas (grades I to III) are alive five years after diagnosis[5,12,41] and 38 percent survive ten years,[12] although several of these have had tumor recurrence. Similar survival rates have been reported in groups of adults and children.[41] For the more malignant glioblastoma multiforme, the results are much worse. Less than 15 percent are alive after two years, and almost no patients survive for more than five years.[1,4,12,37,42]

Ependymomas

Supratentorial ependymomas frequently have no visible relationship to a ventricle and are often partly or extensively cystic. Total extirpation is usually impossible because of their deep location within the cerebrum. Radiation should be given to the residual tumor and probably to the whole CNS as well. The five-year survival rate is 14 to 22 percent.[27,31]

Tumors of the Chiasmal Area

Craniopharyngiomas may become symptomatic at any age but are most often diagnosed in the first two decades. Symptoms may be those of increased intracranial pressure caused by obstruction of the third ventricle, visual field defects due to compression of the optic chiasm, or pituitary hypofunction.

At present there are two schools of thought regarding therapy for craniopharyngioma. Matson[43] was able to completely resect the tumor in the majority of children and none of his patients were given radiotherapy. He stressed the importance of corticosteroid therapy before and during surgery as well as careful observation of the fluid and electrolyte balance. He has not reported the five-year survival rate for his fifty-seven patients, but forty-four children were alive at the time of his last report, with survival times ranging from a few months to seventeen years. Bartlett[44] had less success at complete removal of the tumor, but like Matson he did not include radiotherapy in the primary treatment. The ten-year survival rate for his seventy-three patients will be at best 43 percent.

On the other hand, Kramer[45] feels that radical removal, even if technically feasible, is unnecessary, because radiation therapy, administered after a simple biopsy and cyst decompression, is curative in most patients. The first six children treated with this technique are alive thirteen to fifteen years later and are well except for some minor residual disability, such as a visual defect or the need for hormone replacement therapy. All are working full-time and leading normal lives. Of six more children treated since his initial report, two have died with recurrences but four are well two to five years after radiation.

At the present time it is not clear which approach—primarily surgery or primarily radiotherapy—is better. However, a craniotomy must be done in any case to obtain a biopsy. If it is obvious at craniotomy that the tumor cannot be resected completely and without undue risk, then a biopsy should be done, and if there is a cystic component, fluid may be aspirated to decompress the tumor. Then the tumor should be irradiated. On the other hand, if at craniotomy the tumor appears to be completely resectable, excision should be attempted. Radiotherapy would then be given postoperatively only if the resection were inadvertently subtotal. The endocrinologic and electrolyte status must be followed carefully throughout the primary treatment period and at regular intervals indefinitely. Replacement therapy with thyroid, adrenal, sex and growth hormones is usually necessary.

Optic Nerve Gliomas

These slow-growing tumors are usually astrocytomas of low-grade malignancy. Optic nerve gliomas are more common in children with generalized neurofibromatosis.[46] In 25 percent the tumor is confined to one optic nerve; in the remainder it involves the chiasm, occasionally extending into the other optic nerve as well.

The tumor causes visual field defects, often associated with a decrease in visual acuity. The visual changes are insidious and may progress unnoticed by the child until detected on a routine vision test. Infiltration or compression of the hypothalamus may cause diabetes insipidus, obesity, short stature and precocious puberty, as well as drowsiness, apathy and mental confusion. Exophthalmos may develop if the tumor is intra-orbital. One or both optic foramena may be enlarged on skull x-ray and air ventriculography may demonstrate a mass elevating the floor of the third ventricle. The tumor can best be visualized radiologically by axial tomography of the chiasmal area after injection of air into the basal cistern.[47]

When confined to one optic nerve, the tumor can almost always be totally excised. If the chiasm is involved or if the tumor invades the hypothalamus, total removal is undesirable if not impossible. A craniotomy will reveal whether the tumor is operable, rule out an extrinsic tumor compressing the chiasm, allow definition of the limits of the mass, and permit a biopsy if one can be done without risking further reduction in vision.[48] Occasionally a shunt may be required if the tumor compresses the third ventricle, causing hydrocephalus.

For many years radiotherapy has been the accepted treatment for incompletely resected optic nerve gliomas.[49,50] Recently Hoyt and his associates have challenged the view that radiotherapy is helpful.[48,51] They propose that the tumor growth is self-limiting and that without any treatment the tumor can remain stable or even decrease in size over a period of years.

However, all optic nerve gliomas are not self-limiting. In some patients the vision slowly deteriorates until blindness occurs and a few die, usually from extension of the tumor to involve the hypothalamus and third ventricle. A review of the course of all untreated patients is needed and possibly a prospective randomized study to assess the value of radiation. In the meantime, if children with optic nerve gliomas are not given radiotherapy they should be followed closely with regular assessments of their visual fields and visual acuity, and if there is further deterioration in vision or any evidence of an increase in the size of the tumor, radiotherapy should be started.

If the tumor is confined to a single nerve and completely resected, almost 100 percent of children are cured. When the chiasma is involved and radiotherapy is given, approximately 70 percent of the children will live for many years, the majority of them with useful vision.[49,50]

Diencephalic Syndrome

This syndrome, seen in infants[52,53] is due to a tumor, usually an astrocytoma, arising in the hypothalamus or in the floor of the third ventricle. After initially thriving, the infant gradually becomes extremely emaciated despite a good appetite and apparently adequate caloric intake. Paradoxically these cachectic infants are remarkably cheerful, alert and active. Pallor, nystagmus, excessive sweating, polyuria, hypotension and intermittent vomiting have been reported. Ventriculography reveals a middle mass causing a filling defect in the floor of the elevated third ventricle. The tumor is almost always unrespectable and usually even a biopsy cannot be obtained safely. Irradiation is often followed by a return to normal weight, activity and appearance. Recurrences may occur years later but some children are still alive and well more than ten years after diagnosis.[53]

Tumors of the Pineal Area

Pinealomas are usually found in adolescent boys. "Pinealomas" are of two types: one of pineal origin and the other, more common, an atypical teratoma.[54] Astrocytomas or ependymomas arising in proximity to the pineal gland are capable of producing signs and symptoms identical to pinealomas: paralysis of upward gaze, ptosis, pupillary abnormalities, evidence of increased intracranial pressure and occasionally precocious puberty or sexual hypofunction.

Surgery in the region of the pineal gland is fraught with difficulty[55] and complete resection is usually impossible because the tumor tends to infiltrate adjacent tissue.[56] Pinealomas are sensitive to radiation and surgical removal is usually followed by radiotherapy. If the patient is an adolescent boy with classical symptoms and x-ray findings, the diagnosis is often made clinically, a shunt inserted to relieve the increased intracranial pressure, and radiotherapy given. With this approach, 50 percent may survive five years or more,[5,55,57] with some patients alive fifteen years or more after diagnosis.[55]

Tumors of the Floor of the Third Ventricle

Tumors in this area are usually astrocytomas or atypical teratomas, sometimes called ectopic pinealomas. The patient usually presents with diabetes insipidus, decreased visual acuity, bitemporal hemianopia and signs of hypopituitarism. Hypothalamic involvement may cause pyrexia, drowsiness, somnolence and electrolyte imbalance.

Complete resection is rare because of invasion of vital structures. Local radiotherapy should be given whatever the histopathologic type; if the lesion is an ectopic pinealoma, consideration should be given to radiation of the whole CNS since metastases via the CSF pathway have been reported.[54] Steroid replacement and electrolyte balance must be maintained not only during the initial therapy but indefinitely thereafter. A recent review of the literature reports eight of thirty-six patients alive without evidence of disease 1.6 to 7 years after diagnosis.[54]

Miscellaneous Tumors

Choroid Plexus Papillomas

These rare tumors usually are associated with hydrocephalus due to overproduction of CSF. On pneumoencephalography the tumor can be seen lying within the ventricle. Complete surgical removal will cure the child. Malignant tumors of the choroid plexus are extremely rare and almost always fatal. The value of radiation or chemotherapy is not known.

Meningeal Tumors

Meningiomas are rarely seen in children. They are usually benign and symptoms are caused by compression rather than by invasion of adjacent brain. Treatment is primarily surgical resection, which if complete may result in long-term survival.[15]

Leptomeningeal Sarcomas

These tumors diffusely involve the leptomeninges and tumor cells may seed freely throughout the subarachnoid pathways. Complete surgical resection is not possible. Radiotherapy of the entire CNS may produce prolonged survival.

Melanosarcomas

These tumors may arise in melanin-bearing cells in the meninges and spread throughout the CSF pathway diffusely. Pigmented nevi may be present on the skin. Death usually occurs rapidly, despite surgery, radiotherapy and chemotherapy.

Sarcoma of the Dura

Excision should be as complete as possible followed by radiation of the local area.

Spinal Cord Tumors

Back pain, lordosis, scoliosis, urinary or rectal incontinence, or pain or weakness in one or more extremity may herald a tumor in or adjacent to the spinal cord.

Extradural Tumors

These tumors are usually secondary rather than primary. A paravertebral neuroblastoma or ganglioneuroma may extend through the intervertebral foramina and produce an extradural mass. Metastatic or primary tumors in vertebrae may also result in an extradural mass and compression of the spinal cord.

Treatment depends on the type of tumor. If the tumor is radiosensitive and the signs of cord compression are minimal, then immediate local radiation may be sufficient. However, if the symptoms are progressing rapidly, an emergency laminectomy may be necessary to prevent paraplegia. The tumor can then be partially resected and irradiated. Chemotherapy may be helpful in sensitive tumors, but radiotherapy with or without laminectomy is usually the treatment of choice. For extradural neuroblastomas, laminectomy and radiation therapy are frequently curative, particularly if the child is less than one year old. If the tumor has metastasized from a radiosensitive primary tumor, surgery and radiation are often followed by a significant symptom-free period.

Intradural Tumors (Extramedullary)

Teratomas, lipomas, angiomas, neurofibromas or gliomas of the cauda equina may arise in the subdural space. They are rarely malignant, should be completely resected if possible, and usually give no further problem.

Intramedullary Tumors

Commonly astrocytomas, tumors arising within the cord, are usually benign (grade I or II) but are occasionally more malignant. They are usually unresectable because of their infiltrative nature. A laminectomy allows visualization of the tumor, a biopsy if one can be done without damaging vital pathways, and decompressive aspiration of the tumor if it is cystic. Radiation therapy may retard subsequent growth.

The prognosis depends on the degree of malignancy. The majority of children with tumors of low-grade malignancy survive for ten or more years after diagnosis, although they may have some progression of their neurological findings. A five-year survival rate of 60 percent and a ten-year survival rate of 60 percent and a ten-year survival rate of 52 percent has been reported for thirty intramedullary tumors of the spinal cord treated by irradiation.[5] This series included ependymomas as well as astrocytomas.

Ependymomas

Complete resection is usually possible if the filum terminale or cauda equina is involved, but when the tumor arises within the spinal cord it can rarely be completely resected. Radiotherapy should be directed to the tumor and probably to the whole CNS because of the tendency for seeding via the spinal fluid. Ependymomas of the spinal cord have a better prognosis than those arising elsewhere. Of six children followed for five years or more at the Hospital for Sick Children, four are alive and well, except for some spasticity of the legs in one child. Sixty-five percent of twenty-seven adults and children were alive five years after diagnosis.[58]

CONCLUSION

The diagnosis of a brain tumor in a child is not necessarily catastrophic. If diagnosed early and treated optimally, through the cooperative efforts of a surgeon, radiotherapist and, sometimes, a chemotherapist, the majority of children can be given a significant prolongation of useful active life, and a number of them may be cured. New and more effective chemotherapeutic agents are needed.

REFERENCES

1. Koos, W., and Miller, M.: *Intracranial Tumors of Infants and Children*. St. Louis, C.V. Mosby Company, 1970.
2. Hendrick, E.: Personal communication, 1972.
3. Makeever, L., and King, J.: Medulloblastoma with extracranial metastasis through a ventriculovenous shunt; report of a case and review of the literature. *Am J Clin Pathol, 46*:245-249, 1966.
4. Bloom, H., Wallace, E., and Henk, J.M.: The treatment and prognosis of medulloblastoma in children. *Am J Roentgenol, 105*:43-62, 1969.
5. Bouchard, J.: *Radiation Therapy of Tumors and Diseases of the Nervous System*. Philadelphia, Lea & Febiger, 1966.

6. Russell, D., Rubenstein, L.J., and Lumsden, C.: *Pathology of Tumors of the Nervous System* (3rd ed.). Baltimore, Williams & Wilkins, 1969.
7. Wilson, C., and Hoshino, T.: Current trends in the chemotherapy of brain tumors with special reference to glioblastomas. *J Neurosurg, 31*:589-603, 1969.
8. Norrell, H., and Wilson, C.: Brain tumor chemotherapy with methotrexate given intrathecally; a new technique. *JAMA, 201*:93-95, 1967.
9. Ommaya, A., Rubin, R., Henderson, E. *et al.*: A new approach to the treatment of inoperable brain tumors. *Med Ann DC, 34*:455-458, 1965.
10. Newton, W., Sayers, M., and Samuels, L.: Intrathecal methotrexate (NSC-740) therapy for brain tumors in children. *Cancer Chemother Rep, 52*:257-261, 1968.
11. Lassman, L., Pearce, G., and Gang, J.: Effect of vincristine sulphate on the intracranial gliomata of childhood. *Br J Surg, 53*:774-777, 1966.
12. Sonley, M., Hendrick, E.B., Hoffman, H., and Jenkin, R.: Unpublished data from the Hospital for Sick Children. Toronto, 1972.
13. Lampkin, B.C., Mauer, A.M., and McBride, B.H.: Response of medulloblastoma to vincristine sulfate; a case report. *Pediatrics, 39*:761-763, 1967.
14. Sano, K., Hoshino, T., and Nagai, M.: Radiosensitization of brain tumor cells with a thymidine analogue (bromouridine). *J Neurosurg, 28*:530-538, 1968.
15. Matson, D.: *Neurosurgery of Infancy and Childhood* (2nd ed.). Springfield, Charles C Thomas, 1969.
16. Geisinger, J., and Bucy, P.: Astrocytomas of the cerebellum in children; long-term study. *Arch Neurol, 24*:125-135, 1971.
17. Levy, L., and Elvidge, A.: Astrocytoma of the brain and spinal cord. A review of 176 cases 1940-1949. *J Neurosurg, 13*:413-443, 1956.
18. Bucy, P., and Thieman, P.: Astrocytomas of the cerebellum; a study of a series of patients operated upon over 25 years ago. *Arch Neurol, 18*:14-19, 1968.
19. Schulz, M., Wang, C., Zinninger, G., and Tefft, M.: Radiotherapy of intracranial neoplasma. *Progr Neurol Surg, 2*:318-370, 1968.
20. Jenkin, R.: Medulloblastoma in childhood; radiation therapy. *Can Med Assoc J, 100*:51-53, 1969.
21. Lassman, L., Pearce, G., Banna, M., and Jones, R.: Vincristine sulphate in the treatment of skeletal metastases from cerebellar medulloblastoma. *J Neurosurg, 30*:42-48, 1969.
22. Elsberg, C., and Gotten, N.: The results of conservative compared with radical operations in cerebellar medulloblastomas; an analysis of 23 cases. *Bull Neurol Inst NY, 3*:33-52, 1933.
23. Sayers, M., Newton, W., and Samuels, L.: Intrathecal methotrexate

therapy of brain tumors of childhood. *Ann NY Acad Sci, 159:*608-613, 1969.

24. Paterson, E., and Farr, R.: Cerebellar medulloblastoma; treatment by irradiation of the whole central nervous system. *Acta Radiol, 39:*323-336, 1953.
25. Hope-Stone, H.F.: Results of treatment of medulloblastoma. *J Neurosurg, 32:*83-88, 1970.
26. Jenkin, R.: Personal communication, 1972.
27. Kricheff, I., Becker, M., Schneck, S., and Taveras, J.: Intracranial ependymomas; a study of survival in 65 cases treated by surgery and irradiation. *Am J Roentgenol, 91:*167-175, 1964.
28. Fokes, E., and Earle, K.: Ependymemas; clinical and pathological aspects. *J Neurosurg, 30:*585-594, 1969.
29. Svien, H.J., Gates, E., and Kernohan, J.: Spinal subarachnoid implantation associated with ependymoma. *Arch Neurol Psychiat, 62:*847-856, 1949.
30. Wentworth, P., and Birdsell, D.: Intracranial ependymoma with extracranial metastases; case report. *J Neurosurg, 25:*648-651, 1966.
31. Ringertz, N., and Reymond, A.: Ependymomas and choroid plexus papillomas. *J Neuropathol Exp Neurol, 8:*355-380, 1949.
32. Children's Cancer Group A. Protocol CCA910.
33. Walker, M., and Hurwitz, B.: BCNU (1,3-Bis(2-Chloroetheyl)-1-Nitrosourea NSC-409962) in the treatment of malignant brain tumor; a preliminary report. *Cancer Chemother Rep, 54:*263-271, 1970.
34. Panitch, H., and Berg, B.: Brain stem tumors of childhood and adolescence. *Am J Dis Child, 119:*465-472, 1970.
35. Kernohan, J., and Sayre, G.: Tumors of the central nervous system. *Atlas of Tumor Pathology,* Section 10. Washington D.C., Armed Forces Institute of Pathology, 1952.
36. Ley, A., Giutart, J., and Olivares, C.: Surgical management of intracranial gliomas. *J Neurosurg, 19:*365-374, 1962.
37. Jelsma, R., and Bucy, P.: The treatment of glioblastoma multiforme of the brain. *J Neurosurg, 27:*388-400, 1967.
38. Wilson, C., Boldrey, E.B., and Enot, K.: 1,3-Bis(2-chloroethyl)-1-nitrosourea (NSC-409962) in the treatment of brain tumors. *Cancer Chemother Rep, 54:*273-281, 1970.
39. Childrens Cancer Group A. Protocol CCA-915.
40. Owens, G., Javid, R., Belmusto, L., Bender, M., and Blau, M.: Intra-arterial vincristine therapy of primary gliomas. *Cancer, 18:*756-760, 1965.
41. McCarthy, C.: Results of the surgical management of glial tumors of the brain. In Fields, W., and Sharkey, P. (Eds.): *The Biology and Treatment of Intracranial Tumors.* Springfield, Charles C Thomas, 1962, pp. 434-456.

42. Frankel, S., and German, W.: Glioblastoma multiforme; review of 219 cases with regard to natural history, pathology, diagnostic method and treatment. *J Neurosurg, 15:*489-503, 1958.
43. Matson, D., and Crigler, J.: Management of craniopharyngioma in childhood. *J Neurosurg, 30:*377-390, 1969.
44. Bartlett, J.R.: Craniopharyngiomas; a summary of 85 cases. *J Neurosurg, 34:*37-41, 1971.
45. Kramer, S., McKissock, W., and Concannon, J.P.: Craniopharyngiomas; treatment by combined surgery and radiation therapy. *J Neurosurg, 18:*217-226, 1961.
46. Marsden, H., and Steward, J.K.: *Tumors in Children.* New York, Springer-Verlag, 1968.
47. Harwood-Nash, D.C.: Axial tomography of the optic canals in children. *Radiology, 96:*367-374, 1970.
48. Hoyt, W.F., and Baghdassarian, S.A.: Optic glioma of childhood: Natural history and rationale for conservative management. *Br J Ophthal, 53:*793-798, 1969.
49. Taveras, J., Mount, L., and Wood, E.: The value of radiation therapy in the management of glioma of the optic nerves and chiasm. *Radiology, 66:*518-528, 1956.
50. MacCarty, C., Boyd, A.S., and Childs, D.: Tumors of the optic nerve and optic chiasm. *J Neurosurg, 33:*439-444, 1970.
51. Glaser, J., Hoyt, W., and Corbett, J.: Visual morbidity with chiasmal glioma. *Arch Ophthal, 85:*3-12, 1971.
52. Russell, A.: Diencephalic syndrome of emaciation in infancy and childhood. *Arch Dis Child, 26:*274-278, 1951.
53. Bain, H., Darte, J., Keith, W., and Kruyff, E.: The diencephalic syndrome of early infancy due to silent brain tumor; with special reference to treatment. *Pediatrics, 38:*474-482, 1966.
54. Rubin, P., and Kramer, S.: Ectopic pinealoma; a radiocurable neuroendocrinologic entity. *Radiology, 85:*512-523, 1965.
55. Cummins, F., Taveras, J., and Schlesinger, E.: Treatment of gliomas of the third ventrical and pinealomas, with special reference to the value of radiotherapy. *Neurology, 10:*1031-1036, 1960.
56. Suzuki, J., and Iwabuchi, T.: Surgical removal of pineal tumors (pinealomas and teratomas). *J Neurosurg, 23:*565-571, 1965.
57. Horrax, G.: The diagnosis and treatment of pineal tumors. *Radiology, 52:*186-191, 1949.
58. Barone, B., and Elvidge, A.R.: Ependyomas; a clinical survey. *J Neurosurg, 33:*428-438, 1970.

Chapter 9

MALIGNANT TUMORS OF BONE

Seymour Zimbler

Primary malignant lesions of bone comprise a small but important portion of the overall cancer picture in children. Late diagnoses, difficult treatment programs and devastatingly poor prognoses are major problems for physicians involved in this area.

Accurate diagnosis and treatment require knowledge of bone as a tissue as well as the specific activity of each individual tumor involved. Clinicians such as pediatricians and orthopedic surgeons must cooperate in a team effort with diagnostic radiologists, pathologists, radiotherapists and oncologists in order to achieve the best results possible. Interpretation of x-rays and histologic material must be carried out concurrently, once all clinical information is assembled. Frequently, definitive diagnoses are difficult to reach and experts from other parts of the country must be consulted. Biopsy material should be adequate in amount and representative of the lesion; it must be obtained in an atraumatic manner to minimize cellular emboli and eventual metastases. Operative incision for biopsy purposes must be planned so as not to compromise later, more definitive therapy.

The roles of surgery, radiation therapy and chemotherapy must be established in each individual patient. Scheduling of treatment is crucial in avoiding delay, especially in situations where ablation is to follow a course of radiation therapy. Frequent complete follow-up evaluations are obviously necessary in these situations; again, the team approach seems best. Particular expertise is obviously desirable in the psychologic handling of the young patient and his or her family. This all important but delicate chore is critical to the smooth and rapid completion of a total treatment program. Parents' rapport is enhanced by early and complete understanding of the child's total problem and prognosis as well as the treatment planned. It is our purpose here to review current thinking regarding some of the difficult aspects of malignant bone tumors in children.

OSTEOSARCOMA

Osteosarcoma (osteogenic sarcoma) has been defined by Jaffe[1] as "a specialized connective tissue sarcoma which forms neoplastic osteoid and osseous tissue in the course of evolution." The cells of origin of this tumor may evolve from "primary mesenchyme" or more mature elements of the medullary canal or periosteum of bone.[2] Many authors use the term "osteogenic sarcoma" in the larger sense to encompass all sarcomas originating in skeletal connective tissue.[3-6] Budd and MacDonald[4] subdivided osteogenic sarcoma into osteosarcoma, chondrosarcoma and fibrosarcoma. Their feeling was that the primary mesenchymal stem cell could develop into fibrous tissue, cartilage or bone. However, chondrosarcoma and fibrosarcoma are specific entities which can be separated from the true osteosarcoma by differences in age of occurrence, localization and prognosis, as well as histology. The tumor cells are not bone-forming in these lesions. Our interest in this section is in the true osteosarcoma, arising in the interior of an affected bone and revealing malignant spindle cells which produce tumor-osteoid tissue (Fig. 9-1). Dahlin[7] found three histologic groups within six hundred patients with osteosarcoma: 54.7 percent, osteoblastic; 23.3 percent, fibroblastic; and 22 percent, chondroblastic. He labeled these groups depending on the predominant type of tissue being manufactured by the tumor cells. Excluded from our discussion will be parosteal (juxtacortical osteosarcoma, osteosarcoma of the jawbones, and osteosarcoma occurring in Paget's disease). These are special tumor groups, usually seen in adults and presenting problems other than those of the pediatric ages. The older subclassifications of "central, periosteal, sclerosing, and telangietatic" are not as useful and will not be presented here.[8] They are partially based on radiologic presentation.

Excluding myeloma, osteosarcoma is the most frequently seen primary malignant tumor of bone in all age groups. It is the most

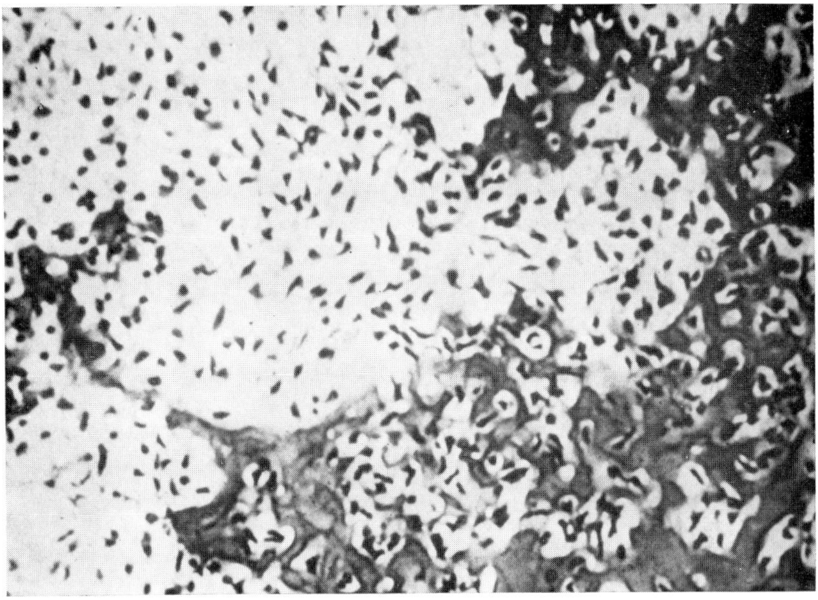

Figure 9-1. Osteosarcoma. This field demonstrates calcification of osteoid matrix. Typical malignant round and spindle cells are seen.

common primary malignancy of bone in children and is estimated to occur in one per one hundred thousand persons in the United States. A Mayo Clinic series found osteosarcoma to be two to eight times more common than other primary malignant bone tumors. This group[8] reviewed 2,276 tumors of which there were 490 osteosarcomas, 218 chondrosarcomas, 58 fibrosarcomata, 70 reticulum cell sarcomata and 141 Ewing's sarcomas.

Osteosarcoma is slightly more common in males (60 percent) and 75 percent of the patients are in the ten to twenty-five age group. Tumors of long bones are almost always found in the metaphyseal regions: the femur is involved in more than 50 percent of the cases. The knee joint area is most commonly involved, with the tibia and humerus as the next most commonly involved bones.

Clinical complaints are usually gradual in onset. Local pain, increasing with activity and more severe with passage of time, is the most common symptom. Limping, or a variation of gait associated with flexion contractures, depends again on the duration of symptoms as well as the close association of tumor with joint capsules such as the knee. Limitation of motion of joints and local tenderness are commonly noted. Increasing masses with superficial venous dilatation in skin are seen in late cases. Minor trauma is a common reason for discovery of a local lesion but has not been implicated in etiology in any series reviewed by us. Pathologic fractures through larger lesions are occasionally the presenting event.

Laboratory values are usually normal in these patients. Occasionally, the serum alkaline phosphatase can be elevated to as much as twice normal values. This will diminish with amputation and radiotherapy but will increase in association with metastases.

Roentgenographic findings in osteosarcoma are usually excellent examples of the true gross pathology. These lesions are solitary, lying toward one end of a long bone and exhibiting some radio-opacity. Opacity can be seen within the soft tissues as well as within the medullary canal; this is caused by so-called "true tumor- bone" (Fig. 9-2). Cortical destruction associated with soft tissue masses are commonly seen. Periosteal new bone formation can be of the Codman's triangle type or appositional (lamellar, "onionskin"). These presentations are due to gradually expanding cortices by tumor pressure. "Sunburst" striations are calcified trabeculae of tumor bone lying in ossifying extracortical tumor tissue; they are not periosteal in origin and lie perpendicular to and long axes of the bone (Fig. 9-3).

Microscopically, osteosarcoma varies depending on the predominant cell type noted. Neoplastic osteoid is present in large or small amounts. Unossified or fibroblastic lesions will have spindle cells in the stroma; chondroblastic lesions will have round shaped cells lying in lacunae. Anaplastic areas can have cells with double or hyperchromatic nuclei. Sarcoma giant cells can be prevalent or occasional. Some highly vascular tumors may show little in the way of new bone formation. More differentiated lesions will show ossification of the stromal tissue with increase in osteoid and intercellular fibrillar "collagenous material" (Fig. 9-4). Cellular

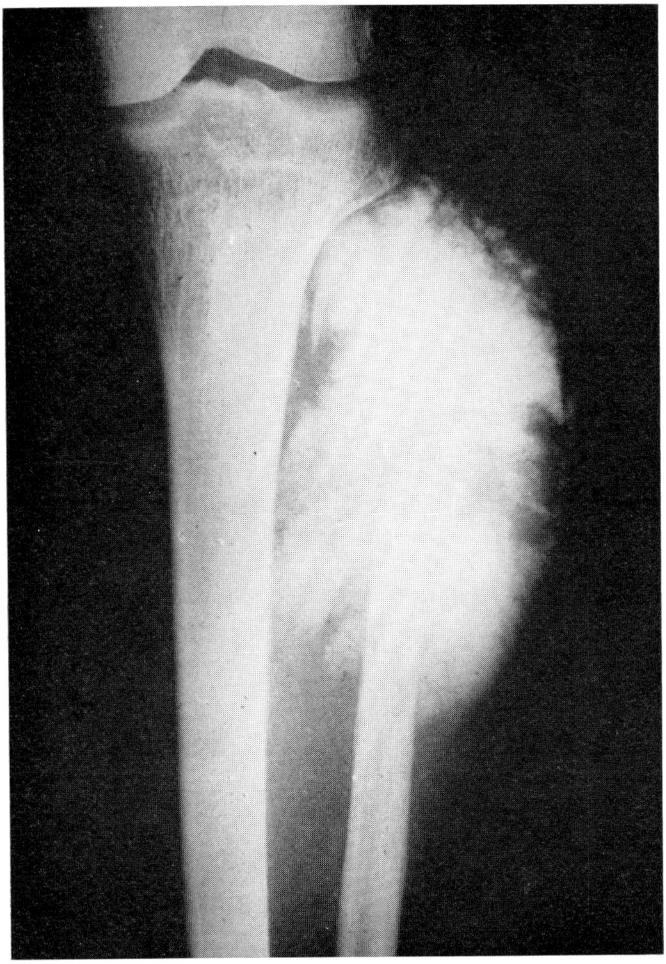

Figure 9-2. Massive extension of osteosarcoma into surrounding soft tissues.

grading of osteosarcoma can be carried out according to the method of Broders.[9] This is set up in grades of I to IV depending on the degree of anaplasia.

Various authors have reviewed factors which could effect the prognosis in this difficult group of patients. Lindbom[10] suggested that women were less likely than men to succumb to osteosarcoma, but this has been disputed by Dahlin[7] and others.[11] Nosanchuk

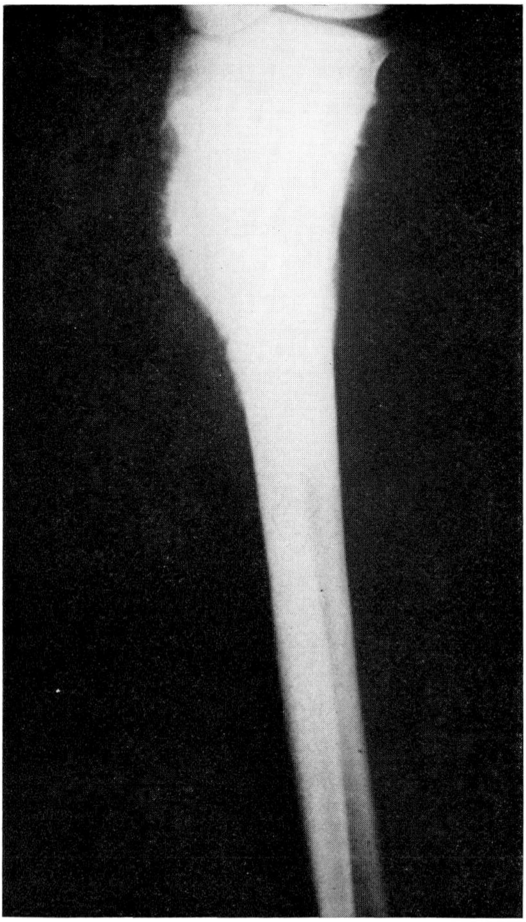

Figure 9-3. Osteosarcoma of the proximal tibia demonstrating "sunburst" striations of tumor bone.

et al.[12] found a slightly better prognosis in older patients as well as in females, but this series included five patients with Paget's disease. The type of tumor involved (osteoblastic, fibroblastic and chondroblastic) did not appear to play a part in the five-year survival figures.[7] Less anaplastic lesions appeared to have a slightly better prognosis but this was again not statistically significant when tested.

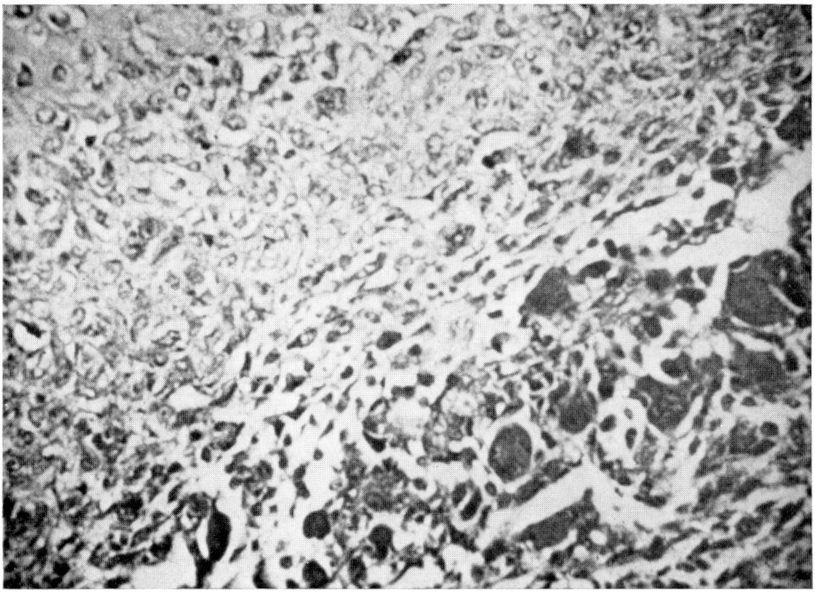

Figure 9-4. Osteosarcoma. This microscopic field reveals sarcoma giant cells as well as a common cellular stromal pattern.

Coventry and Dahlin[8] found a 34.6 percent five-year survival rate for patients with tibial tumors while femoral tumors had only a 17 percent five-year survival. Earlier diagnosis because of the more superficial position of the tibial surface was presented as a possible explanation for this difference in results. None of the thirty patients with osteosarcoma of the innominate bones survived five years in this series.[8] Those patients with longer durations of symptoms prior to treatment may have a slightly improved prognosis.[11] McKenna[3] found that 90 percent of the treatment failures were treated within six months of the onset of symptoms. This may simply represent the potential biological activity of the tumors involved; larger more slowly growing tumors may have a slightly better prognosis.[3] It appears that the type of treatment is the most significant factor determining eventual prognosis. Basically, there have been three major types of treatment programs:

The first major treatment calls for immediate amputation at

the time of biopsy, as advocated at the Mayo Clinic.[7] Amputations are carried out between two tourniquets in an attempt to diminish chances for tumor emboli. This method presupposes that the surgeon obtains excellent, only partially calcified, sections of representative tissue which must then be read by frozen section techniques. Experienced pathological consultation is the necessary ingredient here. In Dahlin's series 20.3 percent of the 408 patients treated, survived more than five years.

The second major treatment includes preoperative megavoltage radiotherapy of 7,000 to 8,000 rads followed by a three to four month observation period, prior to ablation. This method was proposed by Cade in 1951[13] and reported on by Lee and MacKenzie, 1964.[14]

This second group treated only patients with osteosarcoma in situations where no metastases were known. Biopsies were obtained in 146 of 157 cases reported on; these were done by open technique or drill biopsy (trephine technique). Biopsies were sometimes carried out after 1,000 rads had been administered. MeV x-radiation was given by two parallel opposed fields with a tumor dose of 1150 rads per five-day week per total tumor dose of 7,000 to 8,000 rads. A period of observation was then carried out, lasting at least three to four months. Radical amputation would be carried out after this observation period, unless pulmonary metastases were noted or there was an exceptionally good response to x-ray therapy, such as in the upper extremity (adequate function with no disability).

Eighty of 157 patients in this series developed metastases; seventy-five of these in the first five months after x-ray treatment was completed.[14] However, there were 21.8 percent overall five-year survivors in these cases where amputation was carried out. The authors and Sir Stanford Cade[13] feel that this method avoids unnecessary amputation in patients who develop pulmonary metastases; they also point out that their results compare favorably with other more surgically oriented series. Tudway[16] suggested that this method be used for upper extremity lesions only since the extensive radiation frequently made the lower extremity functionless.

The third major treatment method is somewhat similar to the Westminster Hospital series.[14] This involves supravoltage radiation therapy with 1000 rads prebiopsy followed by 6,000 to 8,000 rads post biopsy in a four- to six-week period. Radical amputation is then carried out if no metastases have been found. This treatment schedule has been used primarily in Boston at the Children's Hospital Medical Center. Green[15] stated in 1968 that the results of this method compare favorably with the immediate surgery group.

Chemotherapy has been used extensively in the postbiopsy period, although its individual effect is difficult to evaluate. This method may allow a more rapid removal of the primary tumor but also may result in some unnecessary amputations (75 percent of metastases appear up to five months following cessation of radiation therapy).[14]

There has been some dispute in the literature regarding the appropriate level of amputation. Most reports have favored removal of the joint above the involved bone because of evidence of stump recurrences of tumor when lesser procedures are done. Dahlin[7] reported ten stump recurrences in his series but felt that amputation three inches above the medullary involvement by x-ray evaluation was adequate. Frozen sections should be routinely taken from the distal medullary canal at the time of amputations, if this method is chosen.

Resection of solitary metastases, particularly pulmonary, has been suggested as an attempt to increase survival time. Dahlin[7] reported on fourteen of these patients, two of whom became long-term survivors. Multiple operations were necessary in the other patients with only three others surviving: one, seven and forty-one months after the last pulmonary resection.

Chemotherapy has been utilized only as an adjunct in the therapy of osteosarcoma. Cyclophosphamide (Cytoxan) and actinomycin D have been used in some patients in the postradiation, postamputation phase. Long-term results in these situations are difficult to evaluate. Cyclophosphamide has shown some effect in reducing the size of pulmonary metastases[17] and in our experience has led to several prolonged remissions in patients with documented metastatic disease.

During recent years, radioisotopes such as strontium 85, strontium 87M and gallium 67 have been employed as useful tools both in diagnosis and therapy. Primary bone lesions such as osteosarcoma and Ewing's will pick up these isotopes in substantial amounts. Clinical scanning techniques can then give additional important information regarding size and extent of primary tumors; occult metastases may be noted with techniques of this type. In addition, scanning techniques have proven helpful in evaluating the response of tumor-bearing areas to chemotherapy or radiotherapy.

EWING'S SARCOMA

This lesion was originally described by Ewing in 1921.[18] He felt that the tumor was derived from angioendothelial cells. Others have described the mesenchymal cells of the bone marrow as the basic cells of origin. However, most authors now agree that Ewing's sarcoma is a specific, highly malignant clinicopathologic entity which can be separated on several grounds from reticulum cell sarcoma, metastatic neuroblastoma, eosinophilic granuloma and osteomyelitis. This primary malignant bone tumor is much less common than osteosarcoma. It is more common in males and 95 percent of the cases appear in the four to twenty-five year age group. In some series 50 percent of the tumors originate in a part of an innominate bone; the remainder appear in the femur, tibia, fibula and humerus, in that order.

The most common presenting symptom is local or referred pain of increasing severity over several months. Physical findings include tender, warm masses associated with superficial venous dilatation. Associated systemic signs of fever, anemia, leukocytosis and elevated sedimentation rate are seen in more fulminant cases.

Radiologically, these lesions appear as large or small areas of mottled rarefaction (Fig. 9-5). The tumor itself does not form "new bone" but opacity can occur in certain lesions as a reactive process. Periosteal new bone formation is slight and is secondary to penetration of the cortex by tumor; appositional concentric

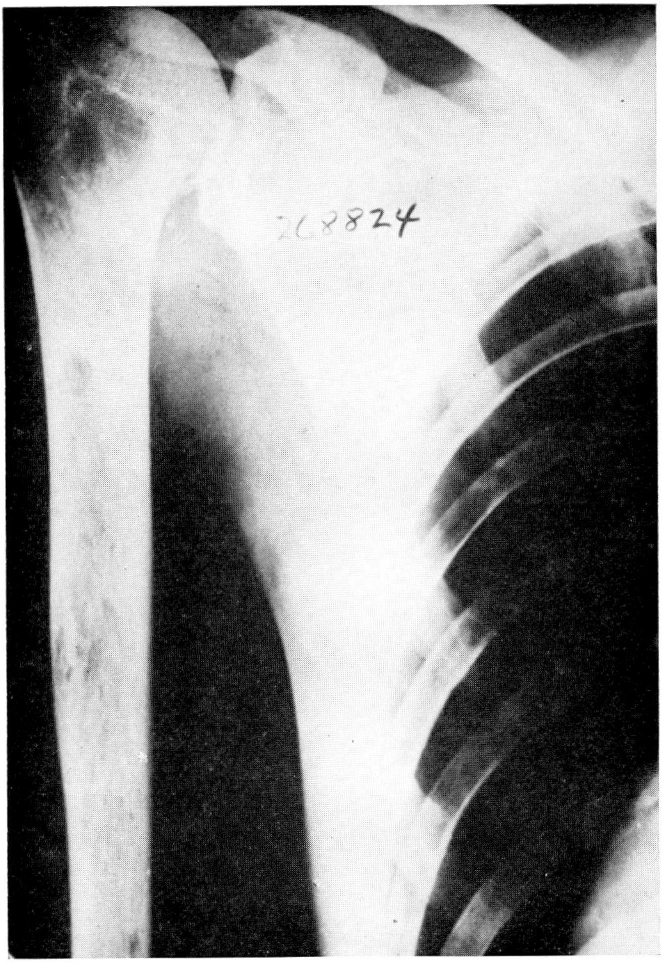

Figure 9-5. This humeral diaphysis shows mottling and rarefaction over a large area due to Ewing's sarcoma.

layers of periosteal new bone can be seen in tubular bones ("onionskin") (Fig. 9-6). Sometimes a large portion of the shaft of a long bone can show just mottling with complete absence of periosteal bone formation.

Grossly, the tissue of Ewing's sarcoma is soft and gray to gray-red in color. It has a fibrous consistency but can be occasionally

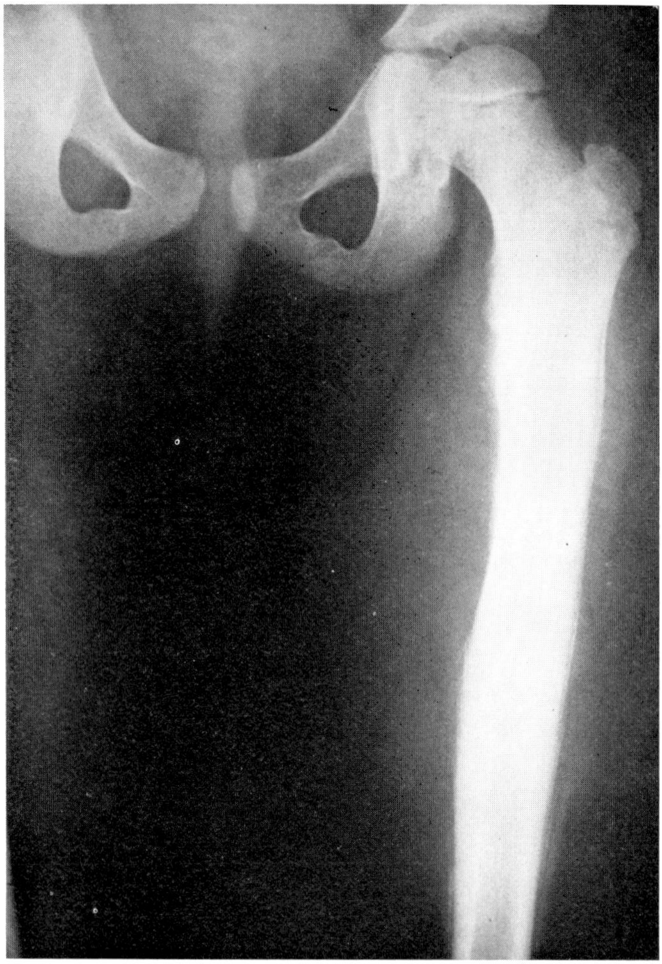

Figure 9-6. Ewing's sarcoma in femoral shaft showing periosteal new bone formation of "onionskin" type.

liquid. Hemorrhage and necrosis are commonly seen within the tumor and can account for sudden increase in the size of masses. Soft, extraosseous tumor is commonly seen in areas where the cortex has broken through. Tumor involvement of almost entire medullary canals of long or flat bones is also quite common; usually this is much more extensive than would be predicted by x-ray examination or changes.

Jaffe[1] has observed wide dissemination of this sarcoma in multiple bones at autopsy. He subscribes to the theory of multicentric origin of Ewing's sarcoma but offers no concrete proof. Lymph nodes are not usually involved with tumor but lungs, liver, heart, spleen, kidneys and thyroid can show extensive involvement.

Microscopically, the cells of the Ewing's sarcoma are found in large or small sheets. The cell nuclei are round or ovoid, usually two to three times as wide as the nucleus of a lymphocyte. Fine chromatin with one or more nucleoli are noted; cell boundaries are indistinct (Fig. 9-7). Nuclear pyknosis and cellular necrosis are seen in many degenerative fields; reactive inflammatory change and hemorrhage are common. Tumor cells are seen lining vascular spaces but also gathering about the degenerating cores of cells, thus stimulating a type of rosette formation; this is an occasional and not too prominent microscopic feature of the tumor. Retic-

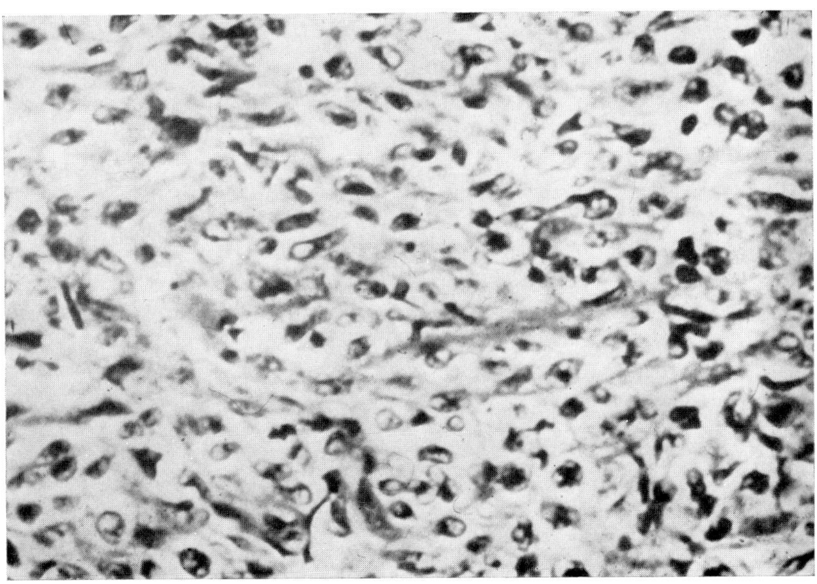

Figure 9-7. Ewing's sarcoma. This high-power view reveals sheets of closely packed nuclei with indistinct cell margins.

ulum cells are also noted but are usually irregularly distributed in these microscopic fields.

The differential diagnosis of the Ewing's sarcoma merits some mention as it is commonly difficult. In children, a solitary eosinophilic granuloma of bone or osteomyelitis can mimic the x-ray picture of the Ewing's sarcoma. Histologic differentiation will not be difficult in these situations. Similarly, an osteolytic or sclerosing type of osteosarcoma can certainly present an x-ray picture quite consistent with the Ewing's sarcoma if appearing in the metaphysis of a long bone. Neuroblastoma, appearing as a solitary bony metastasis, can present histologic diagnostic problems. These usually occur in children under five years old, and demonstration of adrenal masses will certainly help in the diagnosis. Neuroblastoma cells are round with vesicular neuclei; rosettes of tumor cells about central neurofibrils are the characteristic differentiating feature. Reticulum cell sarcoma of bone can also present a similar x-ray picture. The reticulum cell sarcoma will be discussed in more detail later; however, the round cells of this lesion appear quite similar but are larger than those of the Ewing's sarcoma. The cell nuclei in reticulum cell sarcoma are also larger and frequently are indented; reticulum stains show the typical strands about groups of these tumor cells. Schajowicz[19] has demonstrated that tumor cells in Ewing's sarcoma have stainable glycogen while those of reticulum cell sarcoma do not. This has proven to be a helpful histologic differentiation.

As previously inferred, Ewing's sarcoma is a highly lethal lesion; metastases occur rapidly and in a widespread fashion. The possibility of multicentric origin and longitudinal extension within involved bones has led to confusion in establishment of definite treatment programs. Dahlin[20] reviewed 133 patients with Ewing's sarcoma and found that twenty (15 percent) were alive at five years. Ninety-five of the 133 patients reviewed in Dahlin's series were dead within two years of initial diagnosis, fifty-nine of these were in the first year. At ten years, only twelve (10.7 percent) of these patients were surviving. These delayed deaths are characteristic in Ewing's sarcoma and have been noted by other authors.[21] Grouping several reported series together[20-23] revealed that 94 percent of 511 patients reviewed were dead within six to seven months of diagnosis; five-year survival in this group was 6 percent.

There is considerable variation of opinion regarding treatment of Ewing's sarcoma. Dahlin[20] in his report in 1961, pointed out that the large majority of patients with Ewing's sarcoma are eventually treated with irradiation. In this series, eleven of twenty patients who survived five years had as their primary definitive treatment x-ray therapy. However, three of these eleven patients had to undergo amputation for recurrent tumor, three, four and eleven years after the initial radiation. This author (Dahlin) suggests that ablative surgical treatment is more efficacious than radiation. In his series, 35 percent of the five-year survivors were treated with primary amputation. Four of six patients who died late from Ewing's sarcoma received radiation as the primary treatment.

There is no question that radiation alone does not appear to be the complete answer in the treatment of the Ewing's sarcoma. However, most of the major series have used radiation therapy as their primary treatment modality. Undoubtedly, this stems from frustration at the aggressive behavior and widespread appearance of this tumor. There is no large series in the literature featuring amputation therapy alone for Ewing's sarcoma which can be quoted as showing significantly better results than that of radiation or any other measure. There is no question that the primary tumor can be controlled by modern methods of radiation therapy in the doses suggested. However, the early subclinical metastases suggest the usefulness of chemotherapy in addition to radiation. Various agents have been tried and cyclophosphamide (Cytoxan) appears to be the most effective agent. Vincristine, 5-fluorouracil and actinomycin D have also been reported as somewhat useful in the palliative treatment of the Ewing's sarcoma patient.

There have been some encouraging reports in several recent small series of patients treated with combination chemotherapy plus radiotherapy. Hustu *et al.*[30] have used intensive chemotherapy with cyclophosphamide and vincristine concurrently plus high doses of radiotherapy to the primary lesion. They have treated six patients, ages seven to twenty-one years, and four have remained free of metastases. Other chemotherapy study groups have used vincristine and cyclophosphamide in small groups of patients. Roughly, 50 percent of the patients treated are remaining in relatively good condition with their tumor localizing to the primary area. Additional groups of investigators are attempting to use either total body irradiation plus irradiation of the primary lesion or a combination of total body irradiation, irradiation to the lungs and primary irradiation to the lesion in addition to chemotherapy. Certainly, since pulmonary metastases are the predominant area of spread, prophylactic irradiation of the lungs may have some advantage in prolonging the life and comfort of the patient.

Because of these problems with this particular disease, a National Ewing's Sarcoma Study has been set up. An attempt at grouping a large number of cases is being made and control groups with various types of treatment programs are being set up. One control group consists of local radiation therapy to the entire shaft of involved long bones. A midplane dose of 4,000 to 6,000 rads will be given during the four to six weeks after biopsy. Some patients will be treated with radiation alone while others will be treated with local radiation to the tumor area and combination chemotherapy with cyclophosphamide, vincristine and actinomycin D (Cosmegen). Chemotherapy will be continued for fifteen to sixteen months in these patients in an attempt to prevent metastases. Another group of patients will receive local radiation therapy to the tumor, chemotherapy and bilateral pulmonary radiation with a midplane dose of 1200 to 1500 rads to both lung fields. This radiation therapy will be given daily in increments of 100 rads over twelve to fifteen days. Within this study will be a subgroup of patients in whom evidence of early Ewing's sarcoma in long bones will be treated by distal amputations and followed by pulmonary radiation or intensive chemotherapy, or both, with the previously mentioned drugs. A series of this type will certainly help to organize the planning of those physicians in clinical situations.

PRIMARY RETICULUM CELL SARCOMA OF BONE

This lesion has also raised some controversy regarding its presentation as a specific clinical entity. However, most authors in the literature now agree that the tumor has its own individual identifiable characteristics.[24-27] Originally these lesions were confused with Ewing's sarcoma; eventual separation occurred, partially through the obviously improved prognosis in reticulum cell sarcoma.

Reticulum cell sarcoma of bone is more common in males by a ratio of 2:1. At least 50 percent of the patients have been below forty years of age with many in the eleven to twenty year age group. In the condition which we will call "generalized reticulum cell sarcoma," most patients are forty and above. Femur, tibia and humerus are the most commonly affected tubular bones. Pelvic bones, scapula and ribs also are occasionally involved. Diaphyseal lesions are common in the tubular bones.

The clinical presentation of a single lesion of this type can be quite subtle. Local aching, pain with occasional swelling and specific tenderness are common early findings. Symptoms can be mild and intermittent even over periods of months. This fact in itself can help differentiation from Ewing's sarcoma. Pathologic fractures can be the precipitating event prior to definitive diagnosis.

The typical x-ray picture of the early lesion is one presenting osteolysis of the medullary canal of a long bone (Fig. 9-8).[28-29] Irregular areas of radiolucency associated with patches of radiopacity will be found. Cortical destruction or thickening of cortices can occur; there can be some distension of the bony diameter. Periosteal new bone formation occurs but in moderate degree. Non-ossifying extra-osseous masses can develop in longer duration cases.

Grossly, the reticulum cell tissue found in bone is white or gray-white and firm or only slightly friable. Larger tumor masses which cause cortical destruction and extra-osseous lesions will have areas of cyst formation and necrosis within the mass. The basic stromal cell is the round cell with a large single nucleus (larger than in Ewing's sarcoma). The nucleus can be oval or indented; fine chromatin is common and nucleoli can be present (Fig. 9-9). Double nuclei and mitotic figures can be seen but do not dominate the microscopic fields. Reticulum fibers, when stained for,

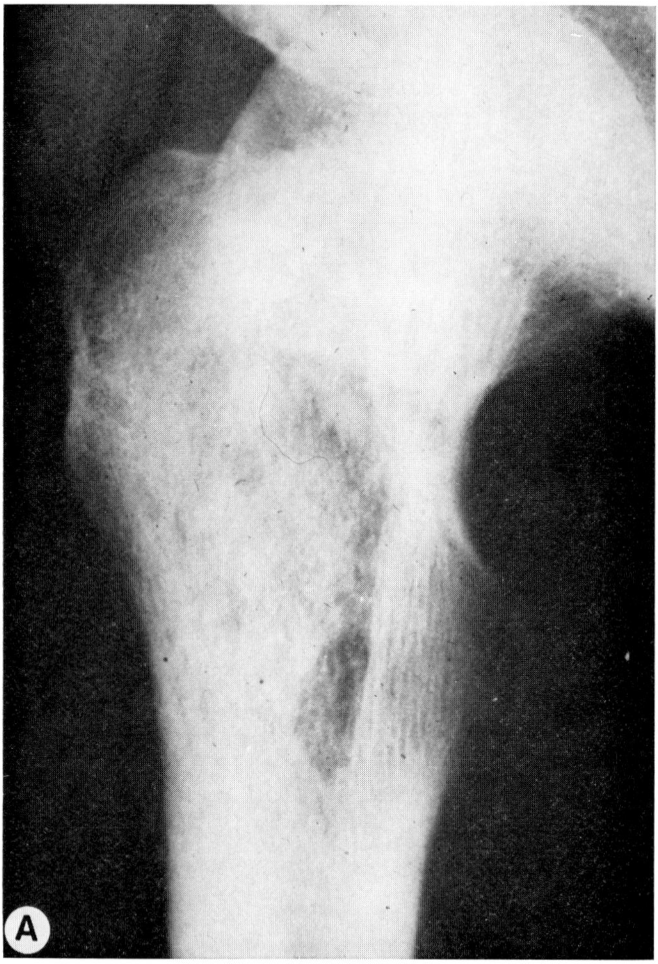

Figure 9-8. Reticulum cell sarcoma. *(A)* An early lesion showing mainly osteolysis. *(B)* A late lesion showing advanced cortical destruction, with patches of dense and lucent bone.

run in threads and strands about groups of tumor cells (Fig. 9-10).

Reticulum cell sarcoma may remain localized to an affected bone for long periods of time. In some cases there can be spread to regional lymph nodes only. These restricted cases in favorable

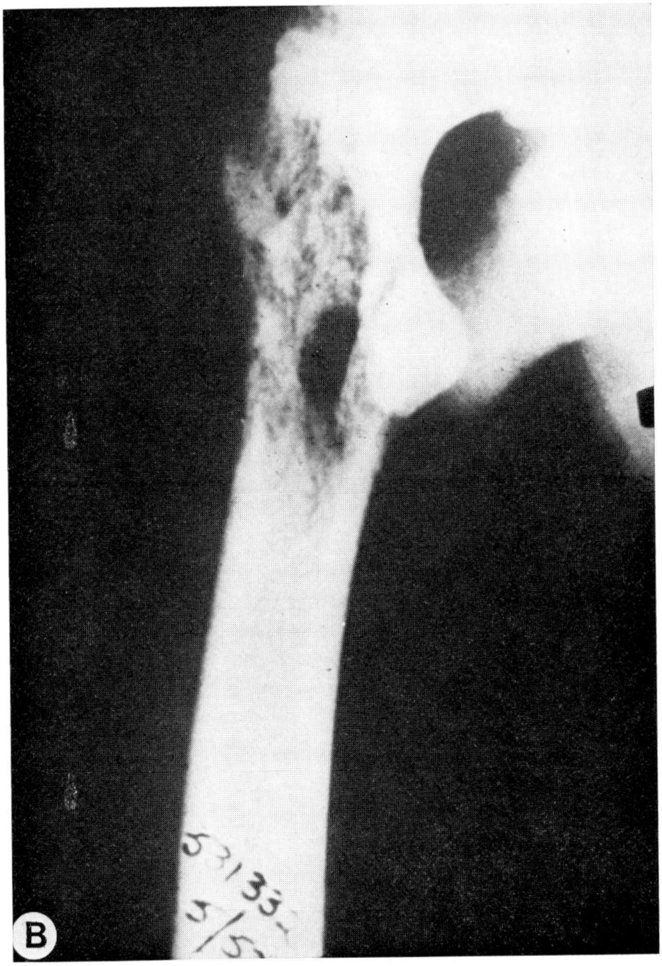

locations will have the best prognosis. Sometimes, however, initial presentation in one single bony site may eventually lead to the more typical widespread picture of generalized reticulum cell sarcoma. Involvement of lymph nodes, spleen, liver and lungs, as well as bone marrow, will occur. Naturally, this generalized type has a poor prognosis.

Most series favor irradiation as primary treatment for the local

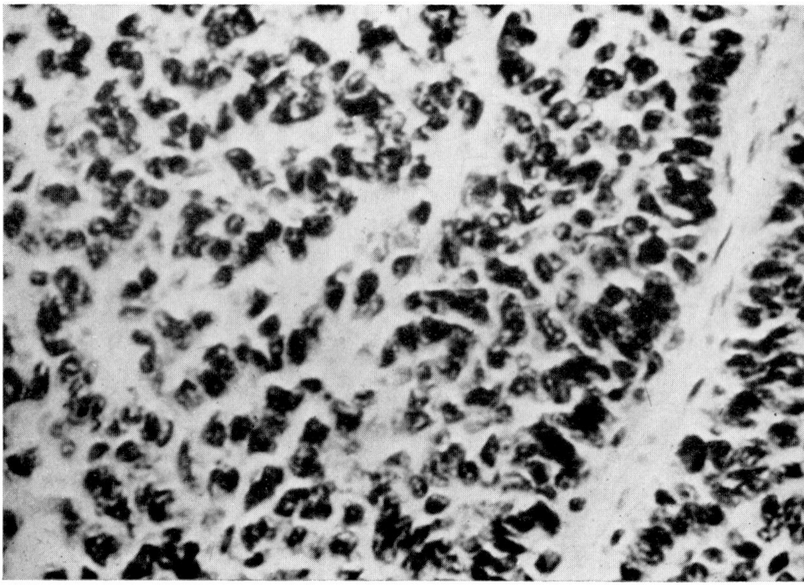

Figure 9-9. Reticulum cell sarcoma. This H and E stain shows stromal cells in clusters. A single large nucleus and prominent nucleolus can be noted.

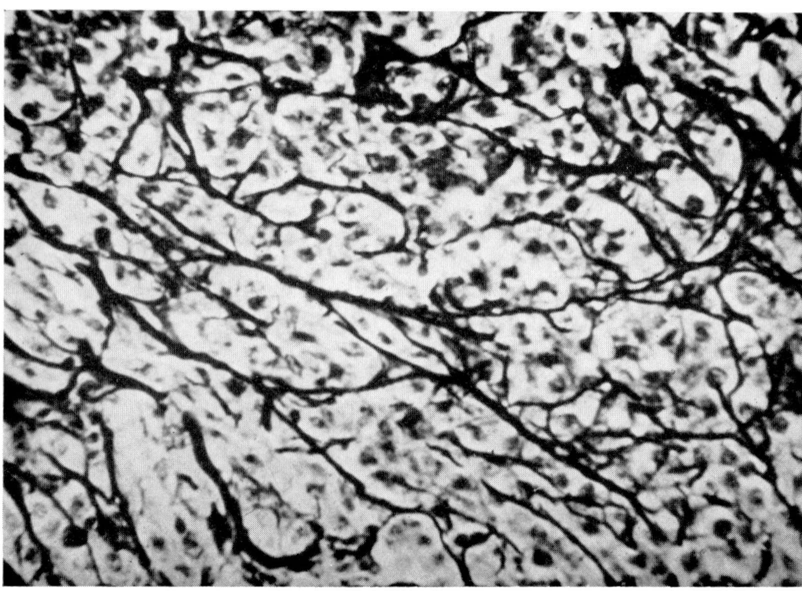

Figure 9-10. Reticulum cell sarcoma. A reticulum stain clearly shows the strands of reticulum fibers about groups of tumor cells.

type of reticulum cell sarcoma of bone. At least 3000 to 4000 rads is delivered locally to the tumor area; this usually results in total tumor destruction and apparent five-year cures. However, late local recurrence is not uncommon in irradiated cases. This has encouraged some groups to favor amputation or wide excision followed by radiation when feasible. However, irradiation and/or surgery has not improved the cure rate beyond 25 percent of cases. Cautious optimism must still be the rule in this disease entity. Combination chemotherapy may play an important role here in improving the survival of patients with apparently isolated single lesions.

In summary, we have presented some pertinent information regarding the most common malignant tumors of bone in childhood. Current thought about diagnosis and therapy as well as etiology has been described. Hopefully, results in the future will be improved by investigations of various groups now attempting to pool their efforts in studying these lesions. In the past, treatment of cases in a haphazard manner has not helped the total prognosis of these particular lesions.

REFERENCES

1. Jaffe, H.L.: *Tumors and Tumorous Conditions of the Bones and Joints.* Philadelphia, Lea & Febiger, 1958, pp. 256-278.
2. Ackerman, L.V., and Spjut, A.J.: *Tumors of Bone and Cartilage.* Section II, Fascicle 4, Washington, D.C., Armed Forces Institute of Pathology, 1962.
3. McKenna, R.J., Schwinn, C.P., Soong, K.: and Higinbotham, N.T.: Sarcomata of the osteogenic series. *J Bone Joint Surg [Am], 48A*:1-26, 1966.
4. Budd, J.W., MacDonald, I.: Modified classification of bone tumors. *Radiology, 40*:486-588, 1943.
5. MacDonald, I., and Budd, J.W.: Osteogenic sarcoma. I. A modified nomenclature and review of 118 five-year cures. *Surg Gynec Obstet, 77*:413-421, 1943.
6. Thomson, A., Turner, R.N., and Warwick, R.: Skeletal sarcomata and giant cell tumor. *J Bone Joint Surg, 37B*:266-303, 1955.
7. Dahlin, D.C., and Coventry, M.B.: Osteogenic sarcoma; a study of 600 cases. *J Bone Joint Surg, 49A*:101-110, 1967.
8. Coventry, M.B., and Dahlin, D.C.: Osteogenic sarcoma. *J Bone Joint Surg, 39A*:714-757, 1957.

9. Broders, A.C.: The microscopic grading of cancer. In Pack, G., and Livingston, E. (Eds.): *Treatment of Cancer and Allied Diseases.* New York, Paul B. Hoeber, 1940, Vol. 1, pp. 19-41.
10. Lindbom, A., Soderberg, G., and Spjut, A.J.: Osteosarcoma; a review of 96 cases. *Acta Radiol, 56:*1-19, 1961.
11. O'Hara, J.M., Hutter, R., Foote, F. *et al.:* An analysis of 30 patients surviving longer than 10 years after treatment for osteogenic sarcoma. *J Bone Joint Surg, 50A:*335-354, 1968.
12. Nosanchuk, J.S., Weatherbee, L., and Brody, G.L.: Osteogeneic sarcoma. *JAMA, 208:*2439-2441, 1969.
13. Cade, S.: Editorial. *Ann R Coll Surg Engl, 9:*211, 1955.
14. Lee, S.E., and Mackenzie, D.H.: Osteosarcoma. *Br J Surg, 51:*252-274, 1964.
15. Green, W.T.: Chapter 36. In *Cancer: A Manual for Practitioners.* Boston, American Cancer Society, 1968, pp. 289-298.
16. Tudway, R.C.: Radiotherapy for osteogenic sarcoma. *J Bone Joint Surg, 43B:*61-67, 1961.
17. Pinkel, D.: Cyclophosphamide in children with cancer. *Cancer, 15:*42, 1962.
18. Ewing, J.: Diffuse endothelioma of bone. *Proc NY Pathol Soc, 21:*17, 1921.
19. Schajowicz, F.: Ewing's sarcoma and reticulum cell sarcoma of bone; with special reference of the histochemical demonstration of glycogen as an aid of differetial diagnosis. *J Bone Joint Surg, 41A:*349-356, 1959.
20. Dahlin, D.C., Coventry, M.B., and Scanlon, P.: Ewing's sarcoma. *J Bone Joint Surg, 43A:*185-192, 1961.
21. Wang, C.C., and Schultz, M.: Ewing's sarcoma; a study of 50 cases treated at the Massachusetts General Hospital, 1930-1952 inclusive. *N Engl J Med, 248:*571-576, 1953.
22. Suit, H.: Ewing's sarcoma; treatment by radiation therapy. In *Tumors of Bone and Soft Tissue.* Chicago, Yearbook Medical Publishers, 1965, pp. 191-200.
23. Geschicter, C., and Copeland, M.: *Tumors of Bone* (3rd ed.). Philadelphia, J.B. Lippincott, 1949, pp. 387-434.
24. Parker, F., and Jackson, H.: Primary reticulum cell sarcoma of bone. *Surg Gynecol Obstet, 68:*45, 1939.
25. Ivins, J.C., and Dahlin, D.C.: Reticulum cell sarcoma of bone. *J Bone Joint Surg, 35A:*835, 1953.
26. Coley, B.L., Higinbotham, N., and Groesbeck, H.: Primary reticulum cell sarcoma of bone. *Radiology, 55:*641, 1950.
27. Valls, J., Muscolo, D., and Schajowicz, F.: Reticulum cell sarcoma of bone. *J Bone Joint Surg, 34B:*588, 1952.

28. Sherman, R.S., and Snyder, R.: The roentgen appearance of primary reticulum cell sarcoma of bone. *Am J Roentgenol, 58:*291, 1947.
29. Wilson, T.W., and Pugh, D.: Primary reticulum cell sarcoma of bone with emphasis on roentgen aspects. *Radiology, 65:*343, 1955.
30. Hustu, O., Holton, C., Jones, D., and Pinkel, D.: Treatment of Ewing's sarcoma with concurrent radiotherapy and chemotherapy. *J Pediatr, 73:*249-251, 1968.

Chapter 10

RETICULOENDOTHELIOSIS

Barbara Jones

The non-lipid reticuloendothelioses have manifestations ranging from benign isolated lesions to widely disseminated malignant disease and a clinical course which may be acute or chronic. The names "Letterer-Siwe disease," "Hand-Schüller-Christian disease," "eosinophilic granuloma of bone," "reticuloendotheliosis" and "histiocytosis X" have been applied to the various clinical entities.

HISTORY

Exophthalmos, diabetes insipidus and osteolytic defects of cranial bones constitute the classic triad of Hand-Schüller-Christian disease. Hand,[1] in 1893, described a three-year-old boy with polydipsia, polyuria and exophthalmos, who at autopsy had a small defect in the right parietal bone, hepatosplenomegaly and generalized lymphadenopathy. He attributed the process to tuberculosis. Three patients of ages four, seven and sixteen years with skull defects were reported by Schüller.[2] The youngest one had diabetes insipidus. The sixteen-year-old had signs suggestive of hypopituitarism. In two of the three patients the skull defects regressed spontaneously. He coined the term "map skull" to describe the x-ray picture. The syndrome was attributed to pituitary dysfunction by both Schüller[3] and Christian.[4] Hand,[5] in 1921, also considered this as a possible explanation for the disorder. Denzer,[6] after reviewing these cases, suggested the eponym

Note: This investigation was supported in part by PHS Grant 07757-07 and PHS Training Grant 08071-05 from the National Cancer Institute.

The author wishes to acknowledge the assistance, in the literature review, of Mr. Lawrence F. Martin, a third-year medical student at West Virginia University, and in the foreign literature translations, of Dr. Counce H. Hancock and Dr. Arthur N. Ward, residents in pediatrics at West Virginia University Hospital.

Hand-Schüller-Christian disease for them. As described by Rowland,[7] the histologic picture is that of an infiltrative process with large, cholesterol-containing histiocytes (foam cells). He concluded that it was a primary lipid disorder.

Letterer,[8] in 1924, and Siwe,[9] in 1933, described young infants with fever, hepatosplenomegaly, lymphadenopathy, purpura and a fulminant, toxic downhill course. Histologic examination of the spleen showed hyperplasia of reticuloendothelial cells without evidence of lipid phagocytosis. Bone lesions and anemia were also observed. Siwe[9] felt the disease occurred exclusively in infants and was neither familial nor hereditary. Abt and Denenholz[10] reviewed published cases between 1924 and 1934, added one of their own, and suggested the eponym Letterer-Siwe's disease.

Otani and Ehrlich[11] and Lichtenstein and Jaffe[12,13] described eosinophilic granuloma limited to one or more bones with no extraskeletal involvement. Histologically, these lesions consist of histiocytes with some evidence of phagocytosis and accumulations of eosinophils.

Wallgren[14] in 1940 reasoned that Letterer-Siwe's disease and Hand-Schüller-Christian disease were merely different clinical manifestations of the same disease process. In reviewing a series of reported cases he noted that foam cells never occurred when the illness lasted less than three months and were always found if it lasted more than twelve months. The rapidity of the course and the organ involvement are age related, with the more fulminant process occurring in young infants. Green and Farber[15] suggested that eosinophilic granuloma of bone represented a variant of Hand-Schüller-Christian disease or Letterer-Siwe's disease.

In 1953, Lichtenstein[16] coined the term "histiocytosis X" to encompass eosinophilic granuloma of bone, Hand-Schüller-Christian disease, and Letterer-Siwe's disease. Some prefer to use the term "reticuloendotheliosis" to connotate these disease entities. This concept has simplified the previously rigid classification of distinct clinical entities but has not augmented our understanding of the basic pathophysiology or etiology.

Lieberman[17] feels that the usage of a unified concept for a broad spectrum of clinical manifestations may lead to therapeutic errors. This should not be a problem as long as therapy is planned for a patient and his problem, rather than assuming a disease entity should be treated with a single form of therapy without consideration of the clinical manifestations in each individual patient.

Etiology

The etiology of the non-lipid reticuloendothelioses is unknown. Many attempts have been made to implicate infectious agents of various types without uniform success. Trauma has also been implicated on occasion. Conceivably, multiple etiologies may produce similar clinical pictures.

MODE OF INHERITANCE

Glass and Miller,[18] in their analysis of deaths due to reticuloendotheliosis, noted that the peak mortality occurred in children under one year of age. Since no other malignancy has a peak at this young an age, they suggested a prenatal origin for this disorder. The acute disease tends to have an onset in early infancy, in fact, eighteen cases of congenital Letterer-Siwe's disease have been reported.[19-29] Two of these had widespread disseminated disease at birth: one was stillborn,[24] and one died shortly after birth.[28] Most of the remainder had skin lesions at birth and subsequently developed systemic disease. No history of maternal infection during pregnancy was noted in these reports.

Of the congenital cases, three were siblings[20]; in another family, one of two involved siblings had an onset at birth.[21] Other familial occurrences involving two or more siblings have been reported. In the analysis of Glass and Miller of 270 deaths due to reticuloendotheliosis, there were five pairs of siblings.[18] An additional eight siblings have been reported.[19-21,30-33] The parents of one family were first cousins,[33] and two abortions preceded the two involved siblings in another family.[32]

In addition to these familial occurrences, concordance in three sets of monozygous twins has been reported.[34-37] Two sets of like-sex twins without zygosity determination also showed concordance.[18,38] Discordance has been reported in one set of monozygous twins[39] and one set of dizygous twins.[40] Juberg reviewed the twin and sibling data and postulated a single autosomal recessive gene "with slightly reduced penetrance."[37]

There have been a number of other reports of familial reticuloendotheliosis which clinically are somewhat different from classical Letterer-Siwe's disease. One complete sibship of five girls, including one set of identical twins, died between the ages of twenty months and four and one-half years. Early, these girls showed failure to thrive, vomiting, eczema, chronic otitis media, and pyogenic abscesses. The terminal picture was one of rapidly progressive lymphadenopathy, hepatosplenomegaly, jaundice and pulmonary infiltrates. Histologically, diffuse reticulum cell infiltrate was seen in the liver, spleen, lungs, lymph nodes, bone marrow, gastrointestinal tract, genitourinary tract and, in two of the five, in the central nervous system.[41]

In large inbred kindred with twelve infants, there were six siblings who died with a disease of the reticuloendothelial system. However, the authors distinguished these cases from Letterer-Siwe's disease because of the prominence of peripheral blood eosinophilia, lack of pulmonary infiltrates, and the occurrence of bone marrow failure.[42] Familial hemophagocytic reticulosis, as described by Farquhar in 1952,[43] is another disseminated disease of the reticuloendothelial system. These infants have hepatosplenomegaly, pancytopenia, recurrent infections and may have jaundice. There is marked proliferation of reticuloendothelial cells and hemophagocytosis. Twelve cases have been reported from five families.[43-48] Another familial disorder referred to as familial lymphohistiocytosis is characterized by hepatosplenomegly, pancytopenia, pneumonitis and meningitis.[49-51] The organ infiltrates consisted of histiocytes and lymphocytes with central nervous system involvement being a prominent feature. Hemophagocytic reticulosis and lymphohistiocytosis may be the same entity.

In spite of these findings, the majority of reported cases of reticuloendotheliosis are not noted to be familial. Very little has been published about possible genetic factors in Hand-Schüller-Christian disease. Forssman[52] reviewed the subject briefly and investigated the possibility of consanguinity in the families of twenty-one patients. No established first cousin or second cousin matings were found, but this possibility could not be eliminated in nine of the families.

With the data presented, it is not possible to derive a single hypothesis regarding the role of inheritance in these disorders. In any one family with multiple cases, the clinical picture and histologic findings are remarkably similar; but significant differences may exist from one family to the next. In any given family, therefore, it can be postulated that we are dealing with a single gene defect. However, taking the group of familial cases as a whole, there are probably several different genes involved; in other words, there is genetic heterogeneity.

The explanation for the sporadic cases remains unsolved from available data. Perhaps there is an as yet unidentified genetic abnormality which predisposes to the development of reticulondotheliosis. There are many examples of this, such as the increased incidence of leukemia in patients with Fanconi's anemia, Bloom's syndrome and trisomy 21, or the predisposition of patients with xeroderma pigmentosa and dyskeratosis congenita to malignancies. The final cancer is several steps removed from the genetic mutation and probably requires environmental effects for expression.

There are two reasons for dwelling on the genetic aspects of these diseases. One is a plea for additional information about pedigrees, paternal consanguinity, early infant deaths and fetal loss. Empiric risk figures would be particularly helpful. The second reason is to provide information for genetic counseling of parents of patients. In such counseling, it is important to adequately and accurately evaluate the family history. In addition, detailed evaluation should be made of the clinical entity in question along with any available histologic data. The recurrence rate in the familial variants tends to be high, and the parents should be so advised.

Age Incidence

The acute disseminated disease (Letterer-Siwe's disease) occurs primarily in infants under two years of age. There is widespread visceral involvement and the course tends to be fulminant and of short duration. Chronic forms (Hand-Schüller-Christian disease) have a peak incidence in the two- to five-year age group. Eosinophilic granuloma of bone occurs most commonly in older children and adults.

PATHOLOGY

The purpose of this report is not to detail the histologic findings in the reticuloendothelioses; such reviews are available elsewhere.[17] Briefly, the primary lesion consists of infiltrates of benign-appearing histiocytes of medium or large size. The cytoplasm has a fine, granular eosinophilic appearance. Evidence of phagocytosis by these histiocytes of cellular material is commonly seen, particularly in areas of necrosis. Mature eosinophils are present in varying numbers along with occasional multinucleated giant cells (Fig. 10-1). In areas of necrosis, neutrophils, lymphocytes and plasma cells may also be seen. All involved organs contain similar infiltrates. In lymph nodes, the architecture is disrupted, thus suggesting a malignant neoplasm. Similar infiltrates

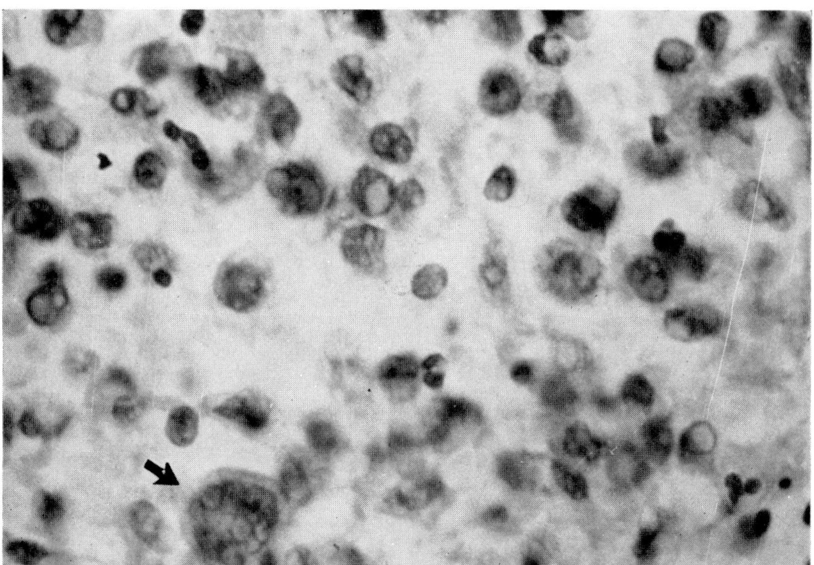

Figure 10-1. High-power view of a polymorphous infiltrate. The infiltrate is principally histiocytic and containing an occasional mutinucleated giant cell (arrow) (×400).

may be seen throughout the reticuloendothelial system. In acute disseminated cases, the infiltrate may be diffuse or show a tendency to form ill-defined aggregates of cells[53]; while in chronic cases, the lesions take on more of a nodular or granulomatous appearance.[54]

Skin lesions may progress from papules to vesicles and then may ulcerate with hemorrhage, crusting and scarring. The histiocytic infiltrate involves the papillary layer of the dermis adjacent to the basal layer of epidermis. Ulceration of the epidermis occurs in some areas (Fig. 10-2). Less exudation and crusting are seen in chronic cases.[55]

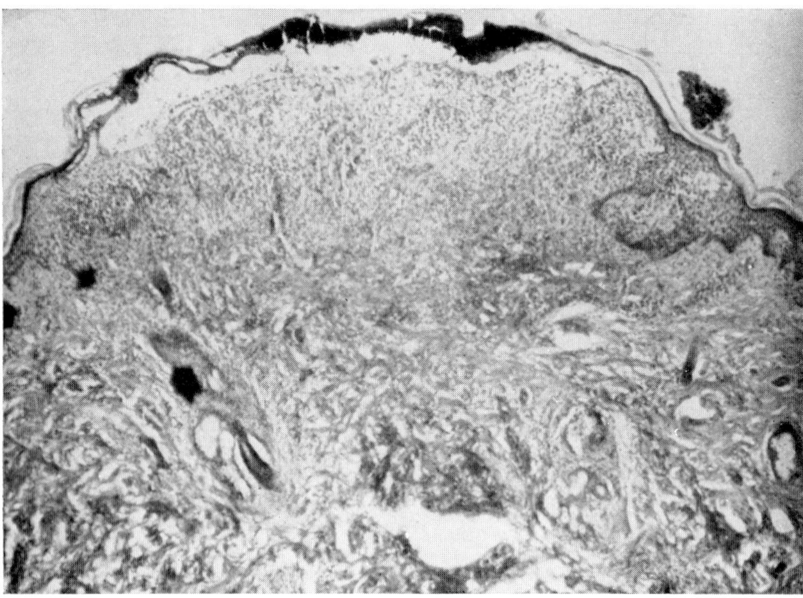

Figure 10-2. Microscopic section of skin lesion showing ulceration of epidermis and dense cellular infiltration of upper dermis.

Lung lesions consist of small, discrete and confluent nodules involving the alveolar septa. Larger nodules destroy or displace lung parenchyma (Fig. 10-3). The nodules consist of histiocytes,

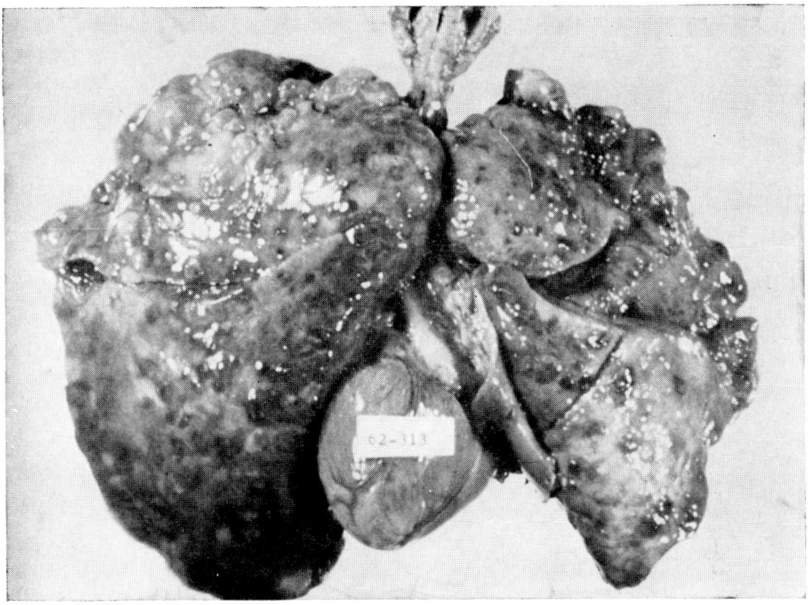

Figure 10-3. Gross appearance of heart and lungs showing multiple diffuse pulmonary nodules.

eosinophils, occasional multinucleated giant cells, and a few lymphocytes and plasma cells. Central necrosis of these nodular lesions leads to cyst formation (Fig. 10-4).[56]

Histologically, bone lesions of solitary eosinophilic granuloma are indistinguishable from those seen in association with widely disseminated disease. Mixtures of histiocytes and eosinophils are present; and in areas of necrosis, the histiocytes may contain cellular debris, hemosiderin granules, leukocytes and red blood cells. Neutrophils, plasma cells and lymphocytes also may be found associated with necrosis. Healing may occur by simple fibrosis. Diffuse bone marrow infiltration occurs infrequently (Fig. 10-5). The gastrointestinal tract may show similar infiltrates involving the mucosa particularly of the jejunum and/or mesenteric lymph nodes. The contour of the intestinal wall may be altered, and interference with absorption may occur.[57]

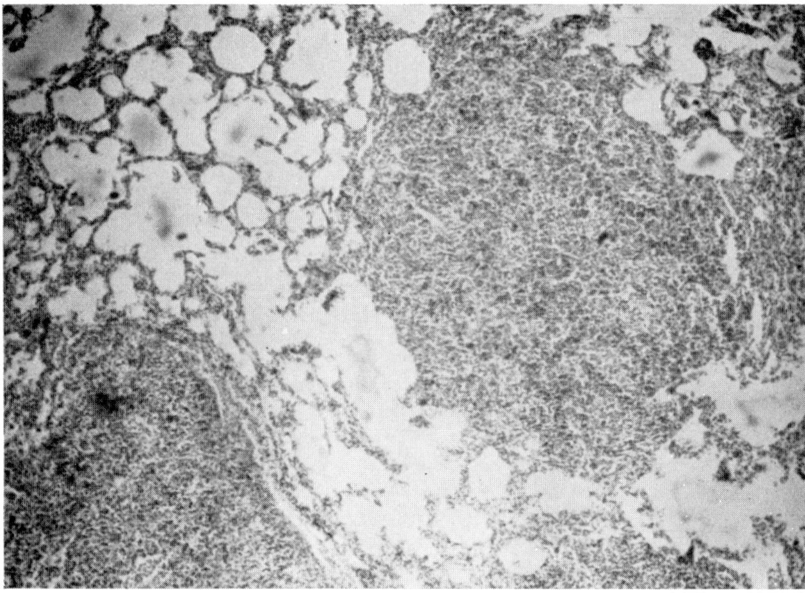

Figure 10-4. Histologic section of lung showing nodular pulmonary infiltrates (×100).

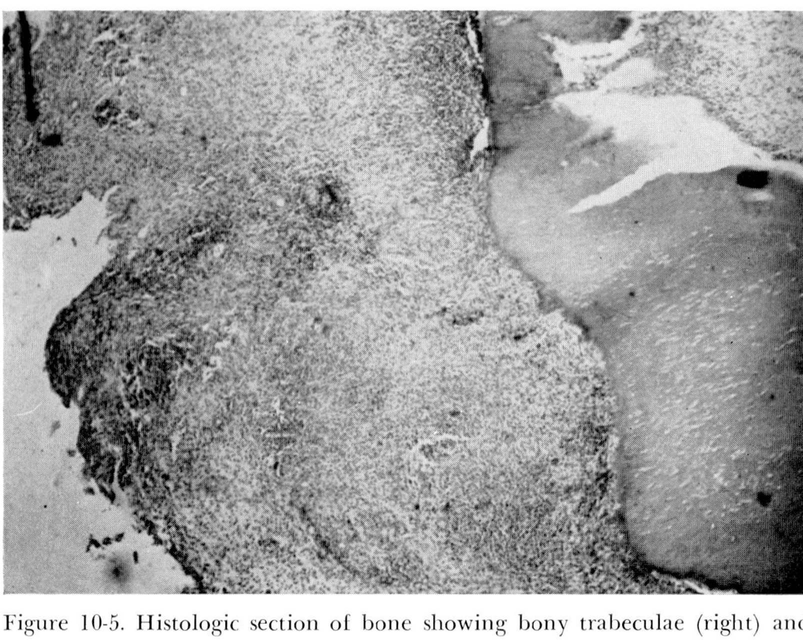

Figure 10-5. Histologic section of bone showing bony trabeculae (right) and marrow space occupied by dense histiocytic infiltrate (×100).

CLINICAL MANIFESTATIONS

Little purpose is served by attempting to use diagnostically a specific eponym concerning a particular patient. Transitional stages[19] are seen between eosinophilic granuloma and Hand-Schüller-Christian disease, as well as between the latter and Letterer-Siwe's disease, which only serve to confuse the clinician. Histologically, the lesions are similar if not identical; and both the prognosis and management are determined in large part by the extent of the involvement and rapidity of progression. Lesions may be limited to one or more bones, skin[26,59-62] or apparently one lymph node.[63] In these instances, the course is benign. Single bone lesions generally occur in older children and adults. Skin lesions may be the only manifestation in infants.

The course may be chronic with bone lesions and a variety of visceral involvement including lung, lymph nodes, diabetes insipidus, gastrointestinal tract and central nervous system. This course is more commonly seen in young children. In very severe cases the disease may follow an acute course with early termination in death, manifesting any combination of the following: hepatosplenomegaly, lymphadenopathy, skin lesions, otitis media, pulmonary involvement, bone lesions, anemia, thrombocytopenia and perhaps leukopenia. This is the usual picture in young infants. Individual organ system involvement will be considered with the understanding that in any one patient, they may occur in a variety of combinations.

Hepatosplenomegaly

Hepatosplenomegaly is common in young infants with the acute picture. Not all infants have this finding; but it is seen less frequently beyond the infant age group. There is frequently an associated pancytopenia with both the anemia and thrombocytopenia having ominous prognostic significance.

Lymphadenopathy

Lymphadenopathy occurs at least twice as frequently as hepatosplenomegaly and may be seen with both acute and chronic disease. Lymphadenopathy is an early finding in acute disease with cervical nodes most commonly involved. The nodes are firm, non tender and do not suppurate.

Bone Lesions

The osteolytic bone lesions may be asymptomatic and discovered by accident on roentgenograms or may present with painful swelling over the involved area. Most frequent sites are the skull, pelvis, femur, ribs and mandible.[64,65] The lesions are sharply demarcated roentgenographically with destruction of bone along the edges (Fig. 10-6). There is no adjacent reaction. In long bones, the shaft is involved with sparing of the epiphyses. Irregular destruction in the long bones may produce a trabeculated or even cystic appearance (Fig. 10-7). Although rare, vertebral lesions have occurred particularly in the dorsal vertebrae. Recently, five instances of cervical spine involvement have been reported, two with neurological deficits.[66] Single or multiple bone lesions may

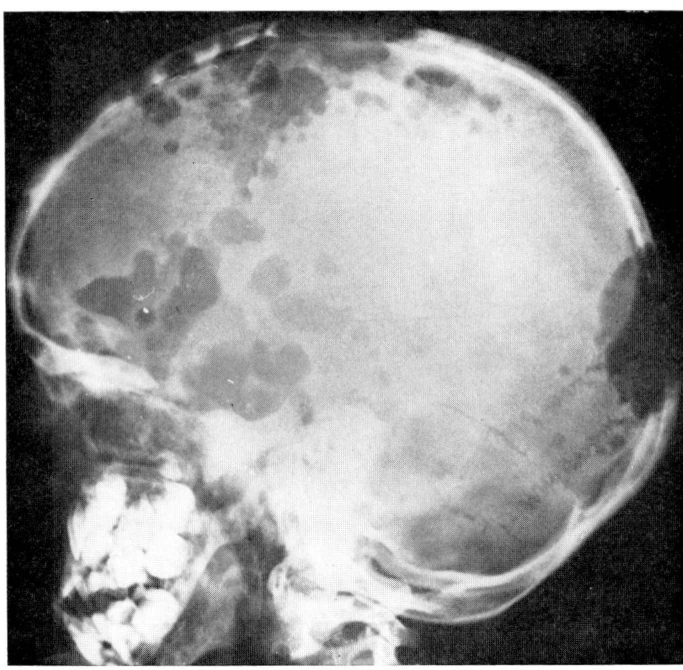

Figure 10-6. Lateral x-ray of the skull showing multiple osteolytic lesions.

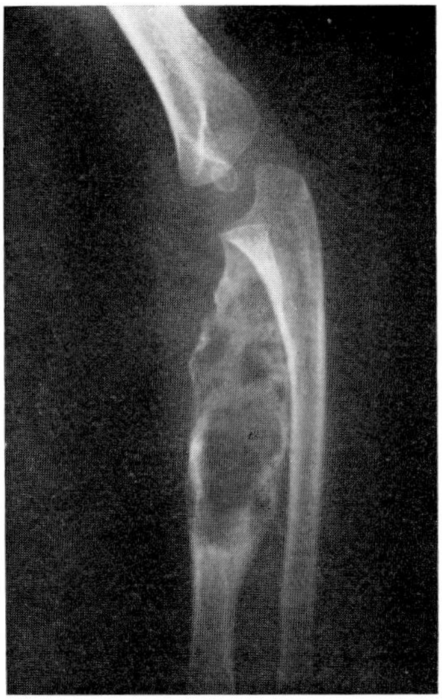

Figure 10-7. Arm showing irregular destructive lesion of radius, giving a cystic appearance.

occur without lesions at other sites, and they may precede or occur concommitantly with visceral manifestations of disseminated disease. Since bone lesions may be asymptomatic and tend to heal spontaneously, they may occur more commonly than the literature would suggest.

Skin

Skin manifestations in histiocytosis X have recently been reviewed.[55] They constitute a very common presenting complaint in acute disseminated disease of young infants and have been present at birth in congenital disease. Altman and Winkelman described five different types of cutaneous lesions in the reticuloendothelioses: (a) diffuse papular scaling eruption (Fig. 10-8), (b) petechial purpura, (c) granulomatous ulcerative lesions (Fig. 10-9), (d) xanthomatous lesions and (e) bronzing of the skin. The petechial purpura is, of course, secondary to thrombocytopenia.[67]

Skin lesions are much less common in the chronic cases and in

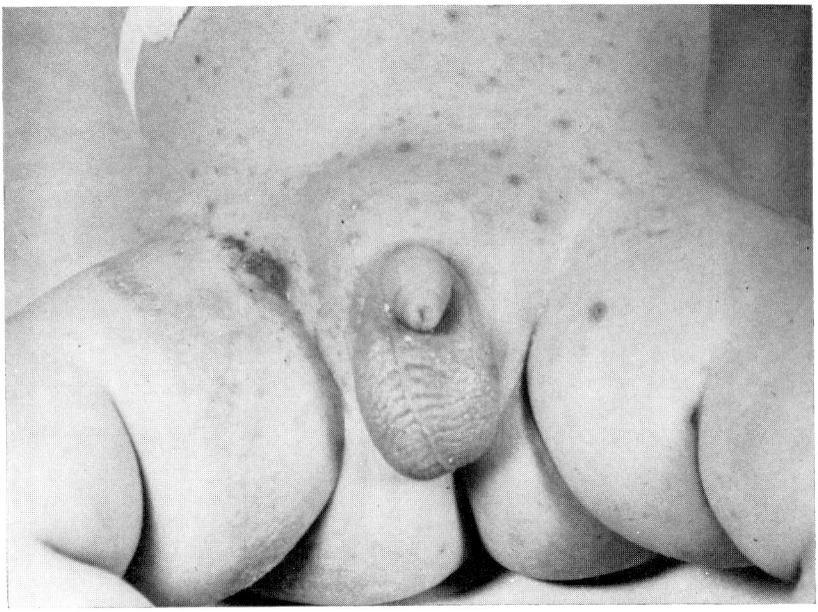

Figure 10-8. Papulovesicular lesions. (Courtesy of *Cutis.*)[26]

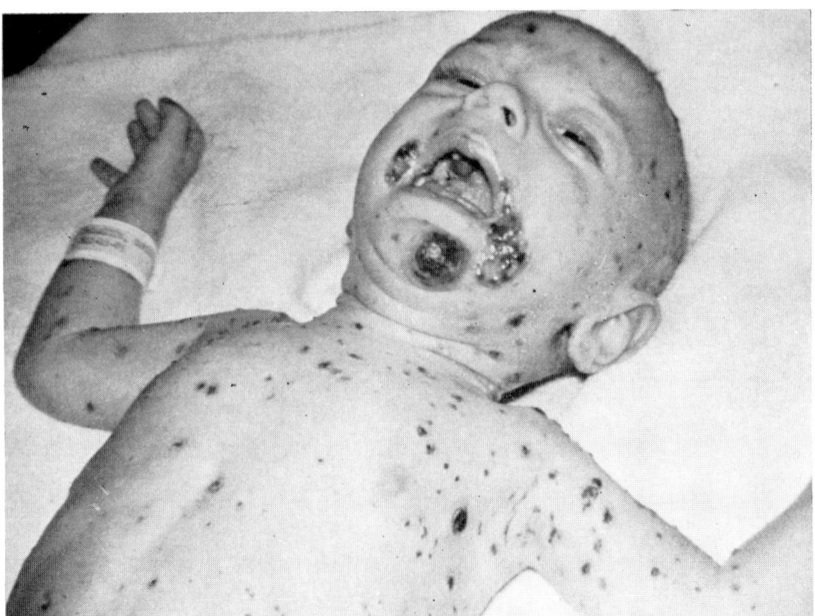

Figure 10-9. A child with multiple small crusted lesions and larger infiltrated and ulcerated areas of chin and palate. (Courtesy of *Cutis.*)[26]

one series only 9 out of 31 patients had such findings.[65] Several cases have been reported with only skin and bone lesions. A few infants, ranging in age from newborns to twenty-two months, have had only skin lesions primarily of the papular or ulcerative type (Fig. 10-10). A mistaken diagnosis of seborrheic dermatitis is often made, and understandably so, in the young infant. The rash has a brownish-yellow papular appearance occurring in crops on the scalp, face, neck and trunk. If it is prominent on the scalp and in the skin folds, it does mimic seborrhea. The papular lesions may then progress to form vesicles or pustules and then ulcerate (Fig. 10-11).

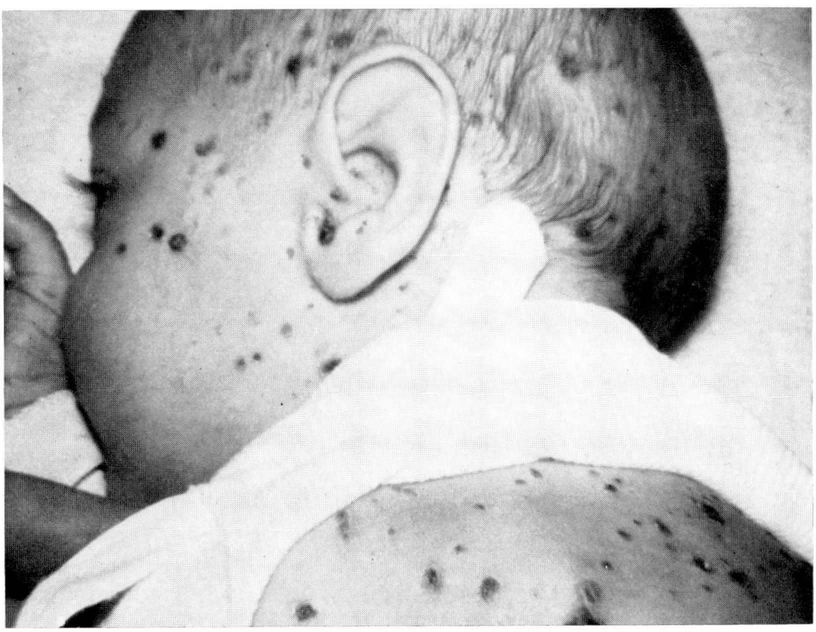

Figure 10-10. Crusted and vesicular lesions. (Courtesy of *Cutis*.)[26]

Gingiva

Granulomatous lesions of the gingiva may occur with or without associated lesions of the mandible or maxilla. The lesions are tender and give rise to feeding problems, particularly in infants. In early infancy, premature eruption of the teeth occurs. Teeth

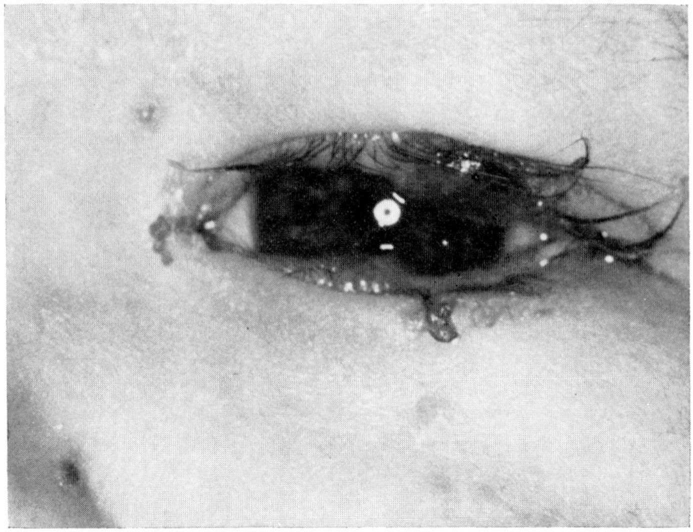

Figure 10-11. Infiltrated eyelid in a child with reticuloendotheliosis. (Courtesy of *Cutis.*)[26]

in the gingival lesions are lost prematurely, especially if underlying bone is eroded.[68]

Otitis Media

Chronic suppurative otitis media is another characteristic finding in the young infant. Smears of the exudate frequently show abnormal histiocytes. Occasionally, soft tissue tumors are seen in the auditory canal.

Pulmonary Lesions

Pulmonary lesions may occur at any age with or without other manifestations of reticuloendotheliosis. Symptomatology may include chronic cough, fatigue, weight loss, respiratory distress or there may be no symptoms.[58,69] Sudden onset of respiratory distress may result from pneumothorax[70] or pneumomediastinum[26] occurring as complications of the primary pulmonary lesions (Fig. 10-12 and 10-13). The earliest roentgenographic picture may be a diffuse reticular pattern or consist of a nodular infiltrate

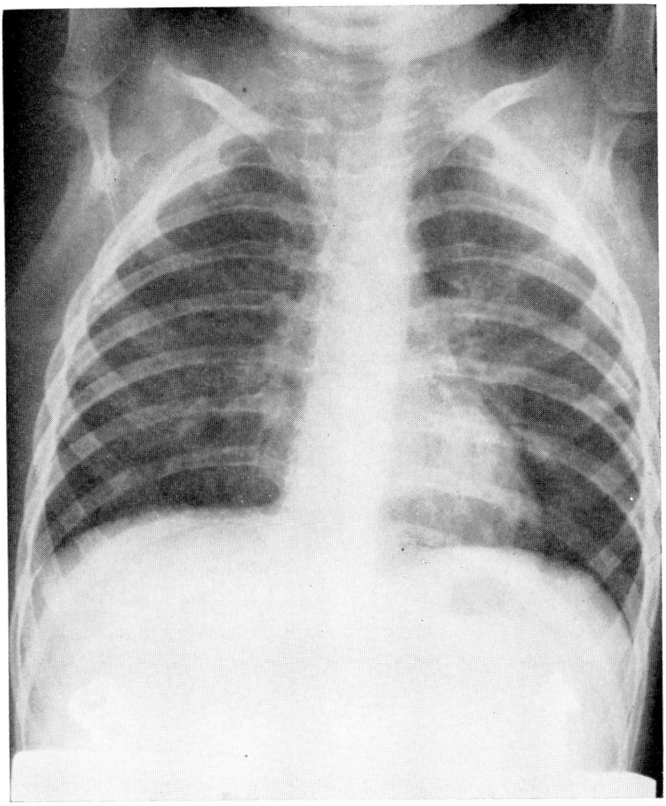

Figure 10-12. Diffuse reticular pulmonary infiltrate.

in the parenchyma as well as on the pleural surfaces (Fig. 10-14). As the disease progresses, diffuse cystic lesions develop which create a honeycomb appearance. Interstitial fibrosis may also develop.[69] With the occurrence of cystic changes, pneumothorax and pneumomediastinum become a very real possibility and the usual precautionary measures should be taken. If the patient is receiving systemic chemotherapy, the pulmonary infiltrates need to be differentiated from such infections as *Pneumocystis carinii* and cytomegalic inclusion disease. Both have occurred in patients receiving immunosuppressive drugs. Long-term methotrexate therapy may produce a diffuse pulmonary infiltration as a toxic manifestation.

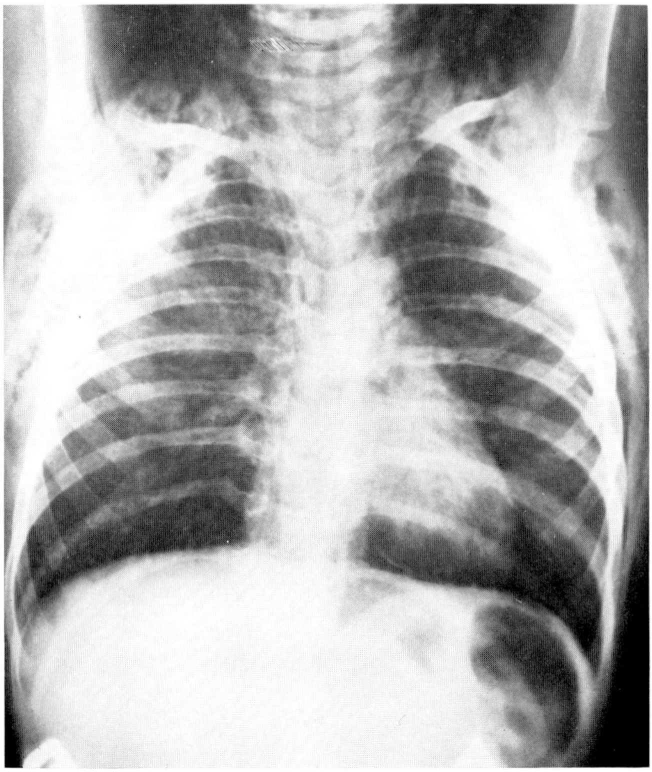

Figure 10-13. Extensive subcutaneous emphysema secondary to pneumomediastinum. Same patient as Figure 10-12, six days later.

Diabetes Insipidus

Diabetes insipidus occurs in about 40 percent of the chronic cases of reticuloendotheliosis and is due to infiltrative lesions of the posterior pituitary and surrounding hypothalamic area. Frequently, there is no discernible destructive bone lesion involving the sella turcica. Polydipsia and polyuria are indicative of the problem and are responsive to Pitressin®. An earlier diagnosis may be made by measuring serum and urine osmolality after salt loading. Usually the Pitressin requirement persists even though other lesions heal spontaneously or respond to therapy.

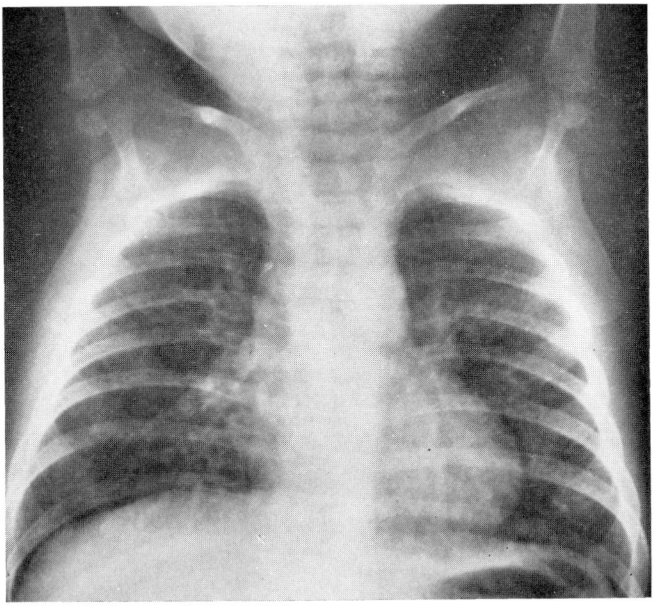

Figure 10-14. Reticular pulmonary infiltrate with suggestive nodular infiltrate.

Central Nervous System

Even though cranial bone lesions and diabetes insipidus are common occurrences, other central nervous system manifestations are unusual in either acute or chronic reticuloendotheliosis judging from the paucity of reports. The insidious onset of increased intracranial pressure and communicating hydrocephalus has been reported. No single lesion accounts for this finding; but hypothalamic lesions, dural or meningeal space obliteration, dural sinus invasion and choroid plexus replacement have been implicated.[71] Intracerebral infiltrates, primarily perivascular, have been reported, but only one of three patients had symptoms referable to the central nervous system—namely, seizures.[58] A similar case report attributed the seizures to fever.[72] Suffice it to say central nervous system involvement should be considered while observing the ongoing course of patients with this disorder.

Exophthalmus

Although exophthalmus is part of the classic triad of Hand-Schüller-Christian disease, it only occurs in about 30 percent of the cases. It may be unilateral or bilateral and is often associated with destructive lesions of orbital and sphenoidal bones.

Gastrointestinal Tract

Diarrhea, vomiting and abdominal distension are common symptoms and may be presenting complaints in infants with acute reticuloendotheliosis. Little emphasis, however, has been placed on intestinal lesions. Two infants had demonstrable abnormalities by barium studies of the gastrointestinal tract, although only one had symptoms. In the one with symptoms, mucosal changes were noted in the duodenal loop and proximal jejunum with complete effacement in some areas and a finely granular pattern elsewhere suggesting hypertrophy or edema of the mucosal wall. The asymptomatic patient showed definite segmentation of distal jejunum and ileum along with minimal coarsening of jejunal mucosa.[57] This prompted the same investigators to examine autopsy material in their institution. Of the acute cases, seven of eleven had intestinal or mesenteric node involvement, or both, and six of these seven had had symptoms related to the gastrointestinal tract. In a literature review, 20 percent of the verified acute cases had similar involvement on autopsy, and in some of these, the presenting complaint was diarrhea.[57] This study has been reviewed in detail because it would appear that too little attention has been given to this aspect of the acute disease, and too often diarrhea and vomiting are regarded as nonspecific symptoms in an acutely ill infant.

DIAGNOSIS

Although the clinical picture is often very typical, a histologic diagnosis is necessary prior to considering therapy. Skin lesions are often the most accessible for biopsy and if present should be diagnostic. Bone lesions in the absence of other findings should be biopsied for definitive diagnosis. The peripheral blood changes are nonspecific. Bone marrow examination is usually normal, but in about 10 percent of cases it will show increased numbers of histiocytes.

Subsequent to establishing a histologic diagnosis, the extent of the disease process should be determined in order to plan appropriate therapy. Roentgenograms of the entire skeleton will permit enumeration of bone lesions. Chest x-ray and barium study of gastrointestinal tract should be performed to identify involvement in these regions. Diabetes insipidus can be diagnosed in the usual manner.

TREATMENT

Solitary eosinophilic granuloma of bone as has been mentioned should be biopsied for accurate diagnosis, and concommitant surgical excision or curettage will usually lead to healing (Fig. 10-15 and 10-16) using bone chips or bone grafts for large lesions.[25,65,73-75] The patient with multiple bone lesions and no other organ involvement presents more of a therapeutic problem. Radiotherapy is frequently effective in doses of 200 to 600 rads with the occasional use of higher doses. The use of this modality needs to be carefully evaluated however, since these are benign lesions and radiotherapy has potential deleterious effects. The symptomatic lesions, which are either not easily accessible to surgical intervention or are too numerous for such an approach, may be considered for this form of therapy. The asymptomatic lesions that are not likely to result in a pathologic fracture may be watched since spontaneous healing may occur. All patients with a solitary bone lesion should be watched for the development of additional lesions, either bone or visceral.

Very little is to be gained by considering the treatment of acute Letterer-Siwe's disease and chronic reticuloendotheliosis (Hand-Schüller-Christian disease) separately. Disseminated disease requires systemic chemotherapy, reserving surgery and radiotherapy for localized areas of involvement which are symptomatic and unresponsive to chemotherapy.

Historically, a variety of treatment modalities have been used with varying success. Antibiotics as the only therapy have been successful on a few occasions. Penicillin, chlortetracycline, strep-

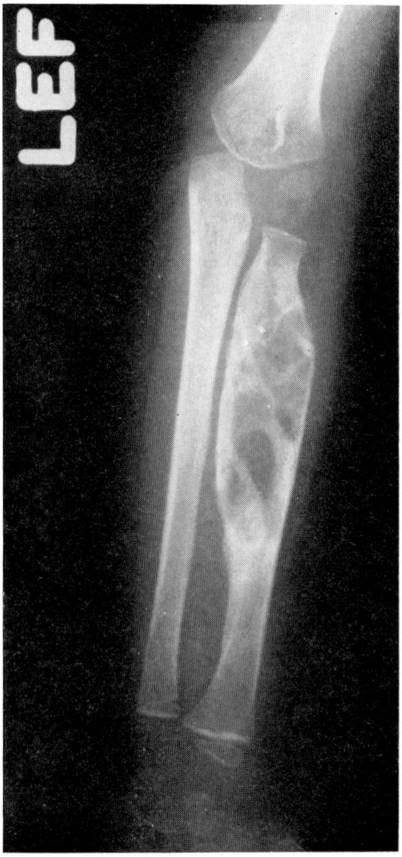

Figure 10-15. Arm showing trabeculated appearance of osteolytic lesion in the radius.

tomycin and chloramphenicol were used in twins, and they were alive and well after seventeen years.[34,35] Streptomycin was used successfully in one patient[76] but was ineffective in another who subsequently responded to chloramphenicol and tetracycline.[77] Sulfonamides and penicillin-controlled infection in one instance, perhaps permitting longer survival, but had no apparent effect on the primary process.[78] In spite of these scattered reports, antibiotics are now used as adjuvant therapy to control secondary infections rather than to treat the primary disease process.

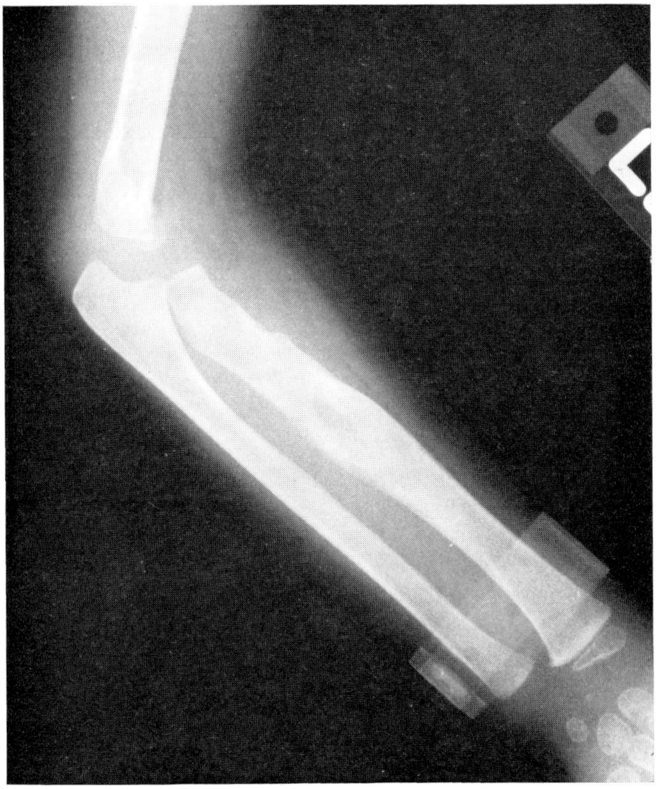

Figure 10-16. Same lesion as shown in Figure 10-15. Healing occurred after surgical curettage.

Corticosteroids have had extensive clinical trial and have often been very effective in controlling the disease.[31,73,79-90] Large doses used for sufficient length of time may result in striking improvement of infants with acute reticuloendotheliosis.[31,82] Improvement has also been noted in both eosinophilic granuloma[84] and Hand-Schüller-Christian disease.[85] Bone lesions frequently respond, but it takes several weeks to a few months to see demonstrable changes by x-ray.[87,90] Skin lesions usually clear promptly and improvement is noted in pulmonary lesions in 50 percent.[73] Nitrogen mustard has had limited use but has been reported to decrease local tumefaction[25,74] and produce regression of gingival lesions, skin rashes, pulmonary infiltrate and possibly bone lesions.[91]

Folic acid antagonists, such as methotrexate, are effective used alone or combined with corticosteroids.[25,74] Dargeon obtained striking results with folic acid antagonists and is of the opinion the only effect steroids added to this was improvement in appetite and nutrition. Bass[31] was more impressed with the role of steroids when the two drugs were given in combination. Using Aminopterin® daily, as a single agent, impressive but short remissions have been reported; more lasting remissions were obtained by alternating high doses of hydrocortisone with Aminopterin in two-week cycle.[92] Similar cyclic therapy with prednisone and methotrexate gave a good response in three of five patients so treated.[73]

Of the newer chemotherapeutic agents, vinblastine sulfate has been the most successful to date. In an early report, three patients received 0.2 to 0.3 mg/kg/week for eight to fifteen weeks with marked improvement.[93] The same investigators later reported the use of this drug in thirty patients using 0.1 to 0.45 mg/kg weekly or biweekly for eight to fifteen doses. Six of seven patients with widely disseminated disease responded, and in three of the six, recovery was dramatic. Eighty-five percent of the thirty patients achieved some improvement.[94] Although these are glowing reports, others have been less successful with vinblastine. Of six patients receiving 2.1 to 0.5 mg/kg weekly, two improved, two showed no change, and two had progressive disease.[95] Two other reports have appeared, one successful, one unsuccessful responses to vinblastine.[96,97] Cyclophosphamide produced clearing of pulmonary infiltrate and lymphadenopathy in one patient who subsequently developed lytic bone lesions which healed completely with vinblastine.[98]

The author has treated two patients with vinblastine. One infant received 4 to 8 mg/m^2/week for six weeks with dramatic regression of skin and gingival lesions. A recurrence four months later again responded to vinblastine.[26] The second infant had received prior therapy with methotrexate, prednisone and vincristine. With the recurrence of adenopathy and skin lesions, he received vinblastine 4 mg/m^2 increasing the dose weekly by 4 mg/

m^2 until 12 mg/m^2 was reached, which was given weekly for six weeks followed by maintenance therapy of 12 mg/m^2 monthly for one year. He has been asymptomatic for three years following discontinuance.

Children's Cancer Study Group A in a prospective study compared the use of vinblastine alone, vinblastine combined with prednisone, and mercaptopurine combined with prednisone. Thirty-five children under two years of age at the time of diagnosis were treated and each of the three regimens was equally effective with one-half to two-thirds of each group showing either a good response or complete remission. The factors important in response were the duration of the disease before therapy and the extent of the disease process. Of eleven patients over two years of age, only one responded.[99]

Vincristine, the other vinca alkaloid, has had more limited trial. An infant with congenital disease was treated with the combination of prednisone, 5 mg/kg/day and vincristine 0.075 mg/kg/week, gradually increasing the dose to 0.150 mg/kg. The total course of therapy was eight weeks. He has remained well over a period of almost two years.[29]

Acute Leukemia Group B has a prospective study in progress comparing the therapeutic efficacy of methotrexate 30 mg/m^2 twice a week plus prednisone 40 mg/m^2/day versus vincristine 2 mg/m^2/week plus the same prednisone dose. Both regimens are effective in some but not all patients treated (Fig. 10-17 and 10-18). At the present time, a statement as to which is preferable cannot be made. Maintenance therapy with methotrexate is also being given to some of the patients to ascertain whether or not maintenance therapy is important in this disease to insure prolonged asymptomatic periods.[100]

Supportive care may be neecssary for many patients with reticuloendotheliosis. The infants with acute disseminated disease frequently required blood and platelet transfusions for their hypersplenism, and on occasion, it would appear that splenectomy is beneficial. A recent report noted the presence of a consumptive coagulopathy in one patient which responded to heparin therapy.[101] Those patients with acute disease and bleeding diatheses

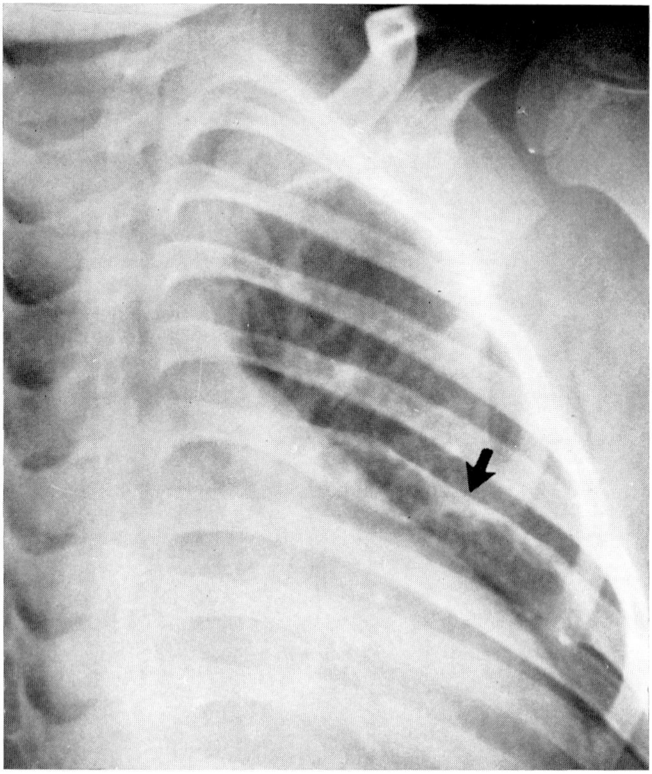

Figure 10-17. Osteolytic lesion of rib (arrow).

should probably be investigated for a consumptive coagulopathy before assuming the bleeding is due to thrombocytopenia. Infections should, of course, be treated appropriately. In those patients receiving chemotherapy, infections due to carinii,[102] cytomegalovirus[103,104] and fungi should be considered in the diagnostic evaluation. Pitressin will control the diabetes insipidus.

PROGNOSIS

Lahey[105] reviewed sixty-nine cases from three institutions with an onset of reticuloendotheliosis between birth and seventeen years of age, excluding patients with solitary bone lesions. Among these patients, the overall mortality rate was 36 percent. The most

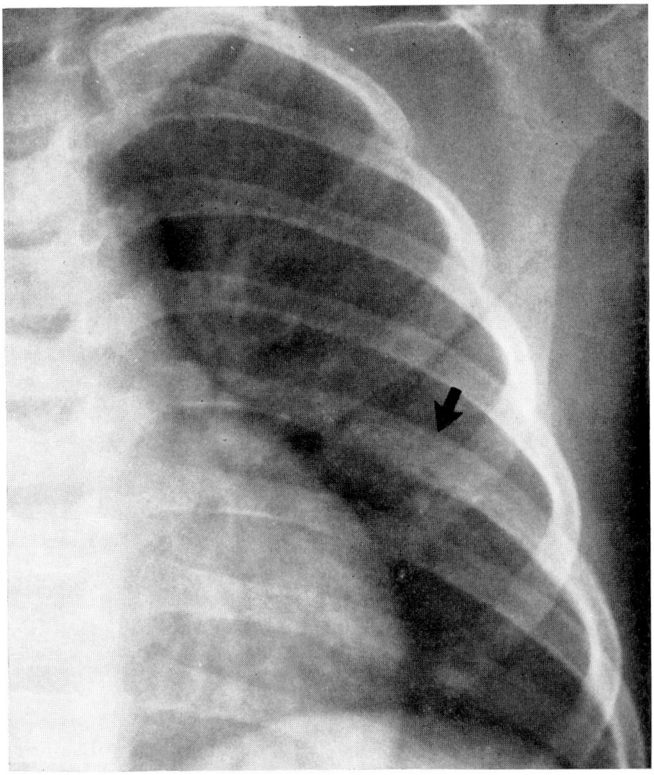

Figure 10-18. Same rib lesion as depicted in Figure 10-17, after patient was treated with methotrexate and prednisone.

important determinant in outcome was the age of onset of the disease. Among those with an onset in the first six months of life, 70 percent died; when the onset was during the first three years of life, 50 percent died. Those patients with pulmonary lesions had a 60 percent mortality. Other significant visceral involvement also indicated an unfavorable prognosis. Skin lesions were also an unfavorable sign, but in cases where the disease is confined to the skin and there is no visceral involvement, the prognosis is excellent. The occurrence of diabetes insipidus has no effect on prognosis.

Doede[106] reviewed ninety-two cases from the literature who had an onset of disease prior to three years of age. Of the eighty-seven followed for over two years, seventeen survived, giving a mortality rate of 76 percent. Both pulmonary lesions and thrombocytopenia were twice as common among those who died as those who survived. Among the cases they reviewed, age was not a factor in survival; but their study was limited to patients under three years of age and in fact, seventy-two of the eighty-seven patients were under one year of age. The effect of therapy on survival is difficult to valuate since any large series of cases covers a wide span of time and a variety of treatment modalities. Doede did find a significantly higher three-year survival among those patients treated with corticosteroids alone, or in combination with other therapy, when compared to all treated patients, untreated patients and treated patients who did not receive steroids. Lahey also found a longer survival among treated versus untreated patients. No attempt was made to analyze the type of treatment. Prospective studies are needed to evaluate the role of various treatment regimens on mortality.

REFERENCES

1. Hand, A.: Polyuria and tuberculosis. *Arch Pediatr, 10:*673-675, 1893.
2. Schüller, A.: Uber Ergenartige Schaldeldefekte im Jugendalter. *Fortschr Roetgenstr, 23:*12-18, 1915.
3. Schüller, A.: Dysostosis hypophysaria. *Br J Radiol, 31:*156-158, 1926.
4. Christian, H.A.: Defects in membranous bones, exophthalmos and diabetes insipidus; an unusual syndrome of dyspituitarism. *Med Clin North Am, 3:*849-871, 1920.
5. Hand, A. Jr.: Defects of membranous bones, exophthalmos and polyuria in childhood; is it dyspituitarism? *Am J Med Sci, 162:*509-515, 1921.
6. Denzer, B.S.: Defects in the membranous bones, diabetes insipidus and exophthalmos. *Am J Dis Child, 31:*480-482, 1926.
7. Rowland, R.S.: Xanthomatosis and the reticuloendothelial system. *Arch Intern Med, 42:*611-674, 1928.
8. Letterer, E.: Aleukämische Retikulose (Ein Beitrag zu den Proliferativen Erkrankugen des Retikuloendothelialapparates). *Frankfurt Z Pathol, 30:*377-393, 1924.
9. Siwe, S.A.: Die Reticuloendotheliose ein neues Krankheitsbied unter den Hepatosplenomegalien. *Z Kinderheilkd, 55:*212-247, 1933.
10. Abt, A.F., and Denenholz, E.J.: Letterer-Siwe's disease: Splenohepatomegaly associated with widespread hyperplasia of nonlipoid-storing

macrophages; discussion of the so-called reticuloendothelioses. *Am J Dis Child, 51*:499-522, 1936.

11. Otani, S., and Ehrlich, J.S.: Solitary granuloma of bone simulating primary neoplasm. *Am J Pathol, 16*:479-490, 1940.
12. Lichtenstein, L., and Jaffe, H.L.: Eosinophilic granuloma of bone; with report of case. *Am J Pathol, 16*:595, 1940.
13. Jaffe, H.L., and Lichtenstein, L.: Eosinophilic granuloma of bone; a condition affecting one, several, or many bones ,but apparently limited to the skeleton and representing the mildest clinical expression of the pedicular inflammatory histiocytosis also underlying Letterer-Siwe disease and Schüller-Christian disease. *Arch Pathol, 37*:99-118, 1944.
14. Wallgren, A.: Systemic reticuloendothelial granuloma; nonlipoid reticuloendotheliosis and Schüller-Christian disease. *Am J Dis Child, 60*: 471-500, 1940.
15. Green, W.T., and Farber, S.: Eosinophilic or solitary granuloma of bone. *J Bone Joint Surg, 24*:499-526, 1942.
16. Lichtenstein, L.: Histiocytosis X. *Arch Pathol, 56*:84-102, 1953.
17. Lieberman, P.H., Jones, C., Dargeon, H., and Begg, C.: A reappraisal of eosinophilic granuloma of bone, Hand-Schüller-Christian syndrome and Letterer-Siwe syndrome. *Medicine, 48*:375-400, 1969.
18. Glass, A.G., and Miller, R.: U.S. mortality from Letterer-Siwe disease, 1960-1964. *Pediatrics, 42*:364-367, 1968.
19. Batson, R., Shapiro, J., Christie, A., and Riley, H.: Acute nonlipid disseminated reticuloendotheliosis. *Am J Dis Child, 90*:323-343, 1955.
20. Hamilton, W.: Congenital Letterer-Siwe disease. *Scott Med J, 6*:575-577, 1961.
21. Rogers, D.L., and Benson, T.: Familial Letterer-Siwe disease. *J Pediatr, 60*:550-554, 1962.
22. Varga, C., Richter, M., and DeSanctis, A.G.: Systemic aleukemic reticuloendotheliosis (Letterer-Siwe disease). *Am J Dis Child, 75*:376-384, 1948.
23. Schafer, E.L.: Nonlipid reticuloendotheliosis, Letterer-Siwe's disease; a report of three cases. *Am J Pathol, 25*:49-83, 1949.
24. Ahnquist, G., and Holyoke, J.B.: Congenital Letterer-Siwe disease (reticuloendotheliosis) in a term stillborn infant. *J Pediatr, 57*:897-904, 1960.
25. Dargeon, H.W.: Considerations in the treatment of reticuloendotheliosis. *Am J Roentgenol, 93*:521-536, 1965.
26. Jones, B., Welton, W.A., and Gilbert, E.F.: Congenital Letterer-Siwe disease, report of three cases. *Cutis, 3*:750-756, 1967.
27. Christie, A., Batson, R., Shapiro, J., Riley, H. *et al.*: Acute disseminated (non-lipid) reticuloendotheliosis. *Acta Paediatr, 43 (Supp 100)*:65-76, 1954.

28. Cohen, D., Mitchell, C.B., and Alexander, J.: Letterer-Siwe disease in a newborn. *Arch Pathol, 81*:347-351, 1966.
29. Hertz, C.G., and Hambrick, G.: Congenital Letterer-Siwe disease. *Am J Dis Child, 116*:533-556, 1968.
30. Reese, A., and Levy, E.: Familial incidence of non-lipoid reticuloendotheliosis (Letterer-Siwe disease). *Arch Dis Child, 26*:578-581, 1951.
31. Bass, M., Sapin, S., and Hodes, H.: Use of cortisone and corticotropin (ACTH) in the treatment of reticuloendotheliosis. *Am J Dis Child, 85*:393-403, 1953.
32. Schoeck, V.W., Peterson, R., and Good, R.: Familial occurrence of Letterer-Siwe disease. *Pediatrics, 32*:1055-1063, 1963.
33. Falk, W., and Gellei, B.: The familial occurrence of Letterer-Siwe disease. *Acta Paediatr, 46*:471-480, 1967.
34. Bierman, H., Lanman, J., Dod, K. *et al.*: The ameliorative effect of antibiotics on nonlipoid reticuloendotheliosis (Letterer-Siwe disease) in identical twins. *J Pediatr, 40*:269-284, 1952.
35. Bierman, H.: Apparent cure of Letterer-Siwe disease seventeen-year survival of identical twins with nonlipoid reticuloendotheliosis. *JAMA, 196*:368-370, 1966.
36. Caldarini, G.: Considerazioni su di una coppia di gamelli affetti da malattia di Letterer-Siwe. *Clin Pediatr (Bologna), 48*:315-332, 1966.
37. Juberg, R.C., Kloepfer, H.W., and Oberman, H.: Genetic determination of acute disseminated histiocytosis X (Letterer-Siwe syndrome). *Pediatrics, 45*:753-765, 1970.
38. Lausecker, H.: Abt-Letterer-Siwesche Krankheit bie Zwillingen. *Wien Klin Wochenschr, 68*:433-435, 1956.
39. Lightwood, R., and Tizard, J.: Recovery from acute infantile non-lipoid reticuloendotheliosis (Letterer-Siwe disease). *Acta Paediatr, 43 (Suppl 100)*:453-468, 1954.
40. Havard, E., Rather, L.J., and Faber, H.: Nonlipoid reticuloendotheliosis (Letterer-Siwe's disease). *Pediatrics, 5*:474-485, 1950.
41. Miller, D.R.: Familial reticuloendotheliosis; concurrence of disease in five siblings. *Pedatrics, 38*:986-995, 1966.
42. Omenn, G.S.: Familial reticuloendotheliosis with eosinophilia. *N Engl J Med, 273*:427-432, 1965.
43. Farquhar, J., and Claireaux, A.: Familial haemophagocytic reticulosis. *Arch Dis Child, 27*:519-525, 1952.
44. Farquhar, J., MacGregor, A., and Richmond, J.: Familial haemophagocytic reticulosis. *Br Med J, 2*:1561-1564, 1958.
45. Marrian, V.J., and Sanerkin, N.: Familial histiocytic reticulosis (familial haemophagocytic reticulosis). *J Clin Pathol, 16*:65-69, 1963.
46. Goodall, H.B., Guthrie, W., and Buist, N.: Familial haemophagocytic reticulosis. *Scott Med J, 10*:425-438, 1965.

47. Bell, R., Grafield, A., Barnes, N., and France, N.: Familial Haemophagocytic Reticulosis. *Arch Dis Child, 43*:601-606, 1968.
48. Varadi, S., Gordon, R., and Abbott, D.: Haemophagocytic reticulosis diagnosed during life. *Acta Haematol (Basel), 31*:349-360, 1964.
49. Nelson, P., Santamaria, A., Olson, R.L., and Nayak, N.: Generalized lymphohistiocytic infiltration. *Pediatrics, 27*:931-950, 1961.
50. MacMahon, H., Bedigel, M., and Ellis, C.A.: Familial erythrophagocytic lymphohistiocytosis. *Pediatrics, 32*:868-879, 1963.
51. Berard, C.W., Cooper, R., Freireich, E., and Rabson, A.: Disseminated histiocytosis associated with a typical lymphoid cells (lymphohistiocytosis). *Cancer, 19*:1429-1437, 1966.
52. Forssman, H., and Rudberg, B.: Study of consanguinity in twenty-one cases of Hand-Schüller-Christian disease. *Acta Med Scand, 168*:427-429, 1960.
53. Kissane, J., and Smith, M.: *Pathology of Infancy and Childhood.* St. Louis, C.V. Mosby Company, 1967, p. 820.
54. Kissane, J., and Smith, M.: *Pathology of Infancy and Childhood.* St. Louis, C.V. Mosby Company, 1967, pp. 938-939.
55. Winkelmann, R.: The skin in histiocytosis X. *Mayo Clin Proc, 44*:535-549, 1969.
56. Keats, T., and Crane, J.: Cystic changes of the lungs in histiocytosis. *Am J Dis Child, 88*:764-771, 1954.
57. Feinberg, S., and Lester, R.: Roentgen examination of the gastrointestinal tract as an and in the diagnosis of acute and subacute reticuloendotheliosis. *Radiology, 71*:525-533, 1958.
58. Rubé, J., de la Pava, S., and Pickren, J.: Histiocytosis X with involvement of brain. *Cancer, 20*:486-492, 1967.
59. Butler, N., and Garretts, M.: Eosinophilic granuloma of skin. *Proc R Soc Med, 46*:276-277, 1953.
60. McCraney, H., and Falk, A.: Eosinophilic granuloma. *Am J Dis Child, 95*:214-216, 1958.
61. Dargeon, H.: *Reticuloendotheliosis in Childhood: A Clinical Survey.* Springfield, Charles C Thomas, 1966, p. 72.
62. Ereaux, L., and Schopflocher, P.: Histiocytosis X in an infant. *Cutis, 3*:223-229, 1967.
63. Morgenfeld, M., and Schajoueicz, F.: Solitary eosinophilic granuloma of lymph node; five-year follow-up. *Pediatrics, 48*:301-305, 1971.
64. Hodgson, J.R., Kennedy, R., and Camp, J.: Reticuloendotheliosis. (Hand-Schüller-Christian disease). *Radiology, 57*:642-652, 1951.
65. Avery, M.E., McAfee, J., and Guild, H.: The course and prognosis of reticuloendotheliosis (eosinophilic granuloma, Schüller-Christian disease and Letterer-Siwe disease). *Am J Med, 22*:636-652, 1957.
66. Davidson, R.I., and Shillito, J.: Eosinophilic granuloma of the cervical spine in children. *Pediatrics, 45*:746-752, 1970.

67. Altman, J., and Winkleman, R.: Xanthomatous cutaneous lesions of histiocytosis X. *Arch Dermatol, 87*:164-170, 1963.
68. Blevins, C., Dahlin, D., Lovestedt, S.A., and Kennedy, R.: Oral and dental manifestations of histiocytosis X. *Oral Surg, 12*:473-483, 1959.
69. Kittredge, R., Geller, A., and Finby, N.: The reticuoendotheliosis in the lung. *Am J Roentgenol, 100*:588-592, 1967.
70. Roland, A., Merdinger, W., and Froeb, H.: Recurrent spontaneous pneumothorax. *N Engl J Med, 270*:73-77, 1964.
71. Feinberg, S., and Langer, L.: Roentgen findings of increased intracranial pressure and communicating hydrocephalus as insidious manifestations of chronic histiocytosis X. *Am J Roengenol, 95*:41-47, 1965.
72. Case Records of the Massachusetts General Hospital; Case 11, 1965. *N Engl J Med, 272*:477-482, 1965.
73. Winkelmann, R., and Burgert, E.O.: Therapy of histiocytosis X. *J Dermatol, 82*:169-175, 1970.
74. Mermann, A., and Dargeon, H.: The management of certain nonlipid reticuloendothelioses. *Cancer, 8*:112-122, 1955.
75. Knighton, R., and Fox, J.: Diagnosis and treatment of eosinophilic granuloma of skull. *JAMA, 162*:1294-1297, 1956.
76. Aronson, R.: Sterptomycin in Letterer-Siwe's disease. *Lancet, 1*:889-890, 1951.
77. Fisher, R.: Multiple lesions of bone in Letterer-Siwe disease; report of a case with culture of paracolon Arizona bacilli from bone lesions and blood followed by response to therapy. *J Bone Joint Surg, 35A*: 445-464, 1953.
78. Holmlund, D.: A case of non-lipoid granulomatosis (Letterer-Siwe disease) observed for 15 years. *Acta Paediatr, 51*:324-330, 1962.
79. Bland, W., Levy, M., and Bassett, S.: A case of Hand-Schüller-Christian syndrome treated with cortisone. *Ann Intern Med, 35*:927-937, 1951.
80. Karlen, K.H.: A case of the Hand-Schüller-Christian disease treated with cortisone. *Acta Paediatr, 41*:282-289, 1952.
81. Bremers, H., George, C., Sunit, C., and Mercer, R.D.: Letterer-Siwe disease. *Arch Dermatol, 66*:291-292, 1952.
82. Cox, P.: Letterer-Siwe disease controlled by cortisone. *Proc R Soc Med, 46*:278-279, 1953.
83. Levin, H.: The use of cortisone in the treatment of reticuloendotheliosis. *J Pediatr, 41*:531-538, 1955.
84. Flosi, A., Assis, L., Bloise, W. *et al.*: Treatment of eosinophilic granuloma by corticotropin; report of 4 cases with disappearance of the bone lesions. *J Clin Endocrinol Metab, 17*:994-1001, 1957.
85. Flosi, A., Assis, L., Bloise, W. *et al.*: Hormonal treatment of Hand-Schüller-Christian disease: Report on a case with disappearance of the bone lesions. *J Clin Endocrinol Metab, 19*:239-247, 1959.

86. Sterky, G.: Non-lipid histiocytosis (systemic reticuloendothelial granuloma). *Acta Paediatr, 48:*421-427, 1959.
87. Avioli, L., Lasersohn, J., and Lopresti, J.: Histicytosis X (Schüller-Christian disease), a clinico-pathological survey; review of ten patients and the results of perdnisone therapy. *Medicine, 42:*119-147, 1963.
88. Koblenzer, P., and Wolman, I.J.: Letterer-Siwe disease. *Arch Dermatol, 90:*337-338, 1964.
89. Goldberg, L., and Diamond, A.: Letterer-Siwe disease. *Arch Dermatol, 92:*561-565, 1965.
90. Prouty, M.: Remission of Letterer-Siwe disease after prednisone therapy. *JAMA, 169:*1877-1879, 1969.
91. Griesemer, R., Letterer-Siwe disease. *Arch Dermatol, 92:*474-476, 1965.
92. Freud, P.: Treatment of reticuloendotheliosis: Use of corticosteroids and antifolic acid compounds. *JAMA, 175:*82-85, 1961.
93. Beier, F., Thatcher, L., and Lahey, M.: Treatment of reticuloendotheliosis with vinblastine sulfate. *J Pediatr, 63:*1087-1092, 1963.
94. Lahey, M.: Vinblastine in the Treatment of Histiocytosis (Abstract). 76th Annual Meeting American Pediatric Society. Atlantic City, April 27-28, 1966, p. 46.
95. Sharp, H., White, J.G., and Krivit, W.: Histiocytosis X treated with vinblastine sulfate (NSC-49842). *Cancer Chemosther Rep, 39:*53-59, 1964.
96. Price, H., and Seligman, E.: Letterer-Siwe disease. *Arch Dermatol, 90:* 366-368, 1964.
97. Siegel, J., and Coltman, C.: Histiocytosis X; response to vinblastine sulfate. *JAMA, 197:*403-406, 1966.
98. Al-Rashid, R.: Successful treatment of an infant with Letterer-Siwe disease with vinblastine sulfate. *Clin Pediatr, 9:*494-496, 1970.
99. Lahey, M.: Comparison of Three Treatment Regimens in Histiocytosis X in Children. (Abstract). Tenth International Cancer Congress. Houston, Texas, 1970, p. 764.
100. Jones, B.: Acute Leukemia Group B. Unpublished data, 1971.
101. Mauger, D.: Letterer-Siwe's disease (acute disseminated histiocytosis X); a case complicated by disseminated intravascular coagulation and responding to heparin therapy. *Pediatrics, 47:*435-437, 1971.
102. Johnson, H., and Johnson, W.: *Pneumocystic carinii* pneumonia in children with cancer; diagnosis and treatment. *JAMA, 214:*1067-1978, 1970.
103. Cangir, A., and Sullivan, M.: The occurrence of cytomegalovirus infections in childhood leukemia. *JAMA, 195:*616-622, 1966.
104. Cangir, A., Sullivan, M., Sutow, W., and Taylor, G.: Cytomegalovirus syndrome in children with acute leukemia: treatment with floxuridine. *JAMA, 201:*612-615, 1967.

105. Lahey, M.: Prognosis in reticuloendotheliosis in children. *J Pediatr, 60:* 664-671, 1962.
106. Doede, K., and Rappaport, H.: Long-term survival of patients with acute differentiated histiocytosis (Letterer-Siwe disease). *Cancer, 20:* 1782-1795, 1967.

Chapter 11

IMMUNOTHERAPY OF CANCER: CURRENT STATUS

EVAN M. HERSH, JORDAN U. GUTTERMAN, GIORA MAVLIGIT

TEN YEARS ago a book on human malignant disease would not have required a chapter on immunology. While tumor antigens and tumor-specific immune responses were recognized in viral- and carcinogen-induced animal tumors, there was essentially no convincing evidence for the same phenomena in human tumors. The few studies which had been done in man were generally ignored; in part because the evidence was circumstantial and in part because there was justifiable criticism of experimental design. A chapter on cancer immunology would also not have been needed because it has only been in the last ten to twenty years that the principles of cell-mediated immunity as applied to transplantation and cancer have been established. The role of cell-mediated immunity in the host control of tumors is now well established. Tumor antigens and tumor-specific immune responses have been identified in the majority of human tumors which have been studied, and exciting preliminary experiments on the immunotherapy of human cancer have been conducted.

The concept that human malignant disease can be treated with immunological methods is at least eighty years old. Shortly after the discovery of antibodies, Erlich hypothesized that patients could be immunized against their own cancers.[1] This idea was strengthened by the finding in the early 1900's that tumor transplants from one animal to another were rejected.[2] However, the

Note: This study was supported by Grant CA 05831 from the National Institutes of Health, Bethesda, Maryland, and Grant ACS-CI-22 from the American Cancer Society.

The authors wish to thank Drs. Emil Frei, III, and Emil J. Freireich for their continuing inspiration and support.

subsequent finding that this rejection was based on tissue histocompatibility[3] and not on tumor antigens led to a thirty-year hiatus in the study of tumor immunity. The observations by Gross in the 1940's[4] and Foley in the 1950's[5] that specific tumor antigens and tumor immunity actually do exist in animal tumor systems eventually led to the resurgence of interest in tumor immunology. The many animal experiments which followed led to the current hope that effective immunotherapeutic methods can be developed to treat human cancer.

During the last five years, tumor-associated cell-surface antigens and specific immune responses to these cell-surface antigens have been identified in a number of human tumors. These immunologic properties were found in sarcomas, malignant melanoma, colon cancer, renal cancer, neuroblastoma and a number of leukemias and lymphomas. On the basis of current knowledge, it seems likely that most if not all human malignant tumors have cell-surface tumor distinctive antigens and elicit tumor distinctive immune responses. This makes it likely that the development of effective immunotherapy is imminent.

The likelihood that effective immunotherapeutic maneuvers can be developed is also made more possible by recent advances in conventional therapy. Thus, approximately 35 percent of all cancer patients with solid tumors are cured by primary surgery[6,7] and the majority who are not cured have a "tumor-free interval" in which the tumor burden is certainly very small. In addition, a large number of patients with nonresectable solid tumors are either cured or brought into temporary complete remission by radiotherapy.[8] Most recently, the efficacy of chemotherapy for a variety of malignant tumors has improved tremendously. Now patients with Wilm's tumor,[9] neuroblastoma,[10] Hodgkin's disease,[11] non-Hodgkin's lymphoma,[12] soft tissue sarcomas such as rhabdomyosarcoma,[13] carcinoma of the breast[14] and acute leukemia[15,16] are brought into complete remission, even from a state of advanced disease, by chemotherapy. Again, while there are almost certainly residual tumor cells left, the tumor burden during remission, is very small. This point is important because of the findings in all animal immunotherapy systems that immunotherapeutic benefits occur with greatest frequency when the tumor burden is reduced to less that 10^5 total residual cells.

PRINCIPLES OF IMMUNOTHERAPY

On the basis of the animal experiments performed to date, a set of guidelines or principles for immunotherapy of human cancer can be established tentatively. These will undoubtedly be replaced by more sophisticated guidelines as our knowledge of human tumor immunology advances. They are as follows:

1. Maximum tumor burden reduction by conventional therapy must precede any immunotherapy approach. This is probably the most important principle. In all animal systems, immunotherapeutic or immunoprophylactic effects can be overcome by a 1 log increase in the tumor cell challenge dose. Thus, an increase in the tumor challenge from 0.1 to 1.0 mg will overwhelm the effects of immunotherapy. The critical number in animal experiments seems to be 10^5 tumor cells. It has been calculated, at least in some human tumors, that there are less than 10^5 tumor cells remaining after complete remission has been achieved.

2. Immunotherapeutic benefits will be achieved only when the host is immunologically competent or when immunocompetence is restored by or concurrent with the immunotherapy. It has been clearly established that immunocompetence and prognosis are closely associated in cancer and that immunological incompetence is associated with progression of disease.[17,18] It has been hypothesized, although not proven, that immunocompetence is needed, because remissions induced by conventional therapy are the result not of therapy alone but also of the adjunctive effects of the host defense mechanisms. Thus, host defense mechanisms would be responsible for the low incidence of metastases after surgery, even though a large number of viable tumor cells are released as the tumor is removed. In patients to be subjected to chemotherapy, host defense status should be evaluated and attempts to correct any deficiency should be made either before or concurrent with the drug treatment. Indeed, nonspecific active immunotherapy with BCG presumably works by the mechanism of augmenting present but inadequate levels of host defense.

3. Since conventional therapy and immunotherapy are likely to be combined in the treatment of some types of malignancy, it is important that the periods of immunosuppression, recovery from immunosuppression and augmentation of immunocompetence following conventional therapy be characterized. Radiotherapy, surgery and chemotherapy all have immunosuppressive properties. It would be pointless to administer active immunotherapy during the period of immunosuppression. Also, following this period of immunosuppression, there is a period of rebound or heightened immunological reactivity. This is likely to be the ideal period for immunotherapy.

4. In passive and adoptive immunotherapy, high specific activity and/or large quantities of reagents are required. Thus, for passive immunotherapy with antiserum, enough specific antibody must be present to attack the majority of the antigenic sites on the tumor cells. Furthermore, if a large amount of non–tumor-specific antibody is present, it may eventuate in more host damage than benefit. For adoptive immunotherapy with specifically sensitized lymphoid cells, the same problem exists. Thus, in animal experiments and *in vitro,* lymphocyte-tumor cell ratios of 100 to 1 at least are required for a sugnificant effect. If immunity is directed against H-2 or HLA as well as tumor antigens, graft-versus-host disease may occur.

5. The timing of immunotherapy is critically important but must be worked out emperically. Thus, in animal immunotherapy experiments, application of the immunotherapeutic treatment is effective at certain times following tumor burden reduction is effective, while at other times it is either ineffective or more important, enhancing of tumor growth. Therefore, clinical protocols must be designed to explore different timing relationships.

6. Another important principle derived from studies in animal systems relates to the sites of immunization for active specific immunotherapy.[19] Thus, Alexander and Hall showed that lymph nodes draining sites of tumor are under constant bombardment with tumor antigen. As a result, they do not release specifically immune immunoblasts into the circulation. Therefore, active im-

munotherapy with patient's tumor cells should be administered in lymphatic drainage areas which are free of tumor.

7. Immunotherapeutic procedures must be designed to augment cell-mediated immunity selectively, since antibody in some tumor systems may be blocking or enhancing rather than cytotoxic. Therefore, it is essential that immunotherapy be evaluated for stimulation of enhancing antibody.

8. Methods must be developed to evaluate anti-tumor host defense mechanisms and these methods must be applied repeatedly during any immunotherapy. This is because current immunotherapy is of marginal benefit. Its failure or success must be evaluated in terms of the effect on cell-mediated and humoral tumor immunity tests *in vitro*. Then clinical success or failure can be evaluated in terms of the effect on host defense mechanisms. Serial evaluation of anti-tumor host defense may also permit and guide the development of better immunotherapeutic methods.

APPROACHES TO IMMUNOTHERAPY

On the basis of animal experiments and preliminary studies of immunotherapy in man, an outline of the current possible approaches to immunotherapy can be made. The following outline includes methods that have been used in man, methods that have only been used in animals, and methods that are theoretically possible but have not yet been used in any system. This outline includes approaches which do not seem desirable and does not indicate the order of importance.

I. Passive immunotherapy*
   A. Xenogenic anti-HLA antibody
   B. Xenogeneic specific anti-tumor antibody
   C. Allogeneic anti-HLA antibody
   D. Allogeneic specific anti-tumor antibody
   E. Radio-labeled specific anti-tumor antibody

*The term "xenogeneic" refers to materials from different species and "allogeneic" refers to materials from an unrelated member of the same species. The word "cells" refers to lymphocytes and/or leukocytes unless otherwise specified.

II. Adoptive immunotherapy
- A. Allogeneic specifically sensitized cells
- B. Allogeneic nonsensitized cells
  1. White cell transfusions
  2. Bone marrow transplants
- C. Extracts of specifically sensitized allogeneic or xenogeneic cells
  1. RNA extracts
  2. Transfer factor
- D. Autologous cells, activated *in vitro* and re-infused
- E. Autologous cells, stored *in vitro* and re-infused after conventional therapy
- F. Autologous cells in the form of lymphoblastoid cell line cells

III. Active immunotherapy
- A. Nonspecific augmentation of immunological reactivity with various adjuvants
  1. BCG and other mycobacterial preparations and extracts
  2. *Corynebacterium parvum* and other bacterial preparations and extracts
  3. Lentinan and other polysaccharide adjuvants
  4. Interferon inducers and interferon
- B. Active specific immunotherapy
  1. Active immunization with unmodified autologous tumor cells
  2. Active immunization with unmodified allogeneic tumor cells
  3. Active immunization with tumor cells modified as follows:
     - a. Neuraminidase-treated
     - b. Iodacetamide or other sulfhydryl active agent-treated
     - c. Coupled to foreign protein or hapten
     - d. Irradiated

4. Active immunization with purified and characterized tumor-specific cell surface antigens, either
    a. Untreated
    b. Treated
    c. Coupled

IV. Combination immunotherapy using two or more of the above outlined methods, either concurrently or sequentially or combined with conventional therapy.

V. Local immunotherapy
    A. With agents or methods that induce delayed hypersensitivity in the lesion
    B. Antiserum injection
    C. Activated lymphocytes injection
    D. Virus inoculation

In animal systems, the most effective methods of demonstrating tumor immunity have involved sensitization of the host before viable tumor cell inoculation. Both nonspecific and tumor specific active immuno-pretherapy are most effective by this schedule. Recent evidence suggests that this type of immuno-pretherapy may be valuable in man. Thus, Davignon found that BCG may be valuable in preventing leukemia in man.[20] In children less than fifteen years old, the incidence of leukemia is 55.87 out of 100,000 in those who have not been vaccinated with BCG and is 23.54 out of 1000,000 in those who have been vaccinated with BCG. This observation needs to be confirmed and extended. One suggestion that it is not correct has already appeared.[21]

PASSIVE IMMUNOTHERAPY

Of the various types of immunotherapy, passive immunotherapy—that is, the administration of antiserum—seems to be the least likely to be successful. This is because it would be very difficult to produce very high titer antisera directed only against the tumor antigens and not against normal host antigens. Furthermore, whenever high titer antisera are produced against tumor cells or tumor cell surface antigens, the possibility of tumor enhancement occurs.[22] Finally, immunoglobulin molecules, being large, tend to enter and leave the circulation slowly. Therefore, only very small tumor cell deposits or tumor cell deposits close to capillaries would be affected. Cells in relatively large solid tumor masses would not be affected by serotherapy. Early attempts at serum therapy, using antiserum produced in animals against human tumors, will not be reviewed here. First, they were not successful and second, they were associated with the development of serum sickness. Finally, they were completely nonspecific, containing antibody against the normal cell surface antigens as well as the tumor antigens.

There have been several recent reports, however, in which the possible use of antiserum has been suggested again. First, good methods have now been developed to produce highly reactive animal antihuman lymphocyte serum.[23] This material is fairly specific to human lymphod cells and can be prepared as pure immunoglobulin. It has been used in the treatment of chronic lymphocytic leukemia.[24] It was fairly well tolerated and did produce a transient reduction in the circulating lymphocyte count. More recently, high titer isoantibody obtained from multiparous or multitransfused subjects has been given to patients with chronic lymphatic leukemia.[25] The use of isoantisera would obviate the problem of immunization against foreign protein, inherent in the use of animal antihuman lymphocyte serum. Again, these transfusions were well tolerated and led to a striking reduction in the circulating leukocyte count. Marrow disease was not affected but lymph node size was reduced. The approach of using antisera to treat acute or chronic leukemia seems of limited value. First, extravascular disease would not be affected in a major way. More important, there is excellent conventional therapy, chemotherapy, which regularly produces complete remission in patients with the leukemias.

There may be some value in more specific serum therapy, under specialized circumstances. In a number of diseases, including melanoma and sarcoma, specific cytotoxic antibodies have been detected either in the patient's serum during remission and in the serum of close relatives. This serum is cytotoxic to the appropriate tumor cells *in vitro,* in the presence of complement. Lewis *et al.* hypothesized that the function of this cytotoxic sera is to prevent metastases by killing cells (through the mechanism of complement mediated cytotoxicity) when they are released into the circulation.[26] Thus, it is reasonable that therapy with this tumor-specific allogeneic serum should be given before, during and immediately after curative surgery or should be given repeatedly in the postsurgical period, when metastatic seeding is most likely to occur. This passive immunotherapy would be expected to increase the surgical cure rate.

ADOPTIVE IMMUNOTHERAPY

During recent years, there have been a number of interesting and provocative studies of adoptive immunotherapy using a variety of methods in man. Many of these studies have been prompted by the initial work of Nadler and Moore, who conducted experiments on adoptive immunotherapy, using the cross-grafting cross-leukocyte transfusion approach.[27] This approach was based on the animal experiments of Alexander and his co-workers, in which allogeneic or even xenogeneic immune leukocytes can induce partial remission in animals bearing chemical carcinogen-induced tumors.[28] Nadler and Moore's studies were done mainly in patients with malignant melanoma, but they also studied patients with breast carcinoma, colon carcinoma, soft tissue sarcomas, osteogenic sarcoma and others. Their accumulating series have been reported several times during the last few years and they have now studied approximately 120 patients.[29] Their approach is to transplant thin sections or minced pieces of solid tumors between a pair of patients, both having the same type of tumor. When evidence of rejection appears (usually at ten days) they begin a series of leukocyte transfusions (collected by plasmapheresis) between the two patients lasting several weeks. All patients studied had metastatic solid tumors. Of the group reported, there have been three complete remissions, two in malignant melanoma and one in osteogenic sarcoma. An additional sixteen patients with melanoma, one with breast carcinoma, two with colon carcinoma and one with soft tissue sarcoma have had partial or mixed responses.

Similar studies were done by Krementz and Samuels.[30] Using the same technique, they studied ten pairs of patients, nine with melanoma and one with renal carcinoma. Of the twenty patients studied, two had objective and very good partial remissions lasting twelve and eight months respectively. Similar studies were also reported by Curtis and Hersh.[31] The rationale for their studies was that they had previously demonstrated that specific immunity to protein antigens could be transferred from immune to non-immune cancer patients using peripheral blood leukocytes.[32] Their experimental design was different from that of Nadler and Moore in that patients were studied in groups of three. Tumor was given from A to B, B to C and C to A, and leukocytes collected with the IBM-NCI Blood Cell Separator were transferred in the opposite direction. Thus, no patients received leukocytes from a donor to whose HLA antigens he had been immunized by a tumor graft. Therefore, immunity to the normal HLA antigens of the leukocyte donor was presumably absent in that specific leukocyte recipient. It was also hoped that the larger number of leukocytes that could be collected with the Blood Cell Separator (up to 5×10^{10} per course) would augment the immunotherapeutic benefit. In total, four pairs of three patients each or twelve patients were studied. In one patient, there was an objective complete remission lasting twelve months. In four additional patients, significant subjective improvement occurred. In the remainder, metastatic tumors were stable or grew during the study period.

Humphrey *et al.* has taken a different approach to adoptive immunotherapy using cross-immunization and cross-transfusion.[33] He immunized with a 20 percent homogenate of the patient's tumor and administered 0.5 ml twice a week for one week and then weekly for at least three weeks. Subsequent to this, ten exchange leukocyte and plasma transfusions were done. As of 1971, Humphrey reported that there have been eight objective tumor regressions in fifty-eight patients studied.

This approach has also been used in acute leukemia.[34] Skurkovich and his colleagues reported studies in twelve children of ages three to ten years with acute leukemia of various types who had active disease and were not on chemotherapy. He immunized pairs of patients with intravenous and intramuscular injections of allogeneic leukemic cells, giving 5 to 500 $\times$ 10^6 cells per injection and a total of two to five injections. Subsequent to this, he administered two to five passive leukocyte and serum transfusions from and to the immunized patients. Over a period of thirty to sixty days, they observed that three patients entered complete remission, five entered partial remission and four failed to respond. The remissions were subsequently maintained with 6-mercaptopurine. Those patients who responded developed positive skin tests to the allogeneic leukemic cells. Negative results have also been reported. Andrews and colleagues studied four patients, two with acute leukemia and two with malignant melanona.[35] Their tumor cells were used to immunize related allogeneic normal human subjects after which large numbers of thoracic duct lymphocytes were transfused from the tumor recipients to the tumor donors. No therapeutic effect was observed.

Adoptive immunotherapy has also been attempted using subcellular fractions rather than intact allogeneic lymphocytes. Studies with transfer factor are worthy of mention. The rationale for using this material was that transfer factor can confer donor-type delayed hypersensitivity on a recipient and that the use of transfer factor avoids the danger of graft-versus-host disease. Brandes *et al.* cross-grafted two patients with malignant melanoma and after immunity had developed, collected leukocytes and prepared transfer factor from each.[36] The transfer factor was administered twice a week for three weeks. A 25 percent tumor regression was observed in one of the two patients. Oettgen and co-workers investigated an interesting use of transfer factor.[37] They hypothesized that tumor-free individuals in the tumor-bearing age range had natural resistance to cancer and that this was based on cell-mediated immunity which could be transferred with transfer factor to cancer-bearing subjects. Transfer factor was therefore prepared from the pooled leukocytes of normal women and administered weekly over a period of up to one year, subcutaneously or intradermally, to five women with metastatic breast cancer. One of the five had a partial regression which lasted six months. The authors concluded that transfer factor could be given safely, could transfer various types of cell-mediated immune responses including tumor immunity, and that its potential as an immunotherapeutic tool should be further explored.

A unique new approach has been proposed by Frenster in which the patient's own leukocytes are used for "adoptive immunotherapy."[38] Frenster and Rogoway based their studies on the observations that mitogen activated lymphocytes can kill target cells *in vitro* and that lymphoblasts released from responding lymph nodes during an immune response, localize to the lungs and gut. The investigators collected 10^8 to 5×10^8 peripheral blood leukocytes from patients with pulmonary metastases of solid tumors. These were activated *in vitro* for twenty-four to forty-eight hours with phytohemagglutinin. The activated cells were washed and re-infused intravenously. No major untoward side effects were noted. Ten patients were studied and objective regression of pulmonary metastases were observed in eight. Metastatic deposits outside of the pulmonary area did not regress and continued to grow.

The idea that allogeneic leukocytes from normal individuals carry some degree of natural tumor immunity or at least can recognize tumor cells *in vivo* (surveillance) has prompted the use of both leukocyte transfusions and bone marrow transplantation therapy in a variety of malignant diseases. Symes and co-workers transfused normal splenic lymphocytes obtained during splenectomy into allogeneic subjects with malignant disease.[39] Only slight responses were observed. In contrast, Schwartzenberg and co-workers studied the effects of transfusions of chronic myelogenous leukemia cells on the status of patients with acute leukemia.[40] Repeated transfusions were given to twenty-one patients. Usually, the CML cells were stored for two hours at 37 C to partially reduce their immunological reactivity so that graft-versus-host disease would not occur. A total of 6 to 98×10^{10} cells were given by repeated daily infusion. Of the twenty-one patients studied, six complete remission were observed. Four lasted less than twenty days, but two were prolonged to three and four months respectively. Only those patients who received more than 10^{11} cells and also only those patients who showed some evidence of graft-versus-host disease achieved remission. This is reminiscent of Boranic and Tonkovic's finding in animals in which cure of acute leukemia was achieved by the appropriately timed and appropriately terminated induction of graft-versus-host disease in the leukemic animal.[41]

The use of graft-versus-host disease in the treatment of acute leukemia has been part of the basis of the interest in bone marrow transplantation therapy in acute leukemia. In addition, it has been hoped that the eradication of the leukemic and normal bone marrow with either chemotherapy or radiotherapy and the subsequent re-population with allogeneic bone marrow might prevent the recurrence of leukemia. One approach to bone marrow transplantation is the use of whole body irradiation.[42] Bone marrow grafts are regularly achieved and these indeed are associated with complete remission. This success is diminished because the morbidity and/or the mortality is high due to infection, hemorrhage and graft-versus-host disease. However, patients who otherwise would have failed to achieve remission, because they were refractory to conventional therapy, benefit by this approach.

Another approach is the cyclophosphamide pretreatment regimen of Santos *et al.*[43] This has also been used by several other investigators.[44] The basic design is to give a unit of whole blood from the potential donor, to stimulate mitosis in the responsive immune clone in the recipient and to follow this in twenty-four hours by a four-day course of cyclophosphamide (at approximately 40 mg/kg/day) to kill that clone. Twenty-four hours after the last dose of cyclophosphamide, the bone marrow infusion is given. The majority of patients so treated do actually achieve a graft. However, in spite of good HLA matching and in spite of supportive care measures, infection, hemorrhage and graft-versus-host disease have claimed a majority of these patients. Recently, Mathé has proposed the use of antilymphocyte serum alone in HLA identical sibling pairs as an ideal preporative to marrow transplantation in patients with acute leukemia.[45] In a small series, he has reported that severe graft-versus-host disease was not a problem, nor did the patients die of early hemorrhage or infection. Salmon and co-workers have developed a hot-pulse thymidine method to eliminate the graft-versus-host disease producing cells which also may be useful to treat the graft cells *in vitro* and prevent subsequent graft-versus-host disease.[46]

Very recently, Thomas has reported a potential limitation on marrow engraftment in patients with acute leukemia.[47] In one subject with acute leukemia, grafted with the normal marrow of a sibling of the opposite sex, the leukemia recurred with the sex chromosome pattern of the donor. Thomas' interpretation of this finding was that a viral agent had re-induced leukemia in the donor cells. However, pretreatment cytogenetics were not available on the recipient. Also, in other instances of recurrent leukemia after cross-sex marrow transplantation, cytogenetic studies revealed that the leukemic cells were of recipient and not donor sex chromosome patterns. This finding does indicate the need for careful follow-up cytogenetic studies in these patients, as well as careful adequate pretherapy cytogenetics.

The efficacy of marrow transplantation in the treatment of acute leukemia is uncertain at this time. The complications are clearly worse than those of conventional chemotherapy and the percentage of remissions is lower. This situation may change when the histocompatibility determinants of graft-versus-host disease in HLA identical siblings are determined and when more specific, less toxic, immunosuppressive therapy is available. Progress should come in this field from those working on tolerance induction and blocking antibodies.

In summary, considerable work utilizing a variety of approaches has been done on adoptive immunotherapy of human neoplasia. These approaches do not fulfill the criteria of acceptable therapy. Thus, the response rates are generally lower than those achieved with conventional therapy. Furthermore, immunological specificity has not been demonstrated and indeed allogeneic leukocyte infusions may simply be nonspecifically augmenting the immune response of the recipient (in a manner similar to that of BCG). Finally, adoptive immunotherapy with bone marrow transplants is both less successful and more toxic than conventional therapy. However, there is still a place for adoptive immunotherapy. It can be used in patients for whom conventional therapy is not suitable. It is possible that some of the modalities could be used in combination with conventional therapy and could be administered between courses of chemotherapy or before or after periods of radiotherapy. It is also possible that adoptive immunotherapeutic maneuvers should be used immediately following surgery, when the number of tumor cells sequestered in the patient is likely to be less than 10^5.

ACTIVE NONSPECIFIC IMMUNOTHERAPY

Active nonspecific immunotherapy is based on the observation that the administration of adjuvants or adjuvant-like materials in animal systems reduces the number of takes of experimental tumors and can actually cause regression of established tumors. In the modern era, active nonspecific immunotherapy is also based on the concept that the host defense mechanisms of the tumor-bearing subjects are diminished. This diminution may be either general or tumor specific, but in either case, a nonspecific immunological activator might augment these deficient responses.

Mathé has done the most extensive work with nonspecific immunotherapy in patients with acute leukemia. In his initial study, he reported striking prolongation of chemotherapy induced but non–chemotherapy-maintained complete remissions in acute leukemia by the administration of either BCG alone, BCG and allogeneic leukemic cells together, or allogeneic leukemic cells alone.[48] The three treatments were equivalent in their effectiveness. The BCG was the Pasteur Institute strain and was administered on top of a scarified area 10 by 10 cm in diameter and at a dose of 75 mg/scarification. This treatment was repeated twice weekly or weekly. In their most current regimen, this group uses the same approach to BCG treatment, but always in combination with other forms of immunotherapy.[49] The British Medical Research Council group has also investigated the use of BCG in the treatment of acute leukemia.[50] To date, their results are negative. Mathé, however, points out that the two regimens (British versus

French) are very different.[51] First, the French give a more prolonged and intensive program of cytoreductive systemic chemotherapy prior to the beginning of immunotherapy. In addition, the French group also uses irradiation of the central nervous system, intrathecal cytosine arabinoside, splenectomy and irradiation of involved lymph nodes prior to immunotherapy. Finally, the British used the Glaxo strain of BCG (administered intradermally) in doses of less than 1 mg/week. Mathé feels that this is inadequate therapy. Proof for this point of view has appeared. Bluming (quoted by Mathé) compared the effects of the British and French methods of BCG immunization using the Glaxo and Pasteur strain of organisms respectively.[51] Only the French method was observed to augment cell-mediated and humoral immune responses.

Other adjuvants of potential value in immunotherapy include *C parvum* and pertussis vaccine. *C parvum* has been used by Mathé and his associates[51] and pertussis vaccine by Guyer and Crowther.[52] The latter group reported sixteen patients with acute leukemia who were brought into complete remission with prednisone and 6-mercaptopurine. This remission was consolidated with five courses of 6-mercaptopurine and methotrexate after which eight underwent repeated inoculations of pertussis vaccine (0.5 ml twice a week, intramuscularly). The results suggested some slight immunotherapeutic benefit in that the treated group had three patients who remained in remission greater than 220 days after the end of treatment, while the nontreated group had only one patient who remained in remission that long. It is interesting to speculate that had the consolidation treatment been more intensive and longer, the immunotherapeutic benefit would have been greater.

C parvum (killed organism vaccine) has also been used in the therapy of metastatic solid tumors given weekly during intensive intermittent chemotherapy and compared to chemotherapy alone.[53] The treated group had a ten-month survival compared to six months in the control. This difference was significant.

Poly-IC has now been added by Mathé as another nonspecific immunotherapeutic agent in his current regimen.[54] This is based on the finding in animal systems, summarized by Gresser,[55] that interferon inducers or interferon itself has anti-tumor properties and can cause animals with lymphomas and other tumors to enter remission.

These early results with nonspecific immunotherapy indicate that it should be considered for use in several groups. First, nonspecific immunotherapy with living organisms should be considered in patients who are apparently free of disease after surgery but who have a high incidence of recurrence. This would include patients with trunk primary melanomas, carcinoma of the lung, carcinoma of the stomach and carcinoma of the breast with axillary metastases. One could devise a schedule of BCG administration or other nonspecific immunotherapy to start some time after the end of surgery and to continue for several months, or perhaps even a year. The end point of the investigation would be a decreased recurrence rate in the treated patients. In addition, nonspecific immunotherapy might be considered for the patients who are brought into complete remission with chemotherapy but who have a relapse rate thereafter. This would include patients with metastatic cancer of the breast, metastatic malignant melanoma, a variety of patients with disseminated malignant lymphomas and, of course, patients with acute leukemia. Finally, nonspecific immunotherapy with killed tubercle bacilli, killed BCG, MER or *C parvum* could be considered, even for patients undergoing active treatment with radiotherapy or chemotherapy. Of course, all of these studies should be done with the appropriate controls and with knowledge that a decreased rather than an increased response rate might result.

ACTIVE SPECIFIC IMMUNOTHERAPY

Active specific immunotherapy by immunization with autologous or allogeneic tumor cells, tumor cell extracts, or other tumor cell preparations either alone or with some type of adjuvant, has been attempted for many years. Until recently, little success was claimed, but in the most recent studies, even when no tumor response was observed, augmentation of tumor-specific immune response occurred. Therefore, there is hope that this approach may be increasingly useful in the future.

The basis for this hope is that spontaneous tumor immunity has been observed in man and that under the appropriate circumstances, this tumor immunity can be demonstrated to be cytotoxic to the patient's own tumor cells. The ultimate hope is that the tumor antigens can be purified, characterized and collected in sufficient quantities so that hyperimmunization can be achieved and tumor immunity can be strengthened to the point where it will effectively operate against large masses of tumor.

Some of the early suggestive work in this area was that of Graham and Graham.[56] They studied active immunotherapy in patients with gynecological cancer, such as ovarian, cervical, corpus or vulval. They made tumor cell suspensions in complete Freund's adjuvant and inoculated 1.5×10^6 fresh uncultured tumor cells on one or more occasions in multiple subcutaneous sites. Other conventional treatment was given if necessary and significant response was taken as an increased survival rate of the treated group. They compared 232 treated patients with 139 controls. At twenty-four months, 13 percent of the treated patients and only 6 percent of the controls survived. If the treated patients were divided into those who had reactions at the immunization site and those who did not, there were 14 percent survivors among the reactors and none among the non-reactors. One of the complications was the severe local reactions which can occur at sites of injection of complete Freund's adjuvant. This can produce lesions which drain for years and this material is currently not approved for human use. The findings of the Grahams have been confirmed and extended by the observations of Hughes *et al.*[57] They prepared an extract of the tumors of patients with advanced malignant melanoma and colon carcinoma by homogenization and sonication. They treated twenty patients by inoculating this material every two weeks in either complete or incomplete Freund's adjuvant or mixed with TAB (typhoid) vaccine. The material was the microsomal faction of the tumor cells. The patients did not receive other therapy during this treatment. There was improved skin reactivity to tumor extract and increased immunofluorescent antibody in these patients and there were three objective, clinically significant, partial remissions.

Active specific immunotherapy of acute leukemia has been investigated extensively by Mathé. He assumed that acute lymphatic leukemia cells share a common cell surface antigen, and therefore he administered pooled allogeneic leukemic cells to his patients as one component of their postchemotherapy immunotherapy.[48] He gave 4×10^7 cells weekly. The cells were irradiated with 4,000 rads before administration. Of patients who received active immunotherapy only, 3 out of 5 were in remission over 130 days compared to 0 out of 10 controls. The current regimen used by Mathé includes active specific immunotherapy combined with several modalities of nonspecific immunotherapy. He still administers 4×10^7 allogeneic leukemic cells per dose, but the schedule is weekly for three doses followed by every other week for three doses and then monthly thereafter. At 480 days after the start of immunotherapy, 83 percent of patients on immunotherapy alone are still in remission compared with 40 percent of those who received immunotherapy plus vincristine or amantadine.[49] Thus, the immunosuppressive effects of vincristine or amantadine may abrogate the immunotherapeutic benefits. Apparently, the cell type of the leukemia also determines the response. Only patients with the more differentiated microlymphoblastic or prolymphocytic types of acute lymphatic leukemia respond to immunitherapy.

Active immunotherapy of acute leukemia has also been administered by Skurkovich.[58] He collected plasma and leukocytes from patients with acute leukemia as they began to enter remission, but before they actually were in remission. He administered the collected plasma intravenously and he administered the collected leukocytes intramuscularly on repeated occasions during remission induction with prednisone and remission maintenance with 6-mercaptopurine. Twenty patients were studied. Their mean remission duration was 491 days compared to 173 days in matched patients treated with chemotherapy only.

Southam has initiated a study of the active specific immunotherapy of osteogenic sarcoma.[59] In this disease, the majority of patients relapse with pulmonary metastases even through they are all or almost all apparently free of disease after surgery. Southam used two forms of active immunotherapy; cell-free extracts of the patients' own sarcoma treated with ultraviolet light or cell suspensions of the patients' own tumor treated with radiation. These materials were given subcutaneously and intravenously weekly until the supply was exhausted. The therapy was started four weeks after amputation if the patient was disease-free at that point. The results were compared to the survival and metastases free interval in historical controls from the same institution. At twenty-four months, 75 percent of the patients treated with the cell-free extract, 45 percent of those treated with irradiated cells and 30 percent of the controls were surviving. At thirty-six months, 33 percent of the patients treated with the cell-free extract, 15 percent of patients treated with irradiated cells, and 15 percent of the controls were free of metastases. These preliminary results call for extension and confirmation.

Several types of tumor cells have been used for immunotherapy. Moore and his colleagues reported that patients repeatedly immunized with cultured solid tumor cells from established cell lines of their original cell type showed some therapeutic benefits.[60,61] Of eighty-five patients with various solid tumors treated, there was one complete remission and three partial remissions. These patients had melanoma or various sarcomas. Various types of modified tumor antigens have also been used for immunotherapy by the active specific approach. Czajkowski used "tumor antigen" coupled by the BDB method to rabbit gamma-globulin and administered it in incomplete Freund's adjuvant to fourteen patients with advanced metastatic disease.[62] Thirteen developed precipitating antibodies to their extract. After this treatment two patients had remissions lasting more than four years. One of these was a squamous carcinoma of the chin with local invasion and the other was a local recurrence of carcinoma of the breast.

This method was used by the Rand group as reported by Ayer.[63] They observed regression of carcinoma *in situ* in six patients. Very few details are available in this report. This approach was extensively explored by Cunningham.[64] He reported studies in forty-two patients with solid tumors. He prepared extracts of the patient's own tumor, coupled it to gamma-globulin by the BDB method, and administered it weekly in incomplete Freund's adjuvant for an average of sixteen weeks. Only one out of forty-two patients had a partial response. This was a patient with squamous carcinoma of the tongue whose oral lesions regressed while other metastatic lesions remained stable.

Most of these reports of benefit from active immunotherapy have not been confirmed nor extended to large numbers of patients. Most suffer from the defect that ancillary immunological studies of a sophisticated nature were not done. These might indicate whether immune responses to tumor were actually changed. Recently, a more hopeful prospect has been suggested by the work of several groups, in which active specific autoimmunization has led to improved specific tumor immunity. For example, Powles and his colleagues immunized patients with acute leukemia with 10^9 irradiated autologous leukemic cells.[65] In 5 out of the 9, the *in vitro* lymphocyte blastogenic response to liquid nitrogen-stored leukemic cells increased over 100 percent. In 4 out of these 5, this increased reactivity was nonspecific, however, in that their allogeneic mixed leukocyte reactivity also increased. Of great interest was the fact that they remained skin test negative after immunization.

Morton has immunized patients with sarcomas with their own tumor cells irradiated with 15,000 rads and mixed with BCG. This led to a marked increase in cytotoxic antibody activity in their serum.[66] Morton, in the same study using the same immunizing material, showed that complement fixing antibody to sarcoma extract also increased dramatically and that skin tests with sarcoma extract changed from negative to positive.[66] Ikonopisov and coworkers actively immunized patients with their own melanoma cells.[67] Dose response studies were done and if the patients were given injections of over 200×10^6 irradiated tumor cells, their cytotoxic antibody levels increased dramatically. These patients had no circulating cytotoxic antibody before immunization because they had active disease. Their cytotoxicity titers peaked at seven days and were gone by fourteen days. Thirteen of twenty-five patients so treated responded. Currie and co-workers from the same group found that this type of immunization increased lymphocyte cytotoxicity against autologous melanoma cells.[68] Before immunization, none of twelve patients had lymphocytes which could carry out cytotoxic reactions. One week later, 5 out of 15 patients were positive. The ideal ratio was at least thirty lymphocytes per tumor cell, and this led to greater than 50 percent killing. No evidence of blocking antibody was detected. All of these studies were conducted in patients with advanced disease, and as would be expected, no therapeutic benefit was observed.

LOCAL IMMUNOTHERAPY

An interesting approach to some problems in cancer therapy has been local immunotherapy. The concept of local immunotherapy is actually approximately sixty years old. This concept is based on the observations by Coley that local and even systemic regression of metastatic solid tumors could be achieved by the direct inoculation of extracts of streptococci and serratia into various human sarcomata.[69] In the modern era, this approach has been most aggressively pursued by Klein.[70,71] He has sensitized patients with DNCB or TEIB and after delayed hypersensitivity developed, he treated their skin tumors with the same sensitizing agent. Tumors treated include epithelioma, basal cell carcinoma, xeroderma pigmentosa, arsenical dermatosis, solar kerotosis and leukoplakia. Ninety percent of squamous epitheliomas and 95 percent of basal cell carcinomas are apparently permanently cured by this treatment. This general approach has been confirmed by Stewart, who treated mycosis fungoides lesions with streptokinase-streptodornase[72]; by Ratner and his associates, who treated mycosis fungoides with DNCB[73]; and by Stjernsward, who used DNCB to treat patients with cutaneous lesions of basal cell carcinoma, mycosis fungoides, reticulum cell sarcomas, malignant lymphoma, malignant melanoma and breast carcinoma.[74] In the latter study, of 19 patients treated, 17 became DNCB-positive and 13 showed excellent regression. These observations have also been confirmed by Cavins who found that 98 percent of lesions treated regressed completely after this type of local therapy.[75]

Living organisms associated with an immune response can also be used in local immunotherapy. Thus, Hunter-Craig found that the local inoculation of vaccinia virus led to complete regression in 6 of 10 and partial regression in 3 of 10 treated lesions of malignant melanoma.[76] Untreated lesions did not regress. No ancillary immunological studies were done. Hunter-Craig's observation confirmed in part, the observations of earlier workers using the same method, although the earlier workers also observed systemic therapeutic benefits. Morton has used the local inoculation of BCG in effective local immunotherapy.[66] He administered on a single occasion, 0.05 to 0.2 ml of Lilly BCG. He observed five responses in eight treated subjects and in two of the eight he observed regression at sites distant from the inoculated lesions. In one of these two, there was a complete remission lasting thirty-seven months. While it is possible that both BCG and vaccinia virus produced their effects by some direct attack on the tumor cells, it is most likely that this effect is achieved by the development and expression of delayed hypersensitivity and the release of lymphocyte cytotoxin at the local site. This would also be the mechanism of the DNCB effect, since only DNCB-positive subjects respond to treatment with DNCB.

This hypothesis was directly confirmed by Cheema and Hersh.[77] They collected autologous lymphocytes from patients with cutaneous metastases of a variety of malignant tumors. These lymphocytes were activated for twenty-four to forty-eight hours *in vitro* with phytohemagglutinin, after which they were washed extensively and inoculated into the lesions. Lesions inoculated with activated lymphocytes regressed dramatically while those inoculated with non-activated lymphocytes regressed only slightly. The mechanism was presumed to be release of lymphocyte cytotoxin from the phytohemogglutin-activated cells. Of interest was the fact that the therapeutic benefit was observed even in patients who were completely anergic. No systemic benefit was noted.

CONCLUSION

There are a variety of potential approaches to the immunotherapy of human cancer. There are many prerequisites and cautions necessary before immunotherapy can become highly effective and widely practical. In spite of the marginal results of immunotherapy reported to date, great enthusiasm for this approach exists, because we can now identify tumor-specific immune responses, and therefore we can measure the effects of therapeutic maneuvers. Immunotherapy is also of great interest today because conventional therapy can reduce the tumor burden to the level at which we know that immunotherapy in animal systems becomes effective. The next ten years of cancer immunology and specifically of cancer immunotherapy appear very bright.

REFERENCES

1. Ehrlich, P.: Uber den jetzigen Stand der Karzinomforschung. In Himmelweit, F. (Ed.): *The Collected Papers of Paul Ehrlich.* London, Pergamon Press, 1957, vol. II, pp. 550-562.
2. Wade, H.: An experimental investigation of infective sarcoma of the dog, with a considertion of its relationship to cancer. *J Pathol Bacteriol, 12:*384-425, 1908.
3. Woglom, W.H.: Immunity to transplantable tumours. *Cancer Rev, 4:* 129-214, 1929.
4. Gross, L.: Intradermal immunization of C_3H mice against a sarcoma not originated in an animal of the same cell line. *Cancer Res, 3:*326-333, 1943.
5. Foley, E.J.: Antigenic properties of methylcholanthrene-induced tumors in mice of the strain of origin. *Cancer Res, 13:*835-837, 1953.
6. *Cancer Facts and Figures, 1970.* New York, American Cancer Society, 1970.
7. Silverberg, E., and Holleb, A.I.: Cancer statistics, 1971. *CA, 21:*13-32, 1971.
8. Schulz, M.D.: Radiation therapy in the clinical management of cancer. *CA, 11:*18-26, 1969.
9. Vietti, T., Sullivan, M.P., Haggard, M.E. *et al.*: Vincristine sulfate and radiation therapy in metastatic Wilms' tumor. *Cancer, 25:*12-20, 1970.
10. Evans, A., Heyn, R., Newton, W., and Leikin, S.: Vincristine sulfate and cyclophosphamide for children with metastatic neuroblastoma. *JAMA, 207:*1325-1326, 1969.
11. DeVita, V.T., Serpick, A., and Carbone, P.: Combination chemotherapy in the treatment of advanced Hodgkin's disease. *Ann Intern Med, 73:*881-895, 1970.
12. Bagley, C., DeVita, V., and Canellos, G.P.: Combination chemotherapy with cyclophosphamide, vincristine, and prednisone in lymphosarcoma. *Proc Am Assoc Cancer Res, 12:*75, 1971.

13. Jacobs, E.M.: Combination chemotherapy of metastatic testicular germinal cell tumors and soft part sarcomas. *Cancer, 25*:324-332, 1970.
14. Cooper, R.: Combination chemotherapy in hormone resistant breast cancer. *Proc Am Assoc Cancer Res, 10*:15, 1969.
15. Aur, R., Simone, J., Hustu, H.O. *et al.*: Central nervous system therapy and combination chemotherapy of childhood lymphocytic leukemia. *Blood, 37*:272-281, 1971.
16. Crowther, D., Bateman, C., Vartan, C. *et al.*: Combination chemotherapy using l-asparaginase, daunorubicin, and cytosine arabinoside in adults with acute myelogenous leukemia. *Brit Med J, 4*:512-517, 1970.
17. Hersh, E.M., Whitecar, J., McCredie, K. *et al.*: Chemotherapy, immunocompetence, immunosuppression and prognosis in acute leukemia. *N Engl J Med, 285*:1211-1216, 1971.
18. Eilber, F., and Morton, D.L.: Impaired immunologic reactivity and recurrence following cancer surgery. *Cancer, 25*:362-367, 1970.
19. Alexander, P., and Hall, J.G.: The role of immunoblasts in host resistance and immunotherapy of primary sarcomata. In Klein, G., and Weinhouse, S. (Eds.): *Advances in Cancer Research*. New York, Academic Press, 1970, vol. 13, pp. 1-38.
20. Davignon, L., Lemonde, P., Robillard, P., and Frappier, A.: B.C.G. Vaccination and leukemia mortality. *Lancet, 2*:638, 1970.
21. Comstock, G.W., Livesay, V., and Webster, R.: Leukaemia and B.C.G. *Lancet, 2*:1062-1063, 1971.
22. Kaliss, N.: Immunological enhancement of tumor homografts in mice. *Cancer Res, 18*:992-1003, 1958.
23. McKenzie, I., Morris, P., Schiff, P. *et al.*: Human antilymphocytic serum; I. Production and *in vitro* testing. *Med J Aust, 1*:203-207, 1969.
24. Tsirimbas, A.D., Pichlmayr, R., Hornung, B. *et al.*: Therapeutische Wirkungen von heterologem antihuman-lymphocytenserum (AHLS) bei chronischer lymphatischer Leukaemie *Klin Wochenschr, 46*:583-586, 1968.
25. Herberman, R.B., Rogentine, G., and Oren, M.E.: Bioassay of antitumor effects of human alloantisera. *Clin Res, 17*:328, 1969.
26. Lewis, M.G., Ikonopisov, R.L., Nairn, R.C. *et al.*: Tumour-specific antibodies in human malignant melanoma and their relationship to the extent of the disease. *Br Med J, 3*:547-552, 1969.
27. Nadler, S.H., and Moore, G.E.: Immunotherapy of malignant melanoma. *Geriatrics, 23*:150-153, 1968.
28. Alexander, P.: Immunotherapy of cancer: Experiments with primary tumours and syngeneic tumour grafts. *Progr Exp Tumor Res, 10*:22-71, 1968.
29. Nadler, S., and Moore, G.E.: Immunotherapy of malignant disease. *Arch Surg, 99*:376-381, 1969.
30. Krementz, E., and Samuels, M.S.: Tumor cross transplantation and cross

transfusion in the treatment of advanced malignant disease. *Bull Tulane U Med Fac, 26:*263-270, 1967.

31. Curtis, J.E.: Adoptive immunotherapy in the treatment of advanced malignant melanoma. *Proc Am Assoc Cancer Res, 12:*52, 1971.
32. Curtis, J.E., Hersh, E.M., and Freireich, E.J.: Antigen-specific immunity in recipients of leukocyte transfusions from immune donors. *Cancer Res, 30:*2921-2929, 1970.
33. Humphrey, L.J., Jewell, W., Murray, D.R., and Griffen, W.: Immunotherapy for the patient with cancer. *Ann Surg, 173:*47-54, 1971.
34. Skurkovich, S., Kisljak, N.S., Machonova, L., and Bengunenko, S.: Active immunization of children suffering from acute leukaemia in acute phase with "live" allogeneic leukaemic cells. *Nature (Lond), 223:* 509-511, 1969.
35. Andrews, G., Congdon, C., Edwards, C. *et al.*: Preliminary trials of clinical immunotherapy. *Cancer Res, 27:*2535-2541, 1967.
36. Brandes, L.J., Galton, D., and Wiltshaw, E.: New approach to immunotherapy of melanoma. *Lancet, 2:*293-295, 1971.
37. Oettgen, H., Old, L., Farrow, J. *et al.*: Effects of transfer factor in cancer patients. *J Clin Invest, 50:*71, 1971.
38. Frenster, J., and Rogoway, W.M.: Clinical use of activated autologous lymphocytes for human cancer immunotherapy. In Cumley, R., and McKay, J. (Eds.): *Oncology 1970.* Chicago, Yearbook Medical Publishers, 1970, pp. 327.
39. Symes, M., Riddel, A.G., Immelman, E., and Terblanche, J.: Immunologically competent cells in the treatment of malignant disease. *Lancet, 1:*1054-1056, 1968.
40. Schwarzenberg, L., Mathé, G., Schneider, M. *et al.*: Attempted adoptive immunotherapy of acute leukaemia by leucocyte transfusions. *Lancet, 2:*365-372, 1966.
41. Boranic, M., and Tonkovic, I.: Time pattern of the antileukemic effect of graft-versus-host reaction in mice. *Cancer Res, 31:*1140-1147, 1971.
42. Buckner, C.D., Epstein, R., Rudolph, R. *et al.*: Allogeneic marrow engraftment following whole body irradiation in a patient with leukemia. *Blood, 35:*741-750, 1970.
43. Santos, G.W., Sensenbrenner, L., Burke, P.J. *et al.*: Marrow transplantation in man following cyclophosphamide. *Transplant Proc, 3:*400-404, 1971.
44. Graw, R., Rogentine, G., Leventhal, B.G. *et al.*: Graft-versus-host reaction complicating HL-A matched bone-marrow transplantation. *Lancet, 2:*1053-1055, 1970.
45. Mathé, G., Amiel, J.L., Schwarzenberg, L. *et al.*: Bone marrow graft in man after conditioning by antilymphocytic serum. *Br Med J, 2:* 131-136, 1970.
46. Salmon, S., Krakauer, R.S., and Whitmore, W.: Lymphocyte stimula-

tion; selective destruction of cells during blastogenic response to transplantation antigens. *Science, 172*:490-492, 1971.

47. Fialkow, P., Bryant, J., Thomas, E.D., and Neiman, P.: Leukaemic transformation of engrafted human marrow cells *in vivo*. *Lancet, 1*: 251-255, 1971.
48. Mathé, G., Amiel, J.L., Schwarzenberg, L. *et al.*: Active immunotherapy for acute lymphoblastic leukemia. *Lancet, 2*:697-699, 1969.
49. Mathé, G., Amiel, J.L., Schwarzenberg, L. *et al.*: Preliminary result of a new protocol for the active immunotherapy of acute lymphoblastic leukaemia; inhibition of the immunotherapeutic effect by vincristine or amantadine. *Rev Europe Etud Clin Biol, 16*:216-224, 1971.
50. Preliminary report of working party on leukaemia in childhood: Treatment of acute lymphoblastic leukaemia; comparison of immunotherapy (B.C.G.), intermittent methotrexate, and no therapy after a five-month intensive cytotoxic regimen (Concord trial). *Br Med J, 4*:189-194, 1971.
51. Mathé, G.: Immunotherapy in the treatment of acute lymphoid leukemia. *Hosp Practice, 6*:43-51, December 1971.
52. Guyer, R., and Crowther, D.: Active immunotherapy in treatment of acute leukaemia. *Br Med J, 4*:406-407, 1969.
53. Israel, L., and Halpern, B.: Le *Corynebacterium parvum* dans les Cancers Avances; Premiere Evaluation de l'activite Therapeutique de Cette Immuno-stimuline. *Nouv Presse Med, 1*:19-23, 1972.
54. Mathé, G., Amiel, J.L., Schwarzenberg, L. *et al.*: Remission induction with poly IC in patients with acute lymphoblastic leukaemia (preliminary results). *Eur J Clin Biol Res, 15*:671-673, 1970.
55. Gresser, I.: Interferon and cancer; therapeutic prospects. *Eur J Clin Biol Res, 15*:23-27, 1970.
56. Graham, J.B., and Graham, R.M.: Autogenous vaccine in cancer patients. *Surg Gynecol Obstet, 114*:1-4, 1962.
57. Hughes, L.E., Kearney, R. and Tully, M.: A study in clinical cancer immunotherapy. *Cancer, 26*:269-278, 1970.
58. Skurkovich, S., Makhonova, L., Reznichenko, F., and Chervonskiy, G.I.: Treatment of children with acute leukemia by passive cyclic immunization with autoplasma and autokeukocytes operated during the remission period. *Blood, 34*:186-197, 1969.
59. Southam, C.M.: Immunotherapeutic trials in sarcoma patients using autogenous tumor vaccines. In *Frontiers in Radiation Therapy and Oncology*. Basel, Karger, 1972, vol. vii.
60. Mendoza, C., Moore, G.E., Watne, A. *et al.*: Immunologic response following homologous transplantation of cultured human tumor cells in patients with malignancy. *Surgery, 64*:897-900, 1968.
61. Moore, G.E.: Cancer immunity. *Tex Med, 64*:54-59, 1968.
62. Czajkowski, N., Rosenblatt, M., Wolf, P., and Vazquez, J.: A new

method of active immunization to autologous human tumour tissue. *Lancet, 2*:905-909, 1967.

63. Ayre, J., and LeGuerrier, J.: Cell regression in carcinoma *in situ* following rand coupled fortified antigen (a cyto-immunologic study.). *Cancer Cytol, 6*:23-27, 1966.
64. Cunningham, T.J., Olson, K., Laffin, R. *et al.*: *Treatment of advanced cancer with active immunization. Cancer, 24*:932-937, 1969.
65. Powles, R.L., Balchin, L., Fairley, G., and Alexander, P.: Recognition of leukaemia cells as foreign before and after autoimmunization. *Br Med J, 1*:486-489, 1971.
66. Morton, D.L., Holmes, E.C., Eilber, F., and Wood, W.: Immunological aspects of neoplasia; a rational basis for immunotherapy. *Ann Intern Med, 74*:587-604, 1971.
67. Ikonopisov, R.L., Lewis, M.G., Hunter-Craig, I. *et al.*: Autoimmunization with irradiated tumour cells in human malignant melanoma. *Br Med J, 2*:752-754, 1970.
68. Currie, G.A., LeJeune, F., and Fairley, G.: Immunization with irradiated tumour cells and specific lymphocyte cytotoxicity in malignant melanoma. *Br Med J, 2*:305-310, 1971.
69. Coley, W.B.: A report of recent cases of inoperable sarcoma successfully treated with mixed toxins of erysipelas and *Bacillus prodigiosus. Surg Gynec Obstet, 13*:174-190, 1911.
70. Klein, E.: Tumors of the skin. X. Immunotherapy of cutaneous and mucosal neoplasms. *NY State J Med, 68*:900-911, 1968.
71. Williams, A., and Klein, E.: Experiences with local chemotherapy and immunotherapy in premalignant and malignant skin lesions. *Cancer, 25*:450-462, 1970.
72. Stewart, T., and Tolnai, G.: The regression of an inflammatory skin lesion by the induction of a delayed hypersensitivity reaction; a case report. *Cancer, 24*:117-121, 1969.
73. Ratner, A.C., Waldorf, D., and Van Scott, E.: Alterations of lesions of mycosis fungoides lymphoma by direct imposition of delayed hypersensitivity reactions. *Cancer, 21*:83-88, 1968.
74. Stjernsward, J., and Levin, A.: Delayed hypersensitivity-induced regression of human neoplasms. *Cancer, 28*:628-640, 1971.
75. Cavins, J.A.: Review of a 3-year experience with topical chemotherapy and immunotherapy of superficial cutaneous neoplasms. *J Surg Oncol, 3*:325-329, 1971.
76. Hunter-Craig, I., Newton, K.A., Westbury, G., and Lacey, B.: Use of vaccinia virus in the treatment of metastatic malignant melanoma. *Br Med J, 2*:512-515, 1970.
77. Cheema, A.R., and Hersh, E.M.: Local tumor immunotherapy with *in vitro* activated autologous lymphocytes. *Cancer* (in Press).

AUTHOR (NAME) INDEX

D

E

F

H

L

M

SUBJECT INDEX

B

D

E

S

T

U

V

Z